Immunodeficiency, Infection, and Stem Cell Transplantation

Guest Editor

NANCY BERLINER, MD

HEMATOLOGY/ONCOLOGY
CLINICS OF NORTH AMERICA

www.hemonc.theclinics.com

Consulting Editors
GEORGE P. CANELLOS, MD
NANCY BERLINER, MD

February 2011 • Volume 25 • Number 1

SAUNDERS an imprint of ELSEVIER, Inc.

W.B. SAUNDERS COMPANY
A Division of Elsevier Inc.

1600 John F. Kennedy Blvd. • Suite 1800 • Philadelphia, PA 19103-2899

http://www.theclinics.com

HEMATOLOGY/ONCOLOGY CLINICS OF NORTH AMERICA Volume 25, Number 1
February 2011 ISSN 0889-8588, ISBN 13: 978-1-4557-0633-4

Editor: Kerry Holland

Hematology/Oncology Clinics (ISSN 0889-8588) is published bimonthly by Elsevier Inc., 360 Park Avenue South, New York, NY 10010-1710. Months of issue are February, April, June, August, October, and December. Business and Editorial Offices: 1600 John F. Kennedy Blvd., Ste. 1800, Philadelphia, PA 19103–2899. Customer Service Office: 3251 Riverport Lane, Maryland Heights, MO 63043. Periodicals postage paid at New York, NY and at additional mailing offices. Subscription prices are $327.00 per year (domestic individuals), $541.00 per year (domestic institutions), $160.00 per year (domestic students/residents), $371.00 per year (Canadian individuals), $662.00 per year (Canadian institutions) $442.00 per year (international individuals), $662.00 per year (international institutions), and $216.00 per year (international and Canadian students/residents). International air speed delivery is included in all *Clinics* subscription prices. All prices are subject to change without notice. **POSTMASTER:** Send address changes to *Hematology/Oncology Clinics of North America*, Elsevier Health Sciences Division, Subscription Customer Service, 3251 Riverport Lane, Maryland Heights, MO 63043. Customer Service (orders, claims, online, change of address): Elsevier Health Sciences Division, Subscription Customer Service, 3251 Riverport Lane, Maryland Heights, MO 63043. Tel: 1-800-654-2452 (U.S. and Canada); 314-447-8871 (outside U.S. and Canada). Fax: 314-447-8029. E-mail: journalscustomerservice-usa@elsevier.com (for print support); journalsonlinesupport-usa@elsevier.com (for online support).

Reprints. For copies of 100 or more, of articles in this publication, please contact the Commercial Reprints Department, Elsevier Inc., 360 Park Avenue South, New York, New York 10010-1710; Tel.: 212-633-3813, Fax: 212-462-1935, E-mail: reprints@elsevier.com.

Hematology/Oncology Clinics of North America is covered in *MEDLINE/PubMed (Index Medicus), EMBASE/ Excerpta Medica,* and *BIOSIS.*

Printed and bound by CPI Group (UK) Ltd, Croydon, CR0 4YY

Transferred to Digital Print 2011

Contributors

CONSULTING EDITORS

GEORGE P. CANELLOS, MD
William Rosenberg Professor of Medicine, Department of Medical Oncology, Dana-Farber Cancer Institute, Boston, Massachusetts

NANCY BERLINER, MD
Chief, Division of Hematology, Brigham and Women's Hospital; Professor of Medicine, Harvard Medical School, Boston, Massachusetts

GUEST EDITOR

NANCY BERLINER, MD
Chief, Division of Hematology, Brigham and Women's Hospital; Professor of Medicine, Harvard Medical School, Boston, Massachusetts

AUTHORS

BARBARA D. ALEXANDER, MD, MHS
Division of Infectious Diseases, Department of Medicine, Duke University Health System, Duke University School of Medicine, Durham, North Carolina

SOWSAN ATABANI, PhD
Department of Infection (Royal Free Campus), University College London; Department of Virology, Royal Free Hampstead NHS Trust, Hampstead, London, United Kingdom

LINDSEY R. BADEN, MD
Assistant Professor of Medicine, Division of Infectious Diseases, Brigham and Women's Hospital; Division of Infectious Diseases, Dana-Farber Cancer Institute; Harvard Medical School, Boston, Massachusetts

EMILY BLUMBERG, MD
Division of Infectious Diseases, Hospital of the University of Pennsylvania, Philadelphia, Pennsylvania

MICHAEL BOECKH, MD
University of Washington, Vaccine and Infectious Disease Institute, Fred Hutchinson Cancer Research Center, Seattle, Washington

M. CAVAZZANA-CALVO, MD, PhD
Developpement normal et pathologique du systeme immunitaire, Inserm U 768; Paris-Descartes University; Department of Biotherapy, Hopital Necker-Enfants Malades, Assistance Publique-Hôpitaux de Paris (AP-HP), Université René Descartes; INSERM, Centre d'Investigation Clinique intégré en Biothérapies, Groupe Hospitalier Universitaire Ouest, AP-HP, Paris, France

AGNIESZKA CZECHOWICZ, PhD
Institute of Stem Cell Biology and Regenerative Medicine, Stanford University School of Medicine, Stanford, California

M. TERESA DE LA MORENA, MD
Associate Professor of Pediatrics and Internal Medicine, Division of Allergy and Immunology, University of Texas Southwestern Medical Center in Dallas, Dallas, Texas

HERMANN EINSELE, PhD
Department of Medicine, University of Wuerzburg, Wuerzburg, Germany

VINCENT C. EMERY, PhD
Department of Infection (Royal Free Campus), University College London, Hampstead, London, United Kingdom

ALAIN FISCHER, MD, PhD
University Paris Descartes, Necker Medical School; Institut National de la Santé et de la Recherche Médicale; Unitéd'Immuno-Hématologie Pédiatrique, Necker Hospital, Assistance Publique-Hôpitaux de Paris, Paris, France

WILHELM FRIEDRICH, MD
Associate Professor, Department of Pediatrics, University of Ulm, Ulm, Germany

RICHARD A. GATTI, MD
Distinguished Professor, Department of Pathology and Laboratory Medicine, Macdonald Research Laboratories, University of California Los Angeles School of Medicine, Los Angeles, California

MICHAEL GREEN, MD, MPH
Professor, Department of Pediatrics and Surgery, Children's Hospital of Pittsburgh, Pittsburgh, Pennsylvania

EYAL GRUNEBAUM, MD
Associate Professor Pediatrics, Division of Clinical Immunology and Allergy, Department of Pediatrics, The Hospital for Sick Children, University of Toronto, Toronto, Ontario, Canada

S. HACEIN-BEY-ABINA, PharmD, PhD
Developpement normal et pathologique du systeme immunitaire, Inserm U 768; Paris-Descartes University; Department of Biotherapy, Hopital Necker-Enfants Malades, Assistance Publique-Hôpitaux de Paris (AP-HP), Université René Descartes; INSERM, Centre d'Investigation Clinique intégré en Biothérapies, Groupe Hospitalier Universitaire Ouest, AP-HP, Paris, France

DAVID HAGIN, MD
Department of Immunology, Weizmann Institute of Science, Rehovot, Israel

MORGAN HAKKI, MD
Division of Infectious Diseases, Oregon Health and Science University, Portland, Oregon

TANZINA HAQUE, PhD
Department of Virology, Royal Free Hampstead NHS Trust, Hampstead, London, United Kingdom

JOHN W. HIEMENZ, MD
Professor of Medicine, Bone Marrow Transplant Program, Division of Hematology/Oncology, University of Florida College of Medicine, Gainesville, Florida

MANFRED HÖNIG, MD
Department of Pediatrics, University of Ulm, Ulm, Germany

JACK HSU, MD
Assistant Professor of Medicine, Bone Marrow Transplant Program, Division of Hematology/Oncology, University of Florida College of Medicine, Gainesville, Florida

NEENA KAPOOR, MD
Professor of Pediatrics, Department of Pediatrics, University of Southern California Keck School of Medicine; Clinical Director, Bone Marrow Transplantation Program, Division of Research Immunology/Bone Marrow Transplantation, Childrens Hospital Los Angeles, Los Angeles, California

DIMITRIOS P. KONTOYIANNIS, MD, ScD
Department of Infectious Diseases, Infection Control and Employee Health, The University of Texas MD Anderson Cancer Center, Houston, Texas

SOPHIA KOO, MD
Clinical and Research Fellow, Division of Infectious Diseases, Brigham and Women's Hospital; Division of Infectious Diseases, Dana-Farber Cancer Institute; Harvard Medical School, Boston, Massachusetts

PER LJUNGMAN, MD, PhD
Department of Hematology, Karolinska University Hospital; Division of Hematology, Department of Medicine Huddinge, Karolinska Institutet, Stockholm, Sweden

FRANCISCO M. MARTY, MD
Assistant Professor of Medicine, Division of Infectious Diseases, Brigham and Women's Hospital; Division of Infectious Diseases, Dana-Farber Cancer Institute; Harvard Medical School, Boston, Massachusetts

MARIAN G. MICHAELS, MD, MPH
Professor, Department of Pediatrics and Surgery, Children's Hospital of Pittsburgh, Pittsburgh, Pennsylvania

RICHARD J. O'REILLY, MD
Chair, Department of Pediatrics; Chief, Pediatric Bone Marrow Transplant Service; Claire L. Tow Chair in Pediatric Oncology Research, Memorial Sloan Kettering Cancer Center, New York, New York

ROBERTSON PARKMAN, MD
Professor of Pediatrics, Division of Research Immunology/BMT, The Saban Research Institute, Childrens Hospital Los Angeles; Department of Pediatrics, Molecular Microbiology and Immunology, University of Southern California Keck School of Medicine, Los Angeles, California

ANNA K. PERSON, MD
Division of Infectious Diseases, Department of Medicine, Duke University Health System, Duke University School of Medicine, Durham, North Carolina

JOEL M. RAPPEPORT, MD
Department of Internal Medicine, Yale University School of Medicine, New Haven, Connecticut

YAIR REISNER, PhD
Chairman, Department of Immunology, Weizmann Institute of Science, Rehovot, Israel

CHAIM M. ROIFMAN, MD, FRCPC, FCACB
Donald and Audrey Campbell Chair of Immunology; Professor of Pediatrics and Immunology, University of Toronto; Director, Canadian Center for Primary Immunodeficiency; Head, Division of Immunology and Allergy, Department of Pediatrics, The Hospital for Sick Children, Toronto, Ontario, Canada

KEVIN SHILEY, MD
Division of Infectious Diseases, Hospital of the University of Pennsylvania, Philadelphia, Pennsylvania

IRVING L. WEISSMAN, MD
Director, Institute of Stem Cell Biology and Regenerative Medicine, Stanford University School of Medicine, Stanford, California

JOHN R. WINGARD, MD
Professor of Medicine, Bone Marrow Transplant Program, Division of Hematology/Oncology, University of Florida College of Medicine, Gainesville, Florida

Contents

The last 40 years has seen the emergence of hematopoietic stem cell transplantation as a therapeutic modality for fatal diseases and as a curative option for individuals born with inherited disorders that carry limited life expectancy and poor quality of life. Despite the rarity of many primary immunodeficiency diseases, these disorders have led the way toward innovative therapies and further provide insights into mechanisms of immunologic reconstitution applicable to all hematopoietic stem cell transplants. This article represents a historical perspective of the early investigators and their contributions. It also reviews the parallel work that oncologists and immunologists have undertaken to treat both primary immunodeficiencies and hematologic malignancies.

It is now more than 40 years since the first successful allogeneic hematopoietic stem cell transplantation (HSCT) for a child with severe combined immunodeficiency (SCID). In the succeeding years, HSCT for SCID patients have represented only a small portion of the total number of allogeneic HSCT performed. Nevertheless, the clinical and biologic importance of the patients transplanted for SCID has continued. SCID patients were the first to be successfully transplanted with nonsibling related bone marrow, unrelated bone marrow, T-cell depleted HSCT, and genetically corrected (gene transfer) autologous HSC. Many of the biologic insights now widely applied to allogeneic HSCT were first identified in the transplantation of SCID patients. This article reviews the clinical and biologic lessons that have been learned from HSCT for SCID patients, and how the information has impacted the general field of allogeneic HSCT.

Curative treatment of Severe Combined Immunodeficiency (SCID) by Hematopoietic Cell Transplantation (HCT) remains a challenge, in particular in infants presenting with serious, poorly controllable complications. In the absence of a matched family donor, HLA-haploidentical transplantation from parental donors represents a uniformly and readily available treatment option, offering a high chance to be successful. Concerning outcomes of HCT in SCID, other important parameters beside survival need to be taken into consideration, in particular the stability and robustness of the graft and its function, as well as potential late complications, related either to the disease or to the treatment.

Since the early 1980s T-cell depletion has allowed haploidentical bone marrow transplantation to be performed in patients with primary immunodeficiency for whom a matched sibling donor was not available, without causing severe graft versus host disease (GVHD). This review article presents the available data in the literature on survival, GVHD, and immune reconstitution in different categories of patients, with special emphasis on the impact of different T-cell depletion methods.

Severe combined immunodeficiency (SCID) is fatal in infancy unless corrected with allogeneic bone marrow transplants (BMT), preferably from a family-related genotypically HLA-identical donor (RID) or phenotypically HLA-matched family donor (PMD). For the majority of SCID patients, such donors are not available; Therefore, parents who are HLA-haploidentical donors (HID) or HLA-matched unrelated donors (MUD) have been used. MUD BMT are associated with increased frequency of acute graft versus host disease, which can be controlled by high doses of steroids. HID BMT are associated with increased frequency of short- and long-term graft failure, need for repeated transplants, fatal pneumonitis, impaired immune reconstitution, and long-term complications, contributing to lower survival. In conclusion, the excellent long-term survival, immune reconstitution, and normal quality of life after MUD BMT suggests that in the absence of RID or PMD, MUD BMT should be offered for patients suffering from SCID.

Replacement of disease-causing stem cells with healthy ones has been achieved clinically via hematopoietic cell transplantation (HCT) for the last 40 years, as a treatment modality for a variety of cancers and immunodeficiencies with moderate, but increasing, success. This procedure has traditionally included transplantation of mixed hematopoietic populations that include hematopoietic stem cells (HSC) and other cells, such as T cells. This article explores and delineates the potential expansion of this technique to treat a variety of inherited diseases of immune function, the current barriers in HCT and pure HSC transplantation, and the up-and-coming strategies to combat these obstacles.

The concept of gene therapy emerged as a way of correcting monogenic inherited diseases by introducing a normal copy of the mutated gene into at least some of the patients' cells. Although this concept has turned out to be quite complicated to implement, it is in the field of primary immunodeficiencies (PIDs) that proof of feasibility has been undoubtedly achieved. There is now a strong rationale in support of gene therapy for at least some PIDs, as discussed in this article.

Hematopoietic stem cell transplantation (HSCT) is a treatment for multiple medical conditions that result in bone marrow failure and as an antineoplastic adoptive immunotherapy for hematologic malignancies. HSCT is associated with profound compromises in host barriers and all arms of innate and acquired immunity. The degree of immune compromise varies by type of transplant and over time. Immune reconstitution occurs within several months after autologous HSCT but takes up to a year or longer after allogeneic HSCT. In those patients who develop chronic graft-versus-host disease, immune reconstitution may take years or may never completely develop. Over time, with strengthening immune reconstitution and control of graft-versus-host disease, the risk for infection dissipates.

The armamentarium of biologic therapies targeting specific elements of the immune system is rapidly expanding. This review describes the spectrum of infectious complications associated to date with each of the immunomodulating biologic therapies approved by the US Food and Drug Administration.

Transplantation increasingly is being used as treatment for children with end-stage organ diseases, hematopoietic rescue from therapy used to treat malignancies, and as cure for primary immune deficiencies. This article reviews some of the major concepts regarding infections that complicate pediatric transplantation, highlighting differences in epidemiology, evaluation, treatment and prevention for children compared with adult recipients.

This article examines the clinical manifestations of and risk factors for cytomegalovirus (CMV). Prevention of CMV infection and disease are also explored. Antiviral resistance and management of CMV are examined.

The herpes viruses are responsible for a wide range of diseases in patients following transplant, resulting from direct viral effects and indirect effects, including tumor promotion. Effective treatments and prophylaxis exist for

THE CLINICS ARE NOW AVAILABLE ONLINE!

Access your subscription at:
www.theclinics.com

Preface

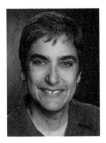

Nancy Berliner, MD
Guest Editor

In this issue of *Hematology/Oncology Clinics of North America*, we are reprinting a selection of articles from three other recent *Clinics* issues that we think will be of special interest to our readers. This is a "hybrid" issue focusing on Immunodeficiency from two different angles.

In the first half of the issue, we present a series of articles on bone marrow transplantation for congenital immunodeficiency syndromes. It includes a brief history of bone marrow transplantation, and articles on the full range of alternative stem cell sources for transplantation for this otherwise fatal disorder. We close this part of the issue with an article summarizing the progress in gene therapy for the disease.

In the second half, we focus on the infectious complications of acquired immunodeficiency associated with stem cell transplantation. There are updates on the natural history of viral, bacterial, and fungal infections that complicate transplantation. In addition, we include a review of the infectious complications of new biologic agents that act to modulate immunity, and a final article focused on immunotherapy and vaccination to prevent posttransplant infections.

Nancy Berliner, MD
Division of Hematology
Brigham and Women's Hospital
Harvard Medical School
Mid-Campus 3
75 Francis Street
Boston, MA 02115, USA

E-mail address:
NBERLINER@PARTNERS.ORG

Hematol Oncol Clin N Am 25 (2011) xiii
doi:10.1016/j.hoc.2010.12.001   hemonc.theclinics.com

A History of Bone Marrow Transplantation

M. Teresa de la Morena, MD[a],*, Richard A. Gatti, MD[b]

KEYWORDS

- Bone marrow transplantation • History
- Primary immunodeficiency diseases

Five decades ago, the concept of bone marrow transplantation to treat humans with inherited diseases of immune function, marrow failure syndromes, and leukemia was met with much skepticism, degrees of enthusiasm, and many disappointments. Transferring what was known from experimental animal models to humans was met with many challenges, and such beginnings were very difficult. Certain death due to the primary disease, characterized the outcomes of individuals who were considered for transplantation. Consequently these patients became the sickest on the medical wards, and the physicians caring for such patients were posed with many questions regarding the benefits of such attempts. One of the major obstacles, graft-versus-host disease (GVHD) was "incomparably more violent than in (inbred) rodents" as stated by Bekkum and van de Vries.[1] Yet through the recognition and subsequent understanding of fundamental immunologic processes, medical resiliency, and the stubborn determination of a few pioneers, bone marrow transplantation changed from an insurmountable therapeutic option for a limited number of patients to a form of therapy for 30,000 to 50,000 people worldwide annually.[2] Hematopoietic stem cell transplantation (HSCT) today is no longer a treatment modality for lethal diseases such as primary immunodeficiency diseases (PIDs) or malignancies but a valid approach of "cellular engineering"[3] for solid tumors, hemoglobinopathies, autoimmune diseases, inherited disorders of metabolism, histiocytic disorders, and other nonmalignancies.[2]

A version of this article was previously published in the *Immunology and Allergy Clinics of North America*, 30:1.

[a] Department of Pediatrics and Internal Medicine, Division of Allergy and Immunology, University of Texas Southwestern Medical Center in Dallas, 5323 Harry Hines Boulevard, Dallas, TX 75390-9063, USA

[b] Department of Pathology and Laboratory Medicine, 675 Charles Young Drive South, Room 4-736, Macdonald Research Laboratories, University of California Los Angeles School of Medicine, Los Angeles, CA 90095-1732, USA

* Corresponding author.

E-mail address: maite.delamorena@utsouthwestern.edu

Hematol Oncol Clin N Am 25 (2011) 1–15

doi:10.1016/j.hoc.2010.11.001

hemonc.theclinics.com

0889-8588/11/$ – see front matter © 2011 Elsevier Inc. All rights reserved.

This article represents a historical perspective of the early investigators and their contributions. It also reviews the parallel work that oncologists and immunologists have undertaken to treat both PIDs and hematologic malignancies.

THE EARLY DAYS

The idea of removing damaged parts of the body and replacing them with healthy organs has been an aim shared by physicians since ancient times. An early discussion on the use of bone marrow was outline in 1896 by Quine in the Chairman's address of the Journal of the American Medical Association, where he discussed the "remedial application of bone marrow extracts."[4] However, the physical consequences of World War II brought research in tissue transplantation to the forefront: skin grafts were needed for burn victims; blood transfusions required careful ABO blood typing and monitoring of blood group antibodies; and high doses of radiation lead to marrow failure and death, with little understanding of radiobiological mechanisms.

By the early 1940s, it was clear that phagocytes were macrophages, antibodies were part of the gamma-globulin fraction of serum proteins (as defined by their electrophoretic mobility),[5] and the "small lymphocytes" were influenced by adrenal hormones.[6] At the request of the Medical Research Council during World War II, Medawar[7] started work on the study of rejection of skin grafts, a priority for the treatment of burn victims. Early versions of immunologic tolerance and alloreactivity were published. In 1945, Ray Owen in Wisconsin, while studying the inheritance of blood group antigens in freemartin cattle, described how fraternal twin cattle were chimeric for 2 blood groups, their own and that of the twin.[8] At the turn of the century, Loeb[9] had been unable to transfer tumors from Japanese waltzing mice to different strains of mice, whereas such tumors grew easily within the inbred strain. To Gorer[10] and subsequently to Snell,[11-13] we owe the identification of the major histocompatibility complex (MHC) genes in rodents (H-2 system in the mouse).

Medawar assimilated this background and provided convincing evidence that graft rejection was an immunologic phenomenon[7] linked to histocompatibility antigens. Subsequently with Billingham and Brent, he designed a series of hallmark experiments, in which he demonstrated the induction of immunologic tolerance.[14] Yet within the first few lines of the article, he cautioned that the experiments described were "…only a 'laboratory' solution of the problem of how to make tissue homografts immunologically acceptable to hosts which would normally react against them."

Massive radiation exposures provided an opportunity to advance therapies for bone marrow failure syndromes and leukemia. A series of critical studies in mice, dogs, and subsequently nonhuman primates that were subjected to high doses of radiation followed by transplantation of marrow grafts provided the basis for understanding concepts of histocompatibility, conditioning, graft-versus-leukemia effect, and GVHD.

Jacobson and colleagues[15] reported that the shielding of spleen, part of the liver, the head, or even 1 hind leg of mice allowed survival after total body irradiation. They also demonstrated similar protection if spleen grafts were transplanted intraperitoneally immediately after radiation exposure. These investigators posited that this phenomenon could be due to "a substance of a non-cellular nature" or that irradiation produced a "toxin" which was "detoxified" by shielding the spleen or the grafting tissues.[15] By 1954, this "humoral" hypothesis was clearly trumped by the "cellular" hypothesis. Barnes and Louitit[16] suggested that living cells were responsible for hematopoietic recovery after radiation. Shortly thereafter, many independent investigators confirmed that after lethal radiation, hematopoietic recovery was dependent upon donor cells.[17-19]

Experienced with marrow transplant work in rodents, Mathé and colleagues[20] in France was faced with the need to rescue 5 subjects who had accidentally been exposed to high doses of radiation. He used bone marrow infusions from different donors. Of the 5 subjects, 4 survived. Subsequently it was recognized that this was because of autologous recovery. His group went on to describe early trials of adaptive immunotherapy with marrow grafts for the management of leukemia patients. Even though all patients died, complete remission from the leukemia was described for several patients for periods of 5 and 9 months before they died of either infection or the secondary disease (today known as GVHD).[21] At around the same time, Thomas and colleagues[22] in the United States attempted human bone marrow transplants for leukemia. Five subjects with end-stage malignancies were infused with marrow from fetuses and adults. These investigators made special efforts to demonstrate that all collections were free of infection and were infused safely in the subjects without immediate transfusion reactions. Unfortunately none of the patients survived. Parenthetically, they also opined that although bone marrow is a source of plasma cells, patients with agammaglobulinemia, which had been recently described by Bruton,[23,24] need not be treated with this modality because these patients did well on infusions of gamma globulin and antibiotics.[22] This remains true today, 50 years later, with the one caveat that some of these patients develop progressive and fatal encephalitis[25] that might be averted by bone marrow transplantation.

As had been previously reported, marrow grafting experiments in dogs were subject to the same consequences as noted in mice: after radiation, the animals could recover promptly if rescued with autologous marrow.[26] In contrast, when allogeneic grafts were used, the graft was rejected, indicative of the immune competence of the animal, or successful engraftment was achieved, followed by lethal GVHD. Most importantly, it was already becoming clear that successful allogeneic marrow transplants, unlike solid organ transplants, depended upon close histocompatibility matching between donor and recipient and, thus, would be limited by the availability of donors. GVHD (the former) and histocompatibility (the latter) represented two hurdles that needed to be surmounted before bone marrow transplantation could be generally applied as a therapeutic modality for many.

THE CHALLENGES OF GVHD

At the same time that these early transplants were being performed for treatment of leukemia, the classification of PIDs was being refined. Attempts to correct lymphopenia with conventional blood transfusions were unsuccessful and often fatal.[27] In 1967, the first symposium on the immunologic deficiencies in man took place in Sanibel Island, Florida.[28] Severe combined immunodeficiency (SCID), until then divided into Swiss type agammaglobulinemia (ie, autosomal recessive) or sex-linked lymphopenic immunologic deficiency, was attributed to thymic dysfunction. However, unlike the situation in DiGeorge syndrome, thymus transplants in SCID were not corrective. DeVries and colleagues[29] suggested that the thymus defect might be secondary and hypothesized that the absence of lymphoid progenitors was the root cause of the combined defect. It made sense then to reconstitute such SCID infants with a source of lymphoid precursors, such as spleen, fetal liver, and bone marrow. Thus, in contrast to patients with leukemia, the main barrier was not rejection of the graft or relapse of leukemia, it was the terrible secondary disease or GVHD (**Fig. 1**).

In August of 1968, an editorial was published by Hong and colleagues,[30] outlining the hazards and potential benefits of blood transfusions in immunologic deficiencies. It was proposed that either "old blood" or irradiated blood products be used in

Graft-versus-Host Reaction

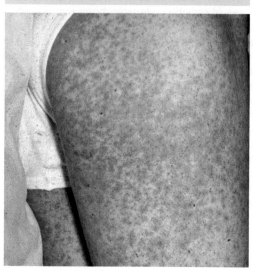

Fig. 1. GVHD in a patient who developed fever, maculopapular rash, hepatosplenomegaly, pancytopenia, and death.

severely immunodeficient patients as a means of preventing GVHD. These authors further hypothesized that if one could find a histocompatible match, the immunologic capacity of the immunodeficient host could potentially be restored.

The first HLA antigens in man were described by Dausset[31] in France, van Rood and colleagues[32] in Holland, Payne and Rolfs[33] and Amos[34,35] in the United States, and Ceppellini and van Rood[36] in Italy. Terasaki and McClellan[37] had developed methodology for a rapidly expanding panel of HLA antigens. A second HLA-Class I locus (HLA-B) had not yet been fully appreciated, most likely because of the high degree of linkage disequilibrium between the closely linked HLA-A and B loci (ie, 1 cM). Continuing studies in mice and dogs consistently demonstrated that if animals were well matched, GVHD could be prevented.[38–40] Occasionally mild reactions occurred, but these were thought to be transient.

With this background of imperfect but rapidly developing knowledge, including the experience being accrued by oncologists,[22,41] a window in history opened when the "right" patient was referred to Robert A. Good, then at the University of Minnesota (discussed in the next section).

RENEWED HOPE FOR SCID PATIENTS

In the late 1950s, X-linked SCID was described (today known as common gamma chain–deficient SCID or γc-SCID). Most likely, this combined immunodeficiency is severe because the defective γ-chain is common to 5 interleukin (IL) receptors (IL-2, IL-7, IL-9, IL-15, and IL-21). Children with this disorder would come to medical attention early in life and die shortly thereafter with recurring and finally overwhelming infections, such as persistent thrush, fatal pneumonias, vaccinia gangrenosa, and susceptibility to *Pneumocystis*. In Sweden at that time, bacille Calmette-Guérin (BCG) vaccination for tuberculosis was mandatory, and about a dozen deaths were recognized related to this immunologic deficiency.[42]

A 5-month-old male child was referred to the University of Minnesota. The baby had previously been diagnosed in Boston as having "thymic alymphoplasia and agamma-globulinemia" (or X-linked SCID). The family history was significant for 11 male deaths over 3 generations. All had died of infections in early infancy (**Fig. 2**).[43] The patient had low serum gamma globulins and was being treated with gamma globulin injections and antibiotics for persistent pneumonia. A chest radiograph revealed absence of thymus. Hematologic studies noted lymphopenia. Antibodies against blood group antigens, diphtheria toxoid, and typhoid antigens were not detected. Cellular responses were absent. Tonsils, adenoids, and peripheral lymph nodes could not be detected.[44]

The most hopeful piece of information was that the child had 4 sisters, for this increased the chances of finding a matched sibling for marrow transplantation. Two forms of histocompatibility testing were developing at the time: (1) serologic typing for HLA (Class I only) and (2) cellular typing by mixed leukocyte cultures (MLCs).

HLA typing was performed by Terasaki at the University of California, Los Angeles. Of all sisters analyzed, 1 was found to be the best match. MLCs, performed by Meuwissen[45] in Minneapolis, demonstrated reactivity to the patient's cells in all 4 sisters; however, 1 sister (sister 3) clearly had a weak reaction (**Fig. 3**). This sister was also ABO incompatible. Making sense of the histocompatibility testing results at that time was a source of considerable discussion and soul-searching, for a misinterpretation of the genetics or biology could result in fatal GVHD reaction: (1) the HLA antigens did not segregate and (2) they did not seem to correlate with the segregation of the MLC results. Only after it was appreciated several years later that 2 serologic loci (HLA-A and HLA-B) existed could a crossover between the 2 loci in the donor cells be postulated to explain the serologic typing.[46] And only when the Class II loci were localized proximal to the Class I region of the MHC on chromosome 6 could one postulate that the crossover between HLA-A and HLA-B in sister 3 would carry with it the Class II region shared between patient and donor on haplotype B (see **Fig. 3**).

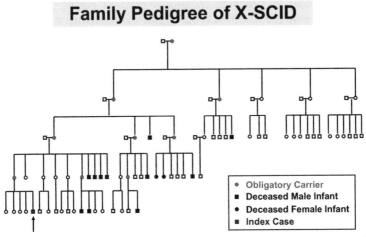

Family Pedigree of X-SCID

- ● Obligatory Carrier
- ■ Deceased Male Infant
- ● Deceased Female Infant
- ■ Index Case

Fig. 2. Patient family pedigree. (*Adapted from* Good RA. Immunologic reconstitution: the achievement and it's meaning. In: Bergsma D, Good RA, editors. Birth defects original articles series, vol. 4. White Plains (NY): The National Foundation-March of Dimes; 1968; with permission.)

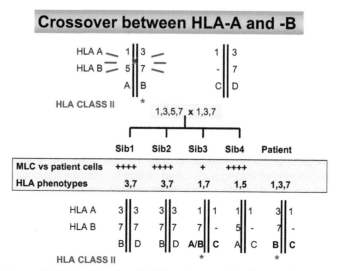

Fig. 3. Histocompatibility testing of an X-SCID patient and family members, using HLA serologic typing and unidirectional MLC. Note that segregation of both HLA haplotyping and MLC reactions were only understandable after a crossover between HLA-A and HLA-B loci was appreciated. Class II loci on haplotype B (*asterisks*) of the patient would have then segregated with the proximal portion of recombinant haplotype B in Sib3, who became the stem cell donor. (*Data from* Gatti RA, Meuwissen HJ, Terasaki PI, et al. Recombination within the HL-A locus. Tissue Antigens 1971;1(5):239–41.)

Driven by the almost certain fatal outcome of the disease in this family without treatment, a decision was made to attempt the bone marrow transplant using the 8-year-old sister 3 as the donor.[44] Both peripheral blood and bone marrow (obtained from iliac crests and tibial bones) were collected from the donor. Peripheral blood was collected 48 hours before collecting the marrow so that a stem-cell–rich fraction of nucleated cells could be prepared by density gradient centrifugation using 5% dextran. The cells were resuspended in donor plasma. In contrast to what was being done for oncologic patients, the infusion of both peripheral blood (5×10^6 lymphocytes/mL) and marrow (total of 10^9 nucleated cells) was given intraperitoneally, primarily to avoid having to filter out bone spicules and thereby reduce the number of cells available for engraftment. (In today's terms, approximately 10×10^6 CD34+ cells were infused into the 7-kg infant, or 1.25×10^6 stem cells/kg.)

One week after the cells were infused, GVHD symptoms appeared, involving the skin, gut, and liver. This was accompanied by a hemolytic anemia thought to be caused by donor/host ABO incompatibility. No immunosuppressive therapies were given because of concern that immunosuppressive drugs would impede stem cell engraftment and because of experimental evidence that a mild GVHD would subside. One week later, the high fever and rash disappeared, and engraftment ensued. Proliferative responses to mitogens normalized, delayed-type hypersensitivity reactions could be demonstrated for the first time, and a bone marrow aspirate showed that 25% of bone marrow cells could be identified as female (donor) by karyotyping.

Despite this early success, 45 days later, the patient developed a severe aplastic anemia. It was speculated that this was GVHD reaction involving the marrow. Donor-specific cytotoxic antibodies were demonstrated. A second bone marrow infusion followed.[45,47] Within 2 weeks, the leukocyte counts improved, GVHD had subsided, and the proportion of erythrocytes with the host's group A type had begun to decline, shifting instead to the donor's group O blood type.[47] Group O cells have persisted to date, and the patient remains cured from his SCID diagnosis. For the first time, both SCID and aplastic anemia had been corrected by bone marrow transplantation and new therapeutic options became available for these disorders. It is also important to recognize that this experience confirmed the proposed model that the central defect in SCID patients resided in their lack of pluripotent stem cells and not a defective thymic microenvironment. A 2-year posttransplant evaluation demonstrated not only a stable immunologic reconstitution but also the transfer of T-cell memory, as evidenced by positive skin tests to mumps, despite that the child had never had mumps; the donor had had mumps shortly before her cells were harvested for transplant.

Bach and colleagues[48] described a 22-month-old boy who was engrafted with bone marrow from a sister to correct for Wiskott-Aldrich syndrome (WAS). In contrast to patients with SCID, patients with WAS have evidence of immunologic function. To overcome the potential for rejection, a conditioning regimen consisting of azathioprine (5 mg/kg) and prednisone (2 mg/kg) was given for 2 days before the transplant. In contrast to the SCID case, the marrow infusion (6.5×10^9) was given intravenously through a femoral line. The patient developed *Staphylococcus aureus* positive intravenous line sepsis and graft failure. A second bone marrow transplant was given 4 days later, consisting of donor-derived peripheral blood mononuclear cells (PBMCs). It was speculated that donor PBMCs induced the expansion of recipient lymphocytes against minor donor HLA antigens. These lymphocytes would be subsequently eliminated by successive doses of cyclophosphamide at specific intervals. The transplanted female marrow initially seemed to engraft successfully. Fifteen years later, the patient was noted to have full T-cell and partial B-cell chimerism but no evidence of hematopoietic engraftment and remained thrombocytopenic.[49]

THE DARK DAYS AND THE DRAWING BOARD

Despite early enthusiasm, the reality was that transplantation for anything other than severe immunodeficiency seemed to be of limited clinical application. An excellent review of all bone marrow transplants attempted between 1939 to 1969 was carefully recorded by Mortimer Bortin.[50] The cases included 73 patients with aplastic anemia, 84 with leukemia, 31 with malignant disease, and 15 with immunodeficiency. Radiation and chloramphenicol were the most important known causes for aplastic anemia. Sixty percent of patients with acute leukemias were children (<18 years). Seven percent of autopsies had pulmonary evidence of marrow emboli. Of 203 transplants, at the time the report was written, 152 patients had died. Taken together, in 125 patients (60%) there was no evidence of engraftment. Evidence of chimerism was recognized in 11. Only 3 patients survived (all were immunodeficient patients and included the 2 patients described earlier). Graft rejection, infection, and GVHD were the main causes of death.

During the 1970s, donor selection, control of GVHD, and conditioning regimens became areas of intense research in preclinical models. MLCs were used for the selection of donors. Weak in vitro responses suggested good compatibility. However, as HLA typing improved, it became apparent that MLC assays were difficult to interpret and were less reliable than what was required for clinical application. Serological testing for HLA-class II antigens was instituted. By the turn of the century serology was largely replaced by molecular identification of histocompatibility antigens. By 1975, Thomas and colleagues[51] published the first of a 2-part medical progress report on bone marrow transplantation. In this excellent synopsis, the authors discussed animal studies, the status of histocompatibility testing, conditioning regimens, techniques for marrow collection, fractionation and infusion, and the level of supportive care necessary for successful bone marrow transplantation.[52,53]

DECADES OF ADVANCES

The 1980s and 1990s saw a rapid increase in the number of transplants performed; national and international bone marrow registries were created, and cord blood was recognized as a source of stem cells. T-cell depletion techniques were introduced for prevention of GVHD, as matched sibling donors were only available 25% of the time, whereas HLA-haploidentical or mismatched family members were readily available. Soybean lectin agglutination coupled with erythrocyte rosetting with sheep red blood cell was developed by Reisner and colleagues[54] and was used successfully in patients with SCID and subsequently in patients with leukemia. Since that time, this approach has allowed for the survival of many infants with SCID[55–58] and continues to be used today in different centers around the world.

Novel methods of T-cell depletion were developed, including counterflow centrifugal elutriation and fractionation on density gradients.[59,60] By 1981, the first clinical trial using antithymocyte globulin was reported.[61] Subsequently monoclonal antibodies were used in vivo and ex vivo for the treatment of marrow grafts for malignancies and PID patients.[62–65] However, with the depletion of T cells, important complications were recognized. These complications were higher incidence of graft failures, delayed immune reconstitution, increased risk of Epstein-Bar virus–associated lymphoproliferative disease, and CMV reactivation, and the overall survival was not significantly improved as compared with non–T-cell-depleted bone marrow.[66]

When CD34 was recognized as a glycoprotein that helped to identify hematopoietic progenitor cells, their isolation from peripheral blood provided another stem cell source. These peripheral blood stem cells (PBSCs) are capable of forming colonies of granulocytes/macrophages, erythrocytes, and other multipotential or immature progenitors.[67] The introduction of growth factors such as granulocyte colony-stimulating factor(filgrastim) and granulocyte/macrophage colony-stimulating factor (sargramostim), plerixafor[68] (a novel molecule that inhibits chemokine receptor CXCR4 binding to stromal cell–derived factor-1), and other agents[69] have contributed to successful mobilization of CD34$^+$ cells into the peripheral circulation and thus their use as a source of hematopoietic stem cells (HSCs). These PBSCs permitted high-dose salvage therapy to patients with refractory malignancies, resulting in prolonged survival and impeding tumor progression.[70] Although PBSCs have become a common source of HSCs for autologous transplants, their role in allogeneic transplants is still unclear.[71–73] Use of PBSCs may be influenced by multiple factors, including preference of the transplant center, primary disease, risk of relapse, graft-versus-leukemia effect, and donor preference. Experience with PBSCs for transplantation in patients with PID is limited.

Umbilical cord blood (UCB) represents another alternative source of HSCs and has become a standard option for both children and adults with hematopoietic disorders and malignancies.[74,75] The advantages include (1) a low rate of viral contamination, (2) lower rates of GVHD, and (3) readily available units.[76] The use of UCB for PID is limited. However 2 single-center experiences have been reported.[77,78] In both series, immunologic reconstitution was demonstrated.

Another promising methodology for HSCT would be to downregulate HLA expression by genetically engineering donor cells, using RNA interference (RNA$_i$). This enables the cells to evade immune recognition.[79] By integrating RNA$_i$ into genomic DNA, a universally accepted and expandable pool of donor cells would become available.

CURRENT STATUS OF SCT FOR PID

There is no doubt that, for the past 4 decades, allogeneic SCT for PID has allowed for survival of patients in whom the natural history of the disease predicted an early death. The Center for International Blood and Marrow Transplant Research (CIBMTR) collects data in collaboration with the European Groups for Blood and Marrow Transplantation (EBMT), the Asia-Pacific Blood Marrow Transplant group (APBMT), and the World Marrow Donor Association (WMDA) along with transplants performed in North and South America. A progress report of comprehensive data as of 2008 is available, including more than 1500 transplants performed around the world for patients with SCID and other PIDs.[2]

SCID represents the group of patients for whom HSCT is now considered standard of care; indeed, this PID has achieved the most successful survival record ranging from 63% to 100% when an HLA-matched sibling donor is available and 50% to 77% when haploidentical or HLA-mismatched donors are used.[58,80–87] The lack of donor availability, variable evidence of long-term immunologic reconstitution, and other limitations have led to the extensive use of unrelated but matched donors as a source of stem cells for SCID. The outcomes have improved over the recent years, with survivals ranging from 63% to 80%.[81,84,85,87,88]

The largest groups of non-SCID patients with primary immunodeficiencies for which SCT has been successful include WAS and chronic granulomatous disease. A collaborative study of the International Bone Marrow Transplant registry analyzed 170 transplants performed for WAS between 1968 and 1996. The overall 5-year probability of survival was 70% (95% confidence interval [CI], 63%–77%). Best outcomes were noted for patients receiving transplants from an HLA-identical sibling, 87% (95% CI, 74%–93%) as compared with 52% (95% CI, 37%–65%) for those receiving from other related donors. Matched unrelated donor transplants demonstrated a 5-year probability of survival of 71% (95% CI, 58%–80%). Of interest, if children receiving matched unrelated donor transplants were transplanted before the age of 5 years, the outcome was similar to HLA-matched sibling transplants.[89]

A more recent long-term outcome analysis for patients who underwent transplant for WAS was performed by the European Society for Immunodeficiencies (ESID) and the EBMT.[90] Included in the study were patients who had survived at least 2 years after HSCT. Survival was similar: 7-year event-free survival of 75%. Yet, a 20% incidence of autoimmunity was associated with mixed chimerism, independent of chronic GVHD. Furthermore, infection related to splenectomy was identified as an iatrogenic complication.[90]

Chronic granulomatous disease, an inherited disease of neutrophil function, is conventionally treated with prophylactic antibiotics and/or interferon therapy.[91] However, long-term follow-up data suggest significant morbidity caused by infection and only 50% to 55% survival through the third and forth decades of life.[92,93] HSCT has been a therapeutic option for the past 2 decades.[94,95] In 2002, the EBMT group reported results of 27 transplants from 1985 to 2000. Almost all (22 of 23) patients survived. These patients had received a myeloablative busulfan-containing conditioning regimen from an HLA-identical donor and achieved full and stable donor chimerism.[96] More recently, excellent survival (90%) after HSCT has been reported by the Newcastle group, with a median 61 months of follow-up.[97]

Disorders such as X-linked lymphoproliferative syndrome,[98] the familial forms of hemophagocytic lymphohistiocytosis,[99] leukocyte adhesion deficiency,[100] CD40 ligand deficiency,[101,102] and immunodysregulation polyendocrinopathy enteropathy X-linked syndrome[103] are within the spectrum of diseases treated with HSCT. Patients with Chédiak-Higashi syndrome have also been treated with HSCT; however, late-onset cognitive impairment has been described 20 years posttransplant.[104]

SUMMARY

The last 40 years has seen the emergence of HSCT as a therapeutic modality for fatal diseases and as a curative option for individuals born with inherited disorders that carry limited life expectancy and poor quality of life. Despite the rarity of many PIDs, these disorders have led the way toward innovative therapies and further provide insights into mechanisms of immunologic reconstitution applicable to all HSC transplants. Critical analysis of outcomes and prospective multicenter clinical trials will be necessary to further our understanding as to best therapeutic approaches for patients with PID, who constitute a very heterogenous group of patients.

REFERENCES

1. Bekkum DW, van de Vries MJ. Radiation chimaeras. London: Logos Press; 1967. p. 277.
2. The Medical College of Wisconsin and The National Marrow Donor Program. Center for International Blood and Marrow Transplant Research (CIBMTR). 2008. Available at: http://www.cibmtr.org/. 2008. Accessed October 28, 2009.
3. Good RA, Kapoor N, Reisner Y. Bone marrow transplantation—an expanding approach to treatment of many diseases. Cell Immunol 1983;82(1):36–54.
4. Quine WME. The remedial application of bone marrow. JAMA 1896;26:1012.
5. Tiselius A, Kabat EA. An electrophoretic study of immune sera and purified antibody preparations. J Exp Med 1939;69:119–31.
6. White TF, Dougherty A. Functional alterations in lymphoid tissue induced by adrenal cortical secretion. Am J Anat 1945;77:81–116.
7. Medawar PB. The experimental study of skin grafts. Br Med Bull 1945;3:79.
8. Owen R. Immunogenetic consequences of vascular anastomoses between bovine twins. Science 1945;28:400.
9. Loeb L. Heredity and internal secretion in the spontaneous development of cancer in mice. Science 1915;42(1095):912–4.
10. Gorer PA. The detection of antigenic differences in mouse erythrocytes by employment of immune sera. Br J Exp Pathol 1936;17:21.
11. Snell GD, Stevens LC. Histocompatibility genes of mice. III. H-1 and H-4, two histocompatibility loci in the first linkage group. Immunology 1961;4:366–79.
12. Snell GD. Histocompatibility genes of the mouse. I. Demonstration of weak histocompatibility differences by immunization and controlled tumor dosage. J Natl Cancer Inst 1958;20(4):787–824.
13. Snell GD, Jackson RB. Histocompatibility genes of the mouse. II. Production and analysis of isogenic resistant lines. J Natl Cancer Inst 1958;21(5):843–77.
14. Billingham RE, Brent L, Medawar PB. Actively acquired tolerance of foreign cells. Nature 1953;172:603–6.
15. Jacobson LO, Simmons EL, Marks EK, et al. Recovery from radiation injury. Science 1951;113:510–1.
16. Barnes DW, Ford CE, Ilbery PL, et al. Tissue transplantation in the radiation chimera. J Cell Physiol Suppl 1957;50(Suppl 1):123–38.

17. Main JM, Prehn RT. Successful skin homografts after the administration of high dosage X radiation and homologous bone marrow. J Natl Cancer Inst 1955; 15(4):1023–9.
18. Ford CE, Hamerton JL, Barnes DW, et al. Cytological identification of radiation-chimaeras. Nature 1956;177(4506):452–4.
19. Crouch BG, Overman RR. Chemical protection against x-radiation death in primates: a preliminary report. Science 1957;125(3257):1092.
20. Mathé G, Jammet H, Pendie N, et al. Transfusions et greffes de moelle osseuse homologue chez des humaine irradies a haute dose accidentellement. Nouvelle rev franc hematol 1959;4:226.
21. Mathe G, Amiel JL, Schwarzenberg L, et al. Adoptive immunotherapy of acute leukemia: experimental and clinical results. Cancer Res 1965;25(9):1525–31.
22. Thomas ED, Lochte HL Jr, Lu WC, et al. Intravenous infusion of bone marrow in patients receiving radiation and chemotherapy. N Engl J Med 1957;257(11): 491–6.
23. Bruton OC. Agammaglobulinemia. Pediatrics 1952;9(6):722–8.
24. Bruton OC, Apt L, Gitlin D, et al. Absence of serum gamma globulins. AMA Am J Dis Child 1952;84(5):632–6.
25. Medici MA, Kagan RM, Menkes J, et al. Chronic progressive panencephalitis in hypogammaglobulinemia: a literature review. In: JMR Foundation, editor. Immunodeficiency. Its nature and etiological significance in human diseases. Tokyo: University of Tokyo Press; 1978. p. 149–60.
26. Mannick JA, Lochte HL Jr, Ashley CA, et al. Autografts of bone marrow in dogs after lethal total-body radiation. Blood 1960;15:255–66.
27. Miller ME. Thymic dysplasia ("Swiss agammaglobulinemia"). I. Graft versus host reaction following bone-marrow transfusion. J Pediatr 1967;70(5):730–6.
28. Bregsma D, Good RA, editors. Immunologic deficiency in man. Birth defects original articles series, vol. 4. White Plains (NY): The National Foundation-March of Dimes; 1968.
29. de Vries MJ, Dooren LJ, Cleton FJ. Graft versus host or autoimmune lesions in the Swiss type of agammaglobulinemia. In: Bergsma D, editor. Immunologic Deficiency in Man. Birth defects original articles series, vol. 4. White Plains (NY): National Foundation-March of Dimes; 1968. p.173.
30. Hong R, Cooper MD, Allan MJ, et al. Immunological restitution in lymphopenic immunological deficiency syndrome. Lancet 1968;1(7541):503–6.
31. Dausset J. [Presence of A & B antigens in leukocytes disclosed by agglutination tests]. C R Seances Soc Biol Fil 1954;148(19–20):1607–8 [in French].
32. van Rood JJ, van Leeuwen A, van Santen MC. Anti HL-A2 inhibitor in normal human serum. Nature 1970;226(5243):366–7.
33. Payne R, Rolfs MR. Fetomaternal leukocyte incompatibility. J Clin Invest 1958; 37(12):1756–63.
34. Amos DB. Genetic and antigenetic aspects of human histocompatibility systems. Adv Immunol 1969;10:251–97.
35. Amos DB, Seigler HF, Southworth JG, et al. Skin graft rejection between subjects genotyped for HL-A. Transplant Proc 1969;1(1):342–6.
36. Ceppellini R, van Rood JJ. The HL-A system. I. Genetics and molecular biology. Semin Hematol 1974;11(3):233–51.
37. Terasaki PI, McClelland JD. Microdroplet assay of human serum cytotoxins. Nature 1964;204:998–1000.
38. Simonsen M. Graft versus host reactions. Their natural history, and applicability as tools of research. Prog Allergy 1962;6:349–467.

39. Good RA, Martinez C, Gabrielsen AE. Progress toward transplantation of tissues in man. Adv Pediatr 1964;13:93–127.

40. Storb R, Epstein RB, Bryant J, et al. Marrow grafts by combined marrow and leukocyte infusions in unrelated dogs selected by histocompatibility typing. Transplantation 1968;6(4):587–93.

41. Thomas ED, Epstein RB, Eschbach JW Jr, et al. Treatment of leukemia by extracorporeal irradiation. N Engl J Med 1965;273:6–12.

42. Good RA, Fisher DW. In: Good RA, Fisher DW, editors. Immunobiology: current knowledge of basic concepts in immunology and their clinical applications. Stamford (CT): Sinauer Associates; 1971. p. 305.

43. Good RA. Immunologic reconstitution: the achievement and it's meaning. In: Bergsma D, Good RA, editors. Birth defects original articles series, vol. 4. White Plains (NY): The National Foundation-March of Dimes; 1968.

44. Gatti RA, Meuwissen HJ, Allen HD, et al. Immunological reconstitution of sex-linked lymphopenic immunological deficiency. Lancet 1968;2(7583):1366–9.

45. Meuwissen HJ, Gatti RA, Terasaki PI, et al. Treatment of lymphopenic hypogammaglobulinemia and bone-marrow aplasia by transplantation of allogeneic marrow. Crucial role of histocompatibility matching. N Engl J Med 1969;281(13):691–7.

46. Gatti RA, Meuwissen HJ, Terasaki PI, et al. Recombination within the HL-A locus. Tissue Antigens 1971;1(5):239–41.

47. Gatti RA, Good RA. Follow-up of correction of severe dual system immunodeficiency with bone marrow transplantation. J Pediatr 1971;79(3):475–9.

48. Bach FH, Albertini RJ, Joo P, et al. Bone-marrow transplantation in a patient with the Wiskott-Aldrich syndrome. Lancet 1968;2(7583):1364–6.

49. Meuwissen HJ, Bortin MM, Bach FH, et al. Long-term survival after bone marrow transplantation: a 15-year follow-up report of a patient with Wiskott-Aldrich syndrome. J Pediatr 1984;105(3):365–9.

50. Bortin MM. A compendium of reported human bone marrow transplants. Transplantation 1970;9(6):571–87.

51. Thomas ED, Storb R, Clift RA, et al. Bone-marrow transplantation (second of two parts). N Engl J Med 1975;292(17):895–902.

52. Gatti RA, Kemple K, Schwartzmann J, et al. HLA-D typing with lymphoblastoid cell lines. VI. Rationale and goals of data reduction. Tissue Antigens 1979;14(3):183–93.

53. Gatti RA, Kempner DH, Leibold W. The role of the MHC antigens in the mature and immature host. Pediatrics 1979;64(5 Pt 2 Suppl):803–13.

54. Reisner Y, Kapoor N, Kirkpatrick D, et al. Transplantation for severe combined immunodeficiency with HLA-A, B, D, DR incompatible parental marrow cells fractionated by soybean agglutinin and sheep red blood cells. Blood 1983;61(2):341–8.

55. O'Reilly RJ, Keever CA, Small TN, et al. The use of HLA-non-identical T-cell-depleted marrow transplants for correction of severe combined immunodeficiency disease. Immunodefic Rev 1989;1(4):273–309.

56. Buckley RH, Schiff SE, Sampson HA, et al. Development of immunity in human severe primary T cell deficiency following haploidentical bone marrow stem cell transplantation. J Immunol 1986;136(7):2398–407.

57. Dror Y, Gallagher R, Wara DW, et al. Immune reconstitution in severe combined immunodeficiency disease after lectin-treated, T-cell-depleted haplocompatible bone marrow transplantation. Blood 1993;81(8):2021–30.

58. Buckley RH, Schiff SE, Schiff RI, et al. Hematopoietic stem-cell transplantation for the treatment of severe combined immunodeficiency. N Engl J Med 1999; 340(7):508–16.
59. de Witte T, Hoogenhout J, de Pauw B, et al. Depletion of donor lymphocytes by counterflow centrifugation successfully prevents acute graft-versus-host disease in matched allogeneic marrow transplantation. Blood 1986;67(5): 1302–8.
60. Lowenberg B, Wagemaker G, van Bekkum DW, et al. Graft-versus-host disease following transplantation of 'one log' versus 'two log' T-lymphocyte-depleted bone marrow from HLA-identical donors. Bone Marrow Transplant 1986;1(2): 133–40.
61. Rodt H, Kolb HJ, Netzel B, et al. Effect of anti-T-cell globulin on GVHD in leukemic patients treated with BMT. Transplant Proc 1981;13(1 Pt 1):257–61.
62. Filipovich AH, McGlave P, Ramsay NK, et al. Treatment of donor bone marrow with OKT3 (PAN-T monoclonal antibody) for prophylaxis of graft-vs.-host disease (GvHD) in histocompatible allogeneic bone marrow transplantation (BMT): a pilot study. J Clin Immunol 1982;2(Suppl 3):154S–7S.
63. Filipovich AH, McGlave PB, Ramsay NK, et al. Pretreatment of donor bone marrow with monoclonal antibody OKT3 for prevention of acute graft-versus-host disease in allogeneic histocompatible bone-marrow transplantation. Lancet 1982;1(8284):1266–9.
64. Martin PJ, Hansen JA, Thomas ED. Preincubation of donor bone marrow cells with a combination of murine monoclonal anti-T-cell antibodies without complement does not prevent graft-versus-host disease after allogeneic marrow transplantation. J Clin Immunol 1984;4(1):18–22.
65. Umiel T, Daley JF, Bhan AK, et al. Acquisition of immune competence by a subset of human cortical thymocytes expressing mature T cell antigens. J Immunol 1982;129(3):1054–60.
66. Ho VT, Soiffer RJ. The history and future of T-cell depletion as graft-versus-host disease prophylaxis for allogeneic hematopoietic stem cell transplantation. Blood 2001;98(12):3192–204.
67. Krause DS, Fackler MJ, Civin CI, et al. CD34: structure, biology, and clinical utility. Blood 1996;87(1):1–13.
68. Cashen AF. Plerixafor hydrochloride: a novel agent for the mobilization of peripheral blood stem cells. Drugs Today (Barc) 2009;45(7):497–505.
69. Greinix HT, Worel N. New agents for mobilizing peripheral blood stem cells. Transfus Apher Sci 2009;41(1):67–71.
70. Kessinger A, Armitage JO, Smith DM, et al. High-dose therapy and autologous peripheral blood stem cell transplantation for patients with lymphoma. Blood 1989;74(4):1260–5.
71. Pidala J, Anasetti C, Kharfan-Dabaja MA, et al. Decision analysis of peripheral blood versus bone marrow hematopoietic stem cells for allogeneic hematopoietic cell transplantation. Biol Blood Marrow Transplant 2009;15(11):1415–21.
72. Gallardo D, de la Camara R, Nieto JB, et al. Is mobilized peripheral blood comparable with bone marrow as a source of hematopoietic stem cells for allogeneic transplantation from HLA-identical sibling donors? A case-control study. Haematologica 2009;94(9):1282–8.
73. Gorin NC, Labopin M, Blaise D, et al. Higher incidence of relapse with peripheral blood rather than marrow as a source of stem cells in adults with acute myelocytic leukemia autografted during the first remission. J Clin Oncol 2009; 27(24):3987–93.

74. Gluckman E, Broxmeyer HA, Auerbach AD, et al. Hematopoietic reconstitution in a patient with Fanconi's anemia by means of umbilical-cord blood from an HLA-identical sibling. N Engl J Med 1989;321(17):1174–8.

75. Gluckman E, Rocha V, Boyer-Chammard A, et al. Outcome of cord-blood transplantation from related and unrelated donors. Eurocord Transplant Group and the European Blood and Marrow Transplantation Group. N Engl J Med 1997; 337(6):373–81.

76. Gluckman E, Rocha V. Cord blood transplantation: state of the art. Haematologica 2009;94(4):451–4.

77. Knutsen AP, Wall DA. Umbilical cord blood transplantation in severe T-cell immunodeficiency disorders: two-year experience. J Clin Immunol 2000;20(6): 466–76.

78. Bhattacharya A, Slatter MA, Chapman CE, et al. Single centre experience of umbilical cord stem cell transplantation for primary immunodeficiency. Bone Marrow Transplant 2005;36(4):295–9.

79. Hacke K, Falahati R, Flebbe-Rehwaldt L, et al. Suppression of HLA expression by lentivirus-mediated gene transfer of siRNA cassettes and in vivo chemoselection to enhance hematopoietic stem cell transplantation. Immunol Res 2009;44(1–3):112–26.

80. Fischer A, Landais P, Friedrich W, et al. Bone marrow transplantation (BMT) in Europe for primary immunodeficiencies other than severe combined immunodeficiency: a report from the European Group for BMT and the European Group for Immunodeficiency. Blood 1994;83(4):1149–54.

81. Antoine C, Muller S, Cant A, et al. Long-term survival and transplantation of haemopoietic stem cells for immunodeficiencies: report of the European experience 1968-99. Lancet 2003;361(9357):553–60.

82. Patel NC, Chinen J, Rosenblatt HM, et al. Long-term outcomes of nonconditioned patients with severe combined immunodeficiency transplanted with HLA-identical or haploidentical bone marrow depleted of T cells with anti-CD6 mAb. J Allergy Clin Immunol 2008;122(6):1185–93.

83. Haddad E, Landais P, Friedrich W, et al. Long-term immune reconstitution and outcome after HLA-nonidentical T-cell-depleted bone marrow transplantation for severe combined immunodeficiency: a European retrospective study of 116 patients. Blood 1998;91(10):3646–53.

84. Roifman CM, Grunebaum E, Dalal I, et al. Matched unrelated bone marrow transplant for severe combined immunodeficiency. Immunol Res 2007; 38(1–3):191–200.

85. Grunebaum E, Mazzolari E, Porta F, et al. Bone marrow transplantation for severe combined immune deficiency. JAMA 2006;295(5):508–18.

86. Railey MD, Lokhnygina Y, Buckley RH. Long-term clinical outcome of patients with severe combined immunodeficiency who received related donor bone marrow transplants without pretransplant chemotherapy or post-transplant GVHD prophylaxis. J Pediatr 2009;155(6):834–40 e1.

87. Mazzolari E, Forino C, Guerci S, et al. Long-term immune reconstitution and clinical outcome after stem cell transplantation for severe T-cell immunodeficiency. J Allergy Clin Immunol 2007;120(4):892–9.

88. Rao K, Amrolia PJ, Jones A, et al. Improved survival after unrelated donor bone marrow transplantation in children with primary immunodeficiency using a reduced-intensity conditioning regimen. Blood 2005;105(2):879–85.

89. Filipovich AH, Stone JV, Tomany SC, et al. Impact of donor type on outcome of bone marrow transplantation for Wiskott-Aldrich syndrome: collaborative study

of the International Bone Marrow Transplant Registry and the National Marrow Donor Program. Blood 2001;97(6):1598–603.

90. Ozsahin H, Cavazzana-Calvo M, Notarangelo LD, et al. Long-term outcome following hematopoietic stem-cell transplantation in Wiskott-Aldrich syndrome: collaborative study of the European Society for Immunodeficiencies and European Group for Blood and Marrow Transplantation. Blood 2008;111(1):439–45.

91. The International Chronic Cooperative Study Group. A controlled trial of interferon gamma to prevent infection in chronic granulomatous disease. The International Chronic Granulomatous Disease Cooperative Study Group. N Engl J Med 1991;324(8):509–16.

92. Liese J, Kloos S, Jendrossek V, et al. Long-term follow-up and outcome of 39 patients with chronic granulomatous disease. J Pediatr 2000;137(5):687–93.

93. Jones LB, McGrogan P, Flood TJ, et al. Special article: chronic granulomatous disease in the United Kingdom and Ireland: a comprehensive national patient-based registry. Clin Exp Immunol 2008;152(2):211–8.

94. Di Bartolomeo P, Di Girolamo G, Angrilli F, et al. Reconstitution of normal neutrophil function in chronic granulomatous disease by bone marrow transplantation. Bone Marrow Transplant 1989;4(6):695–700.

95. Schettini F, De Mattia D, Manzionna MM, et al. Bone marrow transplantation for chronic granulomatous disease associated with cytochrome B deficiency. Pediatr Hematol Oncol 1987;4(3):277–9.

96. Seger RA, Gungor T, Belohradsky BH, et al. Treatment of chronic granulomatous disease with myeloablative conditioning and an unmodified hemopoietic allograft: a survey of the European experience, 1985–2000. Blood 2002;100(13): 4344–50.

97. Soncini E, Slatter MA, Jones LB, et al. Unrelated donor and HLA-identical sibling haematopoietic stem cell transplantation cure chronic granulomatous disease with good long-term outcome and growth. Br J Haematol 2009;145(1):73–83.

98. Hoffmann T, Heilmann C, Madsen HO, et al. Matched unrelated allogeneic bone marrow transplantation for recurrent malignant lymphoma in a patient with X-linked lymphoproliferative disease (XLP). Bone Marrow Transplant 1998;22(6):603–4.

99. Jordan MB, Filipovich AH. Hematopoietic cell transplantation for hemophagocytic lymphohistiocytosis: a journey of a thousand miles begins with a single (big) step. Bone Marrow Transplant 2008;42(7):433–7.

100. Qasim W, Cavazzana-Calvo M, Davies EG, et al. Allogeneic hematopoietic stem-cell transplantation for leukocyte adhesion deficiency. Pediatrics 2009; 123(3):836–40.

101. Isam H, Al-Wahadneh A. Successful bone marrow transplantation in a child with X-linked hyper-IgM syndrome. Saudi J Kidney Dis Transpl 2004;15(4):489–93.

102. Duplantier JE, Seyama K, Day NK, et al. Immunologic reconstitution following bone marrow transplantation for X-linked hyper IgM syndrome. Clin Immunol 2001;98(3):313–8.

103. Rao A, Kamani N, Filipovich A, et al. Successful bone marrow transplantation for IPEX syndrome after reduced-intensity conditioning. Blood 2007;109(1):383–5.

104. Tardieu M, Lacroix C, Neven B, et al. Progressive neurologic dysfunctions 20 years after allogeneic bone marrow transplantation for Chediak-Higashi syndrome. Blood 2005;106(1):40–2.

Hematopoietic Stem Cell Transplantation for Severe Combined Immune Deficiency or What the Children have Taught Us

Joel M. Rappeport, MD[a], Richard J. O'Reilly, MD[b,c,d],
Neena Kapoor, MD[e,f], Robertson Parkman, MD[g,h],*

KEYWORDS

* Severe combined immune deficiency
* Hematopoietic stem cell transplantation • Unrelated • In utero
* Gene transfer

A version of this article was previously published in the *Immunology and Allergy Clinics of North America*, 30:1.

This work was supported by Grant Nos. CA100265 and HL54850 from the National Institutes of Health.

[a] Department of Internal Medicine, Yale University School of Medicine, 333 Cedar Street, New Haven, CT 06510, USA

[b] Department of Pediatrics, Memorial Sloan Kettering Cancer Center, 1275 York Avenue, Box 139, New York, NY 10021, USA

[c] Pediatric Bone Marrow Transplant Service, Memorial Sloan-Kettering Cancer Center, 1275 York Avenue, New York, NY 10065, USA

[d] Pediatric Oncology Research, Memorial Sloan Kettering Cancer Center, New York, NY, USA

[e] Department of Pediatrics, University of Southern California Keck School of Medicine, Los Angeles, CA, USA

[f] Bone Marrow Transplantation Program, Division of Research Immunology/Bone Marrow Transplantation, Childrens Hospital Los Angeles, Los Angeles, 4650 Sunset Boulevard, Mail Stop 62, Los Angeles, CA 90027, USA

[g] Division of Research Immunology/BMT, and The Saban Research Institute, Childrens Hospital Los Angeles, 4650 Sunset Boulevard, Mail Stop 62, Los Angeles, CA 90027, USA

[h] Department of Pediatrics, Molecular Microbiology and Immunology, University of Southern California Keck School of Medicine, Los Angeles, CA, USA

* Corresponding author. Division of Research Immunology/BMT, and The Saban Research Institute, Childrens Hospital Los Angeles, 4650 Sunset Boulevard, Mail Stop 62, Los Angeles, CA 90027.

E-mail address: rparkman@chla.usc.edu

Hematol Oncol Clin N Am 25 (2011) 17–30
doi:10.1016/j.hoc.2010.11.002
0889-8588/11/$ – see front matter © 2011 Elsevier Inc. All rights reserved.

More than 40 years ago, the first successful allogeneic hematopoietic stem cell transplantation (HSCT) was reported by Robert A. Good, MD and his colleagues[1] for a child with severe combined immunodeficiency (SCID). In the succeeding years, HSCT for SCID patients have represented only a small portion of the total number of allogeneic HSCT performed. Nevertheless, the clinical and biologic importance of the patients transplanted for SCID has continued. SCID patients were the first to be successfully transplanted with nonsibling related bone marrow, unrelated bone marrow, T-cell depleted HSCT, and genetically corrected (gene transfer) autologous HSC.[2–5] In addition, many of the biologic insights that are now widely applied to allogeneic HSCT were first identified in the transplantation of SCID patients. Therefore, this article reviews the clinical and biologic lessons that have been learned from HSCT for SCID patients, and how the information has impacted the general field of allogeneic HSCT.

PRELUDES

In 1956 it was established that rodents receiving total body irradiation (TBI) could be rescued from the lethality of bone marrow failure by the infusion of histocompatible bone marrow.[6] In those studies the importance of histocompatibility for the successful rescue of the animals from lethal TBI by the prevention of graft-versus-host disease (GVHD) was identified. In the decade between the biologic reality that the transplantation of bone marrow could rescue irradiated animals and the first successful human allogeneic HSCT, clinical investigators attempted to apply the biologic principles to the treatment of patients. A sentinel event was the irradiation accident that occurred in Yugoslavia in 1959 where 6 patients, who were heavily irradiated, were subsequently treated by the infusion of either fetal liver and spleen cells or unrelated bone marrow cells.[7] No sustained donor hematopoietic engraftment was seen in any patients, although slight increases in donor-type erythrocytes were transiently seen in some patients. The patient with the highest dose of irradiation died whereas the other patients had autologous hematopoietic recovery. Other early attempts included the use of high-dose irradiation/chemotherapy and pooled allogeneic bone marrow for the treatment of related and unrelated patients with acute leukemia. Patients with aplastic anemia were infused with bone marrow from identical twins with some patients having hematopoietic improvement, but it was unclear whether their improvement in hematopoiesis was due to the HSCT or the spontaneous recovery of their underlying aplastic anemia. Many allogeneic recipients developed acute GVHD that had similarities to GVHD seen in rodents following histoincompatible transplants. Thus, clinicians were aware that histocompatibility might improve the likelihood of successful HSCT. During the 1960s, the development of serologic reagents to detect human leukocyte antigen (HLA)-A and HLA-B permitted physicians to determine the class I histocompatibility of potential donors and recipients. The development of the mixed lymphocyte culture (MLC) permitted the determination of class II histocompatibility because no antiserum to HLA-DR existed.

CLINICAL ADVANCES
Allogeneic-Related HSCT

The first successful allogeneic HSCT was a member of a kindred in which 11 male infants had died due to severe recurrent infections during the first year of life.[1] At admission, the child had draining skin pustules, no detectable lymph nodes, and lymphopenia. At that time, no phenotypic assays existed for the enumeration of T lymphocytes, but the diagnosis was confirmed by the absence of cutaneous delayed hypersensitivity as well as functional assays showing that the patient's lymphocytes did not respond to stimulation with either phytohemagglutinin (PHA) or allogeneic cells. HLA-A and -B typing indicated that the patient and a sister were HLA-B identical but differed at one HLA-A antigen; however, the sister did not respond in MLC to stimulation with the patient's cells. The patient was transplanted with a mixture of peripheral blood leukocytes and bone marrow. The cells were given intraperitoneally. A total dose of 3.5×10^8 peripheral blood leukocytes and 1×10^9 nucleated bone marrow cells were given. A week after transplantation, the patient developed an erthymatous rash, which on skin biopsy had histopathological features characteristic of GVHD. Stimulation of the patient's peripheral blood lymphocytes showed the development of large lymphoblasts with a female karyotype, indicating that the circulatory lymphocytes were now responsive to stimulation by PHA and were of donor origin. The patient was challenged with dinitrofluorobenzene and responded to skin testing, demonstrating the development of normal delayed hypersensitivity.

The patient was blood group A and the donor blood group O. The patient's anti-B titers rose, but he developed a Coomb positive hemolytic anemia. Eight weeks after HSCT the patient's platelet and granulocyte counts began to drop, and a bone marrow aspirate showed hypocellularity with both male and female cells. The patient's bone marrow progressed to complete aplasia with all cells being of donor origin.

Three months after the first transplant the patient was transplanted for the second time with 1×10^9 bone marrow cells: 20% into the right ileac marrow space and 80% intraperitoneally. The bone marrow was treated in vitro with a horse antihuman lymphoblast globulin for 2 hours before infusion. By 2 weeks there was an increase in the platelet count, and the white blood cell count began to increase. All bone marrow cells had a female karyotype.[8] The patient is now more than 40 years old, with normal immune and hematopoietic function of donor origin.

The lessons
The authors of the initial report were not able to appreciate the significance of all their clinical and laboratory observations. The patient received peripheral blood T lymphocytes as well as bone marrow cells, and it is likely that the early onset of acute GVHD was due to the large number of donor T lymphocytes given, especially considering that the donor and patient were an HLA-A mismatch. In the second transplant to reduce the probability of GVHD, they tried to reduce the number of T lymphocytes infused by (1) taking smaller bone marrow aspiration to reduce peripheral blood contamination and (2) treating the bone marrow with antiserum to remove T lymphocytes.[9] The patient did not develop any acute GVHD after the second transplant.

Subsequent animal experiments demonstrated that the efficiency of the intraperitoneal injection of HSC was approximately one-tenth that of intravenous injection. The present clinical use of the intravenous route for HSC infusion is based on the canine experiments performed by Thomas and his colleagues. The success of the initial transplants in the SCID patient was, therefore, due to the relatively large number of cells given, the small size of the patient, and the use of a HLA-B identical and MLC nonreactive donor.

The patient developed immune-mediated bone marrow aplasia, which was also seen in some other SCID patients during the 1970s. It is of interest that, although hemolytic anemia has been seen following ABO-incompatible or histoincompatible HSCT in SCID patients in more recent years, rarely has bone marrow aplasia occurred. The reason for this clinical change is unclear. The development of bone marrow aplasia, however, clearly demonstrated that immune cell-mediated events including GVHD can produce severe aplastic anemia, indicating that immunosuppression might have a role in the treatment of aplastic anemia, which was subsequently demonstrated in both animal studies and clinical trials using antithymocyte globulin and other immuno-suppressive agents.[10]

The patient, in addition to being the first patient to have an immune deficiency corrected by HSCT, also represented the first successful treatment of bone marrow failure by allogeneic HSCT. No evidence of donor hematopoietic engraftment occurred following the initial transplant. It is now clear that in SCID patients, no clinically significant donor HSC engraftment occurs without some myelosuppressive therapy. However, once the immune-mediated destruction of the recipient hematopoiesis had occurred and adequate "space" had been developed, it was possible even with the intraperitoneal infusion of donor bone marrow to establish donor-derived hematopoiesis without any chemotherapy. The patient demonstrated what it took another decade to formally prove, that is, that engraftment of donor HSC requires the elimination or reduction of the number of recipient HSC to permit the engraftment of donor hematopoietic cells.[11] The present use of reduced intensity regimens that rely on the engraftment of the donor immune system to eliminate both normal and abnormal (neoplastic) recipient hematopoiesis is a direct descendant of the biologic events that occurred in the first SCID patient.[12]

Related Nonsibling Donors

Because most SCID patients did not have an MLC-nonreactive sibling donor, clinicians began to explore other relatives to see if any potential donors were MLC nonreactive. In a limited number of cases, MLC-nonreactive donors were identified that were successfully used to treat cases of SCID.[2,13] When related donors, who were MLC reactive, were used, patients usually died of acute GVHD, suggesting that MLC nonreactivity (HLA-DR locus identity with modern techniques) was a prerequisite for the successful HSCT of SCID without fatal GVHD. This approach to identifying appropriate donors was subsequently applied to other diseases as well.[14]

The lessons

Differences at single class I alleles do not significantly decrease the overall likelihood of event-free survival, whereas class II differences are almost uniformly associated with poor outcome. Thus, the results from the early transplants for SCID were the basis for focusing on identifying donors who were MLC nonreactive or Class II identical.

Unrelated Donors

Because the majority of SCID patients did not have an MLC-nonreactive related donor, the possibility that an MLC-nonreactive unrelated donor might exist who could be a successful donor was explored. Despite the fact that formal programs to identify unrelated MLC nonreactive donors did not exist, a SCID patient, who had a prevalent haplotype, received 7 transplants from an unrelated individual who was MLC nonreactive.[3] The donor and recipient were HLA-B identical but disparate at one HLA-A antigen. The patient was homozygous for HLA-A1 while the donor was heterozygous (HLA-A1, HLA-A2). At 5 months of age the patient received 10×10^6 bone marrow cells/kg by the intravenous route. The bone marrow had been shipped from Denmark to the United States. Ten days later the patient developed a macular rash consistent with GVHD, and PHA-responsive lymphocytes were detected. Three weeks later the patient received a second infusion of 10×10^6 cells. The patient developed detectable lymph nodes and increasingly severe acute GVHD. At 2 months the circulating donor lymphocytes disappeared, and the patient received a third transplant of

17 × 10^6 cells by the intravenous route. Again the patient developed PHA-responsive donor lymphocytes that persisted for 4 months. A fourth transplant at 13 months of age was performed with 10 × 10^6 bone marrow cells given intravenously. Again there was an increase in PHA-responsive lymphocytes of donor origin, but by 6 months after HSCT the PHA-responsive donor lymphocytes were no longer detected. Therefore, because of the possibility of hybrid resistance, the patient received 2 doses of cyclophosphamide (25 mg/kg) before HSCT, which consisted of 130 × 10^6 cells/kg of fresh bone marrow cells. The patient developed PHA-responsive donor lymphocytes and had in vitro responses to both mitogens and antigens. Donor T lymphocytes but no B lymphocytes were present in the patient's circulation. Three months following the fifth transplant, when the patient was about to be discharged from the hospital, he developed severe aplastic anemia with all detectable residual bone marrow cells being of donor origin. Two months later, without preconditioning, the patient received frozen bone marrow cells from his fifth transplant that did not result in any hematopoietic engraftment. Therefore, 4 months later, after preparation with full doses of cyclosphosphamide (50 mg/kg × 4 days), the patient received 1 × 10^8 bone marrow cells/kg intravenously. At 2 weeks he developed donor hematopoiesis and acute GVHD. All T lymphocytes were of donor origin. B lymphocytes were detected for the first time, with spontaneous rises in his serum immunoglobulin levels. After discharge, all lymphoid and hematopoietic elements were of donor origin by both karyotyping and cell surface antigen analysis.

The lessons

Previous attempts to use unrelated bone marrow to treat aplastic anemia had been unsuccessful. This patient demonstrated that significant pretransplant immunosuppression may be necessary, even in patients with SCID, to achieve successful donor hematopoietic engraftment. The successful treatment of this patient and other SCID patients with unrelated HSCT were a major impetus for the establishment both of the National Donor Marrow Program and the international cooperation that is now available for obtaining unrelated bone marrow, mobilized peripheral blood cells, and cord blood.

Fetal Liver Cells

Based on studies from neonatally thymectomized mice, it was determined that histoincompatible HSCT could be done if the HSC inoculum was devoid of T lymphocytes capable of causing acute GVHD.[15] Clinical investigators, therefore, attempted to identify sources of human HSC that did not contain T lymphocytes. Their attention initially focused on the potential use of fetal liver, which before 14 to 16 weeks of gestational age is a major source of hematopoiesis in the human fetus. Because no T lymphocytes are found in the circulation after 12 weeks of gestation, it was hypothesized that fetal liver obtained from electively aborted fetuses of less than 12 weeks of gestation would not contain significant numbers of T lymphocytes. Therefore, fetal liver cells could be an HSC source devoid of T lymphocytes. HLA typing was not possible before the transplantation of the fetal liver cells. Therefore, questions existed as to whether clinical benefit would be derived from the engraftment of the histoincompatible HSC.[16] Initially, transplants with fetal liver were unsuccessful, possibly due to the use of cryopreserved fetal liver cells in most cases. The first successful immune reconstitution reported using fetal liver cells was achieved in a patient with SCID due to adenosine deaminase (ADA) deficiency.[17] The patient received 25 × 10^8 fetal liver cells intraperitoneally when the patient was 5 months old. IgM-bearing cells were detected 19 days after transplantation, and an increase in T lymphocytes was seen by 40 days.

PHA-responsive cells were present by day 74. The patient developed in vitro proliferative responses to mitogens, specific antigens (candida), and allogeneic lymphocytes. Immunization with φX174 resulted in a low primary IgM response with little IgG production after a repeat immunization. The patient developed appropriate isohemagglutinin antibodies. The patient was taken off replacement immunoglobulin and did well until 1 year of age when he developed nephrotic syndrome, from which he died.

Subsequent SCID patients without ADA deficiency were also transplanted with fetal liver cells. One patient had the correction of his T-lymphocyte immune deficiency after the transplantation of 8.4×8^7 fetal liver cells intraperitoneally at 13 months of age. He developed GVHD, which lasted for 6 weeks, and had the presence of normal numbers of PHA-responsive T lymphocytes by 12 weeks after transplantation. The patient developed a cutaneous response to candida antigen. Serum IgM levels rose to normal levels by 1 year, but he had no detectable IgG, requiring the continued administration of replacement immunoglobulin.[18] However, subsequent series with larger numbers of patients confirmed the potential of fetal liver cells ± fetal thymus to correct T-lymphocyte and sometimes B-lymphocyte immunodeficiencies, but also demonstrated that durable engraftment was less than 30% with a low probably of achieving long-term immune reconstitution.

The lessons

The recipients of fetal liver cells demonstrated that fetal liver cells devoid of T lymphocytes were capable of supporting thymopoiesis without the development of GVHD. The first patient, who developed circulating B lymphocytes, had ADA deficiency. It is now known that cross-feeding can correct ADA deficiency. The investigators could not determine the origin of the circulating B lymphocytes, but they were most likely of recipient origin, while the donor-derived T lymphocytes were the source of ADA. Successful treatment of the ADA-deficient form of SCID with either exogenous enzyme therapy or HSCT results initially in increases in the number of B lymphocytes of recipient origin. Decreased primary and secondary response to φX174 stimulation suggests that there was a lack of normal T- and B-lymphocyte cooperation.

None of the initial recipients of fetal liver cells received any pretransplant chemotherapy.[19,20] Therefore, it is unlikely that HSC engraftment occurred. The cells that gave rise to T lymphocytes of donor origin may thus have been derived from committed lymphoid progenitors (CLP) that were able to migrate to the recipient thymus, induce its differentiation, and differentiate into circulating T lymphocytes of donor origin.[21] The follow-up of the fetal liver recipients should provide important biologic information about the longevity and the breadth of T-lymphocyte immunity derived from CLP.

T-Lymphocyte Depleted HSCT

In 1975 it was first demonstrated in mice that T-lymphocyte depletion of histoincompatible HSC permitted both the hematological and immunologic reconstitution of irradiated mice without GVHD.[22] Attempts were therefore undertaken in humans to eliminate T lymphocytes from histoincompatible bone marrow using a variety of techniques, both physical and biological. The selective separation of T lymphocytes from HSC by albumin density gradients as well as the suicide of donor T lymphocytes after stimulation by recipient antigens were attempted. None of these approaches led to the correction of the immune deficiency of any SCID patients. Most patients had no signs of the engraftment of any donor cells.

The approach to T-lymphocyte depletion that was first shown to be clinically successful was the physical removal of T lymphocytes based on their agglutination with soybean agglutinin (SBA) followed by the physical rosetting of the residual T lymphocytes by sheep red blood cells (E), which had initially been used to immunophenotypically detect T lymphocytes. The combination of SBA agglutination followed by E rosette formation permitted the physical removal of the majority of T lymphocytes from human bone marrow, which could then be used for HSCT. Following preclinical studies in monkeys, patients were treated with HLA haploidentical disparate bone marrow depleted of T lymphocytes.[4,23]

Of the first 6 SCID patients treated with T-lymphocyte depleted MLC-reactive paternal marrow, 5 had durable immune reconstitution, whereas GVHD was limited or nondetectable. None of the patients had chemotherapy before their engraftment. One patient had graft rejection and was successfully retransplanted after pretransplant chemotherapy.

The lessons
The clinical experience confirms the experiments in mice that T-lymphocyte depletion before HSCT could permit the engraftment of histoincompatible HSC without the development of clinically significant or fatal acute GVHD. However, pretransplant immunosuppression is required in some cases to achieve donor immune reconstitution due to the presence of either engrafted maternal T lymphocytes or hybrid resistance. The use of T-lymphocyte depleted HSCT is now in general use for both related and unrelated HSCT.[24]

In Utero HSC Transplantation

A variety of genetic diseases (β- and α-thalassemia, adrenoleukodystrophy, Hurler disease, and so forth) can be cured or stabilized by the postnatal engraftment of normal allogeneic HSC. Some genetic diseases, however, have significant morbidity at the time of birth, suggesting that the engraftment of normal HSC before birth might provide clinical benefit to the patients. Fetuses with hemoglobinopathies have been transplanted in utero with HSC from either fetal liver or T-lymphocyte depleted parental bone marrow without any evidence of sustained hematopoietic engraftment.[25] However, the transplants were performed in fetuses of more than 16 weeks of gestation, by which time the fetuses had T lymphocytes capable of responding to allogeneic cells.[26]

In contrast, 2 SCID patients have been reported who were successfully transplanted with T-lymphocyte depleted parental histoincompatible bone marrow cells.[27,28] In both cases, the genetic basis for the patients' disease was defects in the common γ-chain. The first patient received a total of 18.6×10^6 cells intraperitoneally in 3 injections starting at 16 weeks of gestation. The second patient received 18×10^6 nucleated cells in 2 intraperitoneal injections beginning at 21 weeks of gestation. The clinical outcomes of both patients were similar. Both had PHA-responsive T lymphocytes of donor origin while their B lymphocytes continued to be of recipient origin. In the first case, immunizations were successful with the production of specific antibodies, whereas no information is available about antibody production in the second case. Thus, these patients with the X-linked form of SCID, who have defective natural killer (NK) cells, were able to be successfully engrafted with haploidentical T-cell depleted HSC without the development of any detectable GVHD.

The lessons
In contrast to the SCID patients, the patients with hemoglobinapathies, who have normal immune systems, were not able to be successfully transplanted with haploidentical T-lymphocyte depleted HSC even as early as 16 to 20 weeks of

gestation. It is not clear as to whether the immune reconstitution that occurred in the SCID patients was due to HSC engraftment or whether the T lymphocytes are derived from CLP in the HSC inoculum. Nevertheless, the persistence of the donor lymphoid cells was achieved in the SCID patients. Sustained donor lymphoid or hematopoietic engraftment was not achieved in patients with nonimmune genetic diseases, although one patient may have died of in utero GVHD.[29] Both successfully treated SCID patients had X-linked SCID and, therefore, an absence of functional NK cells and the ability to exhibit hybrid resistance. It would be interesting to know if patients with other forms of SCID, who had normal NK function after birth, could be successfully engrafted in utero.

Genetically Corrected HSC

The identification of the molecular basis of most forms of SCID (common γ-chain deficiency, ADA deficiency, interleukin [IL]-7 receptor deficiency, and so forth) made SCID patients logical candidates for the use of genetically corrected autologous HSC. Murine studies had demonstrated that retroviral vectors could transduce pluripotent hematopoietic stem cells as well as committed lymphoid progenitors. Thus, clinical investigators thought that transplantation of genetically corrected autologous HSC could provide all of the benefits associated with the transplantation of allogeneic HSC without the risks of acute or chronic GVHD.

The first gene to be cloned that was associated with SCID was ADA. Researchers in preclinical studies demonstrated that retroviral vectors containing the human ADA gene could transduce both murine HSC and human mature T lymphocytes.[30] The transduction of mature T lymphocytes normalized their intracellular metabolism, demonstrating that the transduced ADA gene produced adequate levels of functioning enzyme. The first human gene transfer trial was in patients with ADA-deficient SCID, who received their own T lymphocytes that had been transduced in vitro.[31] The patients had had adequate numbers of T lymphocytes for the transduction because they were on enzyme replacement therapy. The patients received multiple infusions of the transduced T lymphocytes. The persistence of the transduced cells could be detected for at least 7 years. It was difficult, however, to determine whether any clinical efficacy was associated with the transduced cells because the patients continued on their exogenous enzyme replacement therapy. However, no toxic effects were assessed with the infusion of the transduced T lymphocytes.

Additional patients were then transplanted with a mixture of transduced bone marrow plus transduced peripheral blood. Different retroviral vectors were used for the 2 transductions so that it would be possible to determine the source of any circulating T lymphocytes.[5] Posttransplant analysis of myeloid cells revealed that all transduced cells contain the vector used to transduce bone marrow cells, whereas all the T lymphocytes early after transplantation were derived from the infused mature T lymphocytes. Over the course of the first year the proportion of T lymphocytes derived from the transduced T lymphocytes decreased, whereas the proportion derived from the transduced bone marrow increased, so that by 1 year all the transduced T lymphocytes contained the bone marrow vector. After the patients had their ADA replacement enzyme therapy discontinued, the frequency of their transduced T lymphocytes was 5% and of the bone marrow precursors 25%. Thus, the patients were able to have significant immune reconstitution following the transplantation of the gene corrected cells with the production of specific antibody and the generation of responses to mitogen stimulation. However, the majority of their immune function was due to nontransduced cells, demonstrating the effect of cross-correction between the transduced and the nontransduced cells.

With the identification of defects in the common γ-chain as the basis for the X-link form of SCID, preclinical research was undertaken to evaluate gene transfer. Using a retroviral vector, French investigators transplanted patients with autologous bone marrow transduced with a retroviral vector containing the human common γ-chain gene. In the majority of patients there was the rapid development of T lymphocytes containing the transduced gene as well as the ability to develop antigen-specific T-lymphocyte proliferation and the production of specific antibodies, so that patients could be removed from immunoglobulin therapy.[32] In comparison with the results with the ADA gene transfer, all of the circulating T lymphocytes contained the transduced gene. Unfortunately, 5 patients have developed acute T-lymphocyte leukemia due to the activation of the *LMO2* gene by the inserted gene.[33] The development of leukemia has resulted in gene transfer trials for X-linked SCID being put on hold.

Because of the limited number of transduced T lymphocytes seen in the patients with ADA deficiency, Italian investigators explored the possibility of pretransplant myeloablative therapy to reduce the number of recipient HSC at the time of transplantation. Patients with ADA deficiency transplanted after reduced doses of busulfan have improved immune reconstitution compared with those with no pretransplant chemotherapy, with a larger percentage of both the myeloid cells and T lymphocytes containing the transduced gene.[34] No cases of leukemia have been seen in the patients receiving gene transfer for ADA deficiency.

The lessons
The major difference between the ADA deficiency and X-linked SCID is that a selective advantage exists in vivo for the transduced T lymphocytes in patients with X-linked SCID, whereas no significant selective advantage for the transduced T lymphocytes exists in patients with ADA deficiency due to the cross-correction of nontransduced T lymphocytes by enzyme replacement or enzyme produced by the transduced cells. Therefore, to increase the frequency of the engraftment of the transduced HSC it was necessary to administer pretransplant myelosuppressive therapy with anti-HSC activity. The use of pretransplant myelosuppressive therapy has the associated risks of neutropenia and thrombocytopenia as well as the possibility of the later development of leukemia. Nevertheless, the use of pretransplant myelosuppressive therapy has resulted in an increased frequency of engraftment of the transduced HSC as well as an increase in the frequency of transduced T lymphocytes. The use of pretransplant myelosuppressive therapy is therefore being entertained for gene transfer trials in which the transduced cells will not have a significant selective advantage, including the hemoglobinopathies.

BIOLOGIC INSIGHTS
HSC Niche

Most patients transplanted for SCID with allogeneic HSC, who did not receive pretransplant myelosuppressive therapy, did not have any evidence of sustained donor hematopoiesis as measured by the presence of donor-specific erythroid antigens or donor-specific HLA antigens on myeloid cells. However, when recipient hematopoiesis is eliminated by either severe GVHD or the administration of pretransplant chemotherapy, donor hematopoiesis was readily achieved after HSCT. Although rare donor-derived CD34+ and myeloid cells have been identified in the marrow of SCID patients after transplantation without pretransplant chemotherapy, the exact biologic nature of the cells is not clear. The absence of the sustained production of mature donor erythroid or myeloid elements indicates that clinically significant donor HSC engraftment cannot occur without the creation of "space." The development of bone marrow aplasia due to GVHD after their successful first transplant indicated that donor HSC engraftment had not occurred in the SCID patient.[8]

The complete correction of patients with Wiskott-Aldrich syndrome occurred only after they had received pretransplant myeloablative therapy in addition to immunosuppressive therapy. The first patient transplanted for Wiskott-Aldrich syndrome had improvement only of his lymphoid function with no correction of his platelet abnormalities after having received only immunosuppressive therapy.[35] Thus, the infusion of allogeneic HSC without HSC-targeted myelosuppression to create marrow space has not resulted in donor HSC engraftment.

Induction of Thymopoiesis

Patients with most forms of SCID are characterized by a thymus that maintains the normal architecture seen in fetuses of less than 12 weeks of gestational age. The fetal thymus is characterized by primarily epithelial elements, small blood vessels, no lymphoid elements and, rarely, Hassel corpuscles. The persistence of the fetal architecture indicates that the migration of prethymic lymphoid cells to the thymus is necessary for the induction of thymic differentiation. In a limited number of cases, patients who have been successfully transplanted have had thymus biopsies done, or have been analyzed at autopsy and have shown the development of normal thymic architecture, including normal lymphoid elements, indicating the inductive influence of the lymphoid precursors.

The fetal thymus first contains lymphoid cells at 12 weeks of gestation, which is 4 to 6 weeks after the development of hematopoiesis in the fetal liver. The transplantation of T-lymphocyte depleted HSC in SCID patients is reproductively characterized by the development of circulating immunophenotypic T lymphocytes 3 months after transplantation,[36] suggesting that it takes the CLP and other HSC-derived cells 3 months to develop into prethymic cells, which can then migrate to the thymus, induce thymic differentiation, and generate mature T lymphocytes. These results in SCID patients indicate that any mature T lymphocytes seen in the peripheral blood of HSCT recipients earlier than 3 months after HSCT are due to the homeostatic expansion of the mature T lymphocytes present in the HSC inoculum rather than thymopoiesis.

Duration of the Immune Correction in SCID Patients

An area of ongoing controversy is the duration of the correction of the immune deficiency of patients with SCID following HSCT. Although some SCID patients have functional B lymphocytes, all forms of SCID are characterized by the absence of functional antigen-specific T lymphocytes. Antigen-specific T-lymphocyte function after successful HSCT is due to donor-derived T lymphocytes. When unmodified HSC is used for transplantation, the initial donor-derived T lymphocytes are derived from the mature lymphocytes contained in the HSC inoculum. Starting 3 months after transplantation there is an increasing contribution from thymopoiesis. It is possible to quantitate recipient thymopoiesis by T-cell receptor excision circles (TREC) analysis as well as the immunophenotypic characteristics of naïve recent thymic emigrant (CD4+, CD45RA+) cells. Patients successfully transplanted with T-lymphocyte depleted HSC have the development of T lymphocytes between 3 and 6 months after HSCT. Recipient thymopoiesis peaks 1 year after transplantation.[37] Differences may then occur between patients who have received pretransplant myelosuppression and those who did not receive chemotherapy. Patients who did not receive pre-HSCT chemotherapy and who do not have detectable HSC engraftment have a slow decrease in their thymopoiesis, with a resultant decrease in TREC-positive T lymphocytes and PHA stimulation, as might be expected if the number of CLP capable of entering the thymus decreased due to their lack of self-renewal. Patients who receive chemotherapy and have HSC engraftment have the ongoing production of new CLP capable of supporting recipient thymopoiesis, and the ongoing production of new T lymphocytes. It will be interesting to compare these 2 groups for the persistence of antigen-specific T-lymphocyte responses to infectious antigens, particularly herpes papilloma virus (HPV), because there has been an increased incidence of HPV infections in the long-term recipients who did not receive pretransplant chemotherapy.[38]

Maternal T-Lymphocyte Chimerism

Many SCID patients, especially those with X-linked SCID, are born with circulating T lymphocytes of maternal origin. Rarely do patients have clinical acute GVHD. Some defects in maternal T-lymphocyte function have been identified, including the inability to respond to allogeneic cells.[39] Nevertheless, the presence of maternal T lymphocytes without the presence of acute GVHD raises questions as to the mechanism of the tolerance that had been generated.

Mechanism of Tolerance

The successful HSCT of SCID patients with histoincompatible HSC, either haploidentical parents or incompatible fetal liver, demonstrated that successful HSC engraftment can occur without fatal GVHD. Studies of the successful recipients have revealed several mechanisms of tolerance, including clonal deletion and the presence of IL-10 producing regulatory T lymphocytes.[40,41]

HLA Restriction of Antigen-specific T-Lymphocyte Function

When the first successful fetal liver transplants were performed, Zinkernagel predicted that the recipients of the histoincompatible HSC would fail to achieve the functional reconstitution of T-lymphocyte immunity and would continue to have opportunistic infections because the histoincompatibility between the fetal liver cells and the recipient thymic epithelial cells would result in a lack of development of HLA-restricted antigen-specific T-lymphocyte function.[16] Surprisingly, the patients successfully transplanted with fetal liver cells did develop antigen-specific T-lymphocyte immunity and did not develop clinical opportunistic infections.[42] Subsequent murine experiments demonstrated that histoincompatible HSC could develop into antigen-specific T lymphocytes, restricting the recipient epithelial cell histocompatibility antigens.

The studies of the emergence of antigen restriction after haploidentical T-lymphocyte depleted transplantation for SCID gave additional insights into the development of major histocompatibility complex antigen restriction of human T-lymphocyte function.[43] The evaluation of antigen-specific T-lymphocyte clones during the first 2 years after HSCT demonstrated that the T-lymphocyte clones were restricted by the recipient HLA antigens. However, with time the antigen specificity broadened, and some T-lymphocyte clones restricted by the disparate parental haplotype were identified, suggesting that the T lymphocytes could also be restricted by the HLA alleles of the disparate donor haplotype. The patient who had received pretransplant myeloablative therapy had myeloid cells of donor origin, suggesting that donor antigen-presenting cells were present in the recipient thymus and controlled the development of T-lymphocyte histocompatibility restriction.

SUMMARY

In addition to being curative therapy, HSCT for SCID patients has provided major insights into the immunobiology of allogeneic HSCT, as well as leading the clinical breakthroughs that have resulted in expanding the pool of potential donors for HSCT for non-SCID diseases.

ACKNOWLEDGMENTS

The authors wish to thank Manuela Alvarez-Wilson for her assistance in the preparation of this article.

REFERENCES

1. Gatti RA, Meeuwissen HJ, Allen HD, et al. Immunological reconstitution of sex-linked lymphopenic immunological deficiency. Lancet 1968;2:1366–9.
2. Copenhagen Study Group of Immunodeficiencies. Bone-marrow transplantation from an HLA-A-nonidentical but mixed-lymphocyte-culture identical donor. Lancet 1973;2:1146–50.
3. O'Reilly RJ, Dupont B, Pahwa D, et al. Reconstitution in severe combined immunodeficiency by transplantation of marrow from an unrelated donor. N Engl J Med 1977;297:1311–8.
4. Reisner Y, Kapoor N, Kirkpatrick D, et al. Transplantation for SCID with HLA-1, B, D/DR incompatible marrow fractionated by soy bean agglutinin and sheep red blood cells. Blood 1983;61:341–8.
5. Bordignon C, Notarangelo LD, Nobili N, et al. Gene therapy in peripheral blood lymphocytes and bone marrow for ADA-immunodeficient patients. Science 1995;270:470–4.
6. Ford CE, Hamerton JL, Barnes DWH, et al. Cytological identification of radiation chimaeras. Nature 1956;177:452–4.
7. Jammet H, Mathé G, Pendic B, et al. Etude de six cas d'irradiation totale aiguë accidentelle [Study of six cases of accidental total body irradiation]. Rev Fr Etud Clin Biol 1959;4:210–25 [in French].
8. Meuwissen HJ, Gatti RA, Terasaki PI, et al. Treatment of lymphopenic hypogammaglobulinemia and bone-marrow aplasia by transplantation of allogenic marrow. Crucial role of histocompatibility matching. N Engl J Med 1969;281: 691–7.
9. Park BH, Biggar WE, Good RA. Paucity of thymus-dependent cells in human marrow. Transplantation 1972;14:284–6.
10. Speck B, Gluckman E, Haak HL, et al. Treatment of aplastic anaemia by antilymphocyte globulin with or without marrow infusion. Clin Haematol 1978;7:611–21.
11. Parkman R, Rappeport J, Geha R, et al. Complete correction of the Wiskott-Aldrich syndrome by allogeneic bone marrow transplantation. N Engl J Med 1978;209:921–7.
12. Maris MB, Niederwieser D, Sandmaier BM, et al. HLA-matched unrelated donor hematopoietic cell transplantation after nonmyeloablative conditioning for patients with hematologic malignancies. Blood 2003;102:2021–30.
13. Vossen JM, de Koning J, van Bekkum DW, et al. Successful treatment of an infant with severe combined immunodeficiency by transplantation of bone marrow cells from an uncle. Clin Exp Immunol 1973;13:9–20.
14. Beatty PG, Clift RA, Mickelson EM, et al. Marrow transplantation from related donors other than HLA-identical siblings. N Engl J Med 1985;313:765–71.
15. Yunis EJ, Good RA, Smith J, et al. Protection of lethally irradiated mice by spleen cells from neonatally thymectomized mice. Proc Natl Acad Sci U S A 1974;71(6): 2544–8.

16. Zinkernagel RM. Thymus function and reconstitution of immunodeficiency. N Engl J Med 1978;198:222.
17. Keightley R, Lawton AR, Cooper MD. Successful fetal liver transplantation in a child with severe combined immunodeficiency. Lancet 1975;2:850–3.
18. Buckley RH, Whisnant JK, Schiff RI, et al. Correction of severe combined immunodeficiency by fetal liver cells. N Engl J Med 1976;297:1076–81.
19. O'Reilly RJ, Kapoor N, Kirkpatrick D. Fetal tissue transplants for severe combined immunodeficiency- their limitations and functional potential. In: Seligmann M, Hitzig WH, editors. Primary immunodeficiencies INSERM symposium No. 16. N Holland (Dutch): Elsevier; 1980. p. 419–33.
20. O'Reilly J, Pollack MS, Kapoor N, et al. Fetal liver transplantation in man and animals. In: Gale RP, editor, Recent advances in bone marrow transplantation. UCLA symposia on molecular and cellular biology, vol. 7. New York: Alan R. Liss, Inc; 1983. p. 799.
21. Mebius RE, Miyamoto T, Christensen J, et al. The fetal liver counterpart of adult common lymphoid progenitors gives rise to all lymphoid lineages, CD45+CD4+CD3− cells, as well as macrophages. J Immunol 2001;166:6593–601.
22. Boehmer H, Sprent J, Nabholz M. Tolerance to histocompatibility determinants in tetraparental bone marrow chimeras. J Exp Med 1975;141(2):322–34.
23. Reisner Y, Kapoor N, Kirkpatrick D, et al. Transplantation for acute leukemia with HLA-A and -B nonidentical parental marrow cells fractionated with soybean agglutinin and sheep red cells. Lancet 1981;2:327–31.
24. Papadopoulos EB, Carabasi MH, Castro-Malaspina H, et al. T-cell-depleted allogeneic bone marrow transplantation as postremission therapy for acute myelogenous leukemia: freedom from relapse in the absence of graft-versus-host disease. Blood 1998;91:1083–90.
25. Flake AW, Zanjani ED. In utero transplantation for thalassemia. Ann N Y Acad Sci 1998;850:300–11.
26. Carr MC, Stites DP, Fudenberg HH. Dissociation of responses to phytohaemagglutinin and adult allogeneic lymphocytes in human foetal lymphoid tissues. Nature New Biol 1973;241(113):279–81.
27. Flake AW, Roncarolo M-G, Puck JM, et al. Treatment of X-linked severe combined immunodeficiency by in utero transplantation of paternal bone marrow. N Engl J Med 1996;335:1806–10.
28. Wengler GS, Lanfranchi A, Frusca T, et al. In-utero transplantation of parental CD34 haematopoietic progenitor cells in a patient with X-linked severe combined immunodeficiency (SCIDXI). Lancet 1996;348:1484–8.
29. Bambach BJ, Moser HW, Blakemore K, et al. Engraftment following in utero bone marrow transplantation for globoid cell leukodystrophy. Bone Marrow Transplant 1997;19:399–402.
30. Kantoff PW, Kohn DB, Mitsuya H, et al. Correction of adenosine deaminase deficiency in cultured human T and B cells by retrovirus-mediated gene transfer. Proc Natl Acad Sci U S A 1986;83:6563–7.
31. Blaese RM, Culver KW, Miller AD, et al. T lymphocyte-directed gene therapy for ADA-SCID: initial trial results after 4 years. Science 1995;270:475–80.
32. Hacein-Bey-Abina S, Le Deist F, Carlier F, et al. Sustained correction of X-linked severe combined immunodeficiency by ex vivo gene therapy. N Engl J Med 2002;346:1185–93.
33. Hacein-Bey-Abina S, von Kalle C, Schmidt M, et al. A serious adverse event after successful gene therapy for X-linked severe combined immunodeficiency. N Engl J Med 2003;348:255–6.

34. Aiuti A, Slavin S, Aker M, et al. Correction of ADA-SCID by stem cell gene therapy combined with nonmyeloablative conditioning. Science 2002;296:2410–3.
35. Bach FH, Alberini RJ, Anderson JL, et al. Bone marrow transplantation in a patient with the Wiskott-Aldrich syndrome. Lancet 1968;2:1364–6.
36. O'Reilly RJ, Keever CA, Small TN, et al. The use of HLA non-identical T-cell depleted marrow transplants for correction of severe combined immunodeficiency. Immunodefic Rev 1989;1:273–309.
37. Patel DD, Gooding ME, Parrott RE, et al. Thymic function after hematopoietic stem-cell transplantation for the treatment of severe combined immunodeficiency. N Engl J Med 2000;342:1325–32.
38. Neven B, Leroy S, Decaluwe H, et al. Long-term outcome after hematopoietic stem cell transplantation of a single-center cohort of 90 patients with severe combined immunodeficiency. Blood 2009;113:4114–24.
39. Pollack MS, Kirkpatrick D, Kapoor N, et al. Identification by HLA typing of intra-uterine-derived maternal immunodeficiency. N Engl J Med 1982;307:662–6.
40. Rosenkrantz K, Keever C, Bhimani K, et al. Both ongoing suppression and clonal elimination contribute to graft-host tolerance after transplantation of HLA mismatched T cell-depleted marrow for severe combined immunodeficiency. J Immunol 1990;144:1721–8.
41. Bacchetta R, Bigler M, Touraine JL, et al. High levels of interleukin 10 production in vivo are associated with tolerance in SCID patients transplanted with HLA mismatched hematopoietic stem cells. J Exp Med 1994;179:493–502.
42. Roncarolo MG, Yssel H, Touraine JL, et al. Antigen recognition by MHC-incompatible cells of a human mismatched chimera. J Exp Med 1988;168(6):2139–52.
43. Geha RS, Rosen FS. The evolution of MHC restrictions in antigen recognition by T cells in a haploidentical bone marrow transplant recipient. J Immunol 1989;143:84–8.

HLA-haploidentical Donor Transplantation in Severe Combined Immunodeficiency

Wilhelm Friedrich, MD*, Manfred Hönig, MD

KEYWORDS

- Hematopoietic cell transplantation • HLA-haploidentical
- Severe combined immunodeficiency

Treatment of severe combined immunodeficiency (SCID) by hematopoietic cell transplantation (HCT) changed profoundly in the early eighties when Reisner and colleagues[1] developed a procedure to efficiently reduce the number of T cells contained in marrow grafts responsible for graft-versus-host disease (GVHD), opening the possibility to prevent this complication after HLA-mismatched donor transplantation. The procedure used soybean agglutination in combination with sheep red blood cell rosette formation to fractionate bone marrow cells and provided precursor cell–enriched grafts with drastically reduced T-cell numbers. Reisner and colleagues[2] and, subsequently, several other groups[3–9] were able to demonstrate the potential of T-cell–depleted, HLA-haploidentical parental donor transplants to establish stable immunologic reconstitution in SCID patients with significantly reduced risk for acute and chronic GVHD. Newly developed donor T cells were found to be tolerant to cells of the HLA-haploidentical recipient. Other subsequently developed technologies for T-cell depletion of marrow grafts took advantage of lymphocyte-specific monoclonal antibodies, and more recently, antibodies directed at CD34$^+$ are used to purify CD34$^-$ expressing hematopoietic progenitor cells by positive selection from peripheral blood after their mobilization by granulocyte colony-stimulating factor (GCSF). In patients with SCID, for whom HCT represented the only available curative therapy, these advances led to profound changes in the prognosis of this otherwise lethal disorder, which became uniformly treatable regardless of the availability of a matched family donor. Over the last years, HCT from unrelated matched donors also has been

A version of this article was previously published in the *Immunology and Allergy Clinics of North America*, 30:1.
Department of Pediatrics, University of Ulm, Eythstrasse 24, 89075 Ulm, Germany
* Corresponding author. Universitäts-Kinderklinik, Eythstrasse 24, 89075 Ulm, Germany.
E-mail address: wilhelm.friedrich@uniklinik-ulm.de

Hematol Oncol Clin N Am 25 (2011) 31–44
doi:10.1016/j.hoc.2010.11.003
0889-8588/11/$ – see front matter © 2011 Elsevier Inc. All rights reserved.

markedly advanced, and both approaches now are well established in the treatment of the disorder. In this review, several pertinent findings in SCID patients undergoing HLA-haploidentical HCT are discussed, and several unresolved issues, such as the nonuniformity of B-cell reconstitution, graft resistance, the role of conditioning, and long-term immune reconstitution, are addressed.

SPECIFIC ASPECTS OF HCT IN SCID

In contrast to other disorders, the profound immunodeficiency in SCID minimizes the risk of immunologic graft rejection, conceptually eliminating the need for immunosuppressive conditioning before transplantation. This approach of transplanting SCID patients without conditioning, providing a significant advantage because of the reduced toxicity of the procedure, has been widely explored in HLA-identical and HLA-nonidentical transplantation. Because the recipient's hematopoietic system remains intact, there is no advantage for donor precursor cells to engraft and to replace this system, and indeed, evidence for sustained or substantial marrow engraftment by donor cells is usually lacking.[10–13] Nevertheless, lymphocytes of donor origin develop, in contrast to other blood cells, which remain of recipient origin. The potential of HCT to induce stable immune reconstitution in the absence of marrow engraftment raises the obvious question regarding the underlying mechanisms of lymphocyte development in the absence of progenitor cell engraftment in the marrow.

DIFFERENT OUTCOMES AFTER HLA-IDENTICAL AND HAPLOIDENTICAL HCT WITHOUT CONDITIONING

The outcome of HCT in SCID when performed without conditioning differs substantially depending on whether nonmanipulated grafts from HLA-identical donors or manipulated, T-cell depleted grafts from HLA-nonidentical donors are used. Mature donor T cells contained in the graft have the capacity to undergo marked proliferation and expansion in the recipient, giving rise to an initial wave of T cells early after transplantation. These T cells are responsible for induction of GVHD but also are potentially beneficial and protective, in particular if GVHD is limited or absent, as is commonly the case in SCID patients after sibling transplantation. The scenario obviously is different after HLA-haploidentical transplantation, where this effect of expanding mature T cells is abolished. Development of T cells after T-cell depleted transplantation depends solely on de novo maturation in the thymus. This maturation process is slow. Newly differentiated T cells appear in the circulation only several months after transplantation. In contrast to early developing T cells, which carry predominantly a memory phenotype, newly differentiated T cells disclose a naive phenotype and are rich in a cell marker, the so called T-cell receptor excision circle (TREC), which indicates their recent thymus emigration.[14] These cells are furthermore characterized by a diverse receptor repertoire, in contrast to the more skewed repertoire of early T cells arising by expansion.[15,16] Simultaneously with the delayed development of naive T cells, the previously small thymus characteristic for SCID enlarges in size, as easily visualized by ultrasonography.[17] Notably, after transplantation of unmanipulated grafts, a similar kinetics of slow development of naive T cells is observed.[17] It is also interesting that T-cell development is similarly delayed in other congenital disorders after HLA-haploidentical, T-cell depleted transplantation, such as infantile osteopetrosis and Wiskott-Aldrich syndrome.[18,19] Furthermore, in SCID patients receiving cytoreductive conditioning before transplantation for reasons that are discussed in more detail later in the article, the kinetics of slow T-cell reconstitution is not altered.[17]

The distinct pattern of T-cell reconstitution after HLA-identical and after HLA-haploidentical, T-cell–depleted transplantation is demonstrated in **Fig. 1**.

Patients remain profoundly immunodeficient for a prolonged period after HLA-haploidentical HCT because it takes up to 4 months until T cells become demonstrable, in contrast to patients after sibling transplantation, in whom early-appearing donor T cells can be effective to control and prevent infections.

Another marked difference after transplantation of grafts with and without T-cell depletion regards reconstitution of humoral immunity. Whereas transplantation of nonmanipulated grafts from HLA-identical donors commonly results in sustained B-cell reconstitution with detection of donor B cells in the circulation, patients after HLA-haploidentical, T-cell–depleted transplantation, when performed without cytoreductive conditioning, commonly fail to develop effective B-cell immunity. With rare exceptions, B cells of donor origin remain absent, as most evident in patients with B− SCID, who fail to develop circulating B cells. In most patients with B+ SCID, autologous B cells persist as expected but fail to become functional, as elegantly shown in a study by White and colleagues.[20] Only exceptionally, such as in patients with IL7R deficiency, CD3 deficiency, and adenosine deaminase (ADA) deficiency, has the functional maturation of autologous B cells after effective T-cell reconstitution been observed. Because in the absence of conditioning, as noted earlier, evidence of substantial engraftment of donor precursor cells in the marrow is usually lacking after both HLA-identical and HLA-nonidentical transplantation, this discrepancy in humoral reconstitution requires an explanation. Graft manipulation and depletion of T cells usually also lead to drastic reduction of B-cell numbers in the grafts. As one possible explanation, it is conceivable that donor B cells arising after HLA-identical transplantation are derived from the pool of donor B cells contained in nonmanipulated grafts. The longevity of mature B cells and their potential to undergo extensive homeostatic

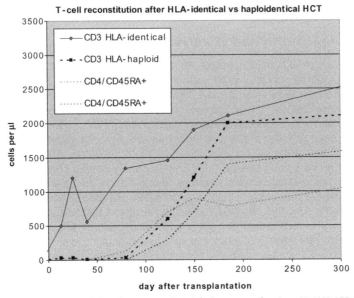

Fig. 1. Different kinetics of development of CD3$^+$, but not of naive CD4/CD45RA$^+$ T cells after HLA-identical sibling transplantation and HLA-haploidentical, T-cell–depleted transplantation in 2 SCID patients.

proliferation analogous to T cells is well established in murine models and recently also in man,[21,22] and it is conceivable that transfer of mature donor B cells into allogeneic hosts may be effective to establish stable long-term humoral immunity. Nevertheless, the heterogeneity of B-cell reconstitution remains incompletely understood and requires further studies.

Although most patients develop normal and sustained T-cell functions after HLA-haploidentical transplantation without conditioning, a proportion of patients fail to do so, showing either complete graft failures or subnormal T-cell reconstitution. Complete graft failure has been common in particular in ADA deficiency, in SCID patients characterized by the presence of poorly functional T cells, such as in Omenn syndrome, and in SCID patients with functional NK-cell systems. This experience again is in contrast to the outcome after nonmanipulated, HLA-identical sibling transplants, which almost uniformly, regardless of the underlying variant of SCID, will lead to engraftment and development of T-cell immunity. The less-uniform reconstitution after HLA-haploidentical transplantation may be because of several factors restricting T-cell development. One factor may be the absence of an engraftment-facilitating effect mediated by mature donor T cells. Also persistent viral disease, such as cytomegalovirus infections, may suppress lymphoid differentiation and cause poor reconstitution. Furthermore, in certain SCID variants, the environment of the thymus may limit homing of donor precursor cells to specific niches, as has been demonstrated in relevant murine SCID models.[23] The most important factor for subnormal T-cell reconstitution probably is GVHD and its treatment, a complication that may also be induced by maternal T cells secondary to an intrauterine maternofetal transfusion and that may take a subclinical course.[24] Furthermore, graft resistance may be mediated by NK cells, which function in subgroups of SCID patients. Importantly, graft failures can usually be overcome by using pretransplant cytoreductive conditioning. Because this approach also allows marrow engraftment of precursor cells and as a consequence donor B-cell development, conditioning has been used in a significant proportion of patients before initial transplantation.

SURVIVAL AND COMPLICATIONS IN SCID PATIENTS AFTER HLA-HAPLOIDENTICAL HCT

The exploration of HLA-haploidentical HCT in the treatment of SCID has resulted in a series of larger single- and multicenter studies, the latter in particular by groups collaborating in the European Group for Blood and Marrow Transplantation (EBMT) who established the Stem Cell Transplantation for Immunodeficiencies (SCETIDE) registry.[25–29] In the following sections, several issues of HLA-haploidentical HCT are addressed based on these studies, including survival, immune reconstitution, complications, and late outcome.

A multicenter study published in 2003 analyzed the outcome after HCT in patients with primary immunodeficiencies treated in Europe between 1968 and 1999.[25] The study included 475 patients with SCID. Donors in 294 of these cases were HLA-haploidentical parents. The majority (207 cases) had received pretransplant conditioning, consisting mostly of busulfan (8 mg/kg) and cyclophosphamide (200 mg/kg). The 3-year survival rate after HLA-haploidentical transplantation was 54%, which was significantly lower compared with a survival rate of 77% in patients after HLA-identical HCT ($P = .002$) reported in the same study. Importantly, survival rates after haploidentical transplantation have improved significantly over time, from about 50% during the initial period up to 80% during the more recent period, as shown in **Fig. 2**, where survival data of a more recent EBMT survey are demonstrated. It was also noted that the variant of SCID had an impact on survival after HLA-haploidentical HCT, because cases of

5-year survival after HLA-haploidentical HCT according to time period (EBMT/SCETIDE 2007)

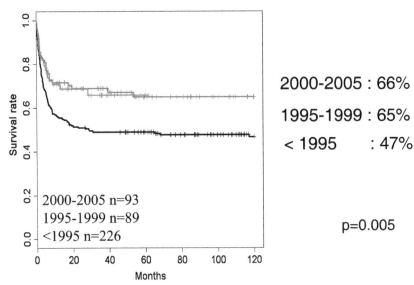

2000-2005 : 66%

1995-1999 : 65%

< 1995   : 47%

p=0.005

Fig. 2. Survival after HLA-haploidentical HCT in SCID according to year of transplantation. (*Data from* EBMT/SCETIDE registry.)

B– SCID tended to have a poorer prognosis than those of B+ SCID, confirming similar observations in a previous analysis.[29] In the former group, the use of conditioning before HCT was found to result in better survival, whereas in cases of B+ SCID, survival was not affected by conditioning. For patients with ADA deficiency (n = 26) and for patients with reticular dysgenesis (n = 8), 3-year survival rates were 30%.

In a separate study of 10 patients with reticular dysgenesis, cytoreductive conditioning before HLA-haploidentical HCT was found mandatory to obtain reconstitution of both lymphoid and myeloid functions in this disorder.[30]

Independent predictors of poorer outcome, besides underlying variants of SCID, were the presence of pulmonary infection at transplantation, absence of a protected environment, and occurrence of acute GVHD (grade II or higher). The study also revealed that the incidence of GVHD had decreased over time, from 35% to 40% before 1996 to 22% thereafter ($P<.001$), possibly related to the use of more stringent methods for T-cell depletion, a factor that partly accounted for the observed better survival with time. The main causes of death were infections (56%), GVHD (25%), and B-cell lymphoproliferative syndrome (5%).

In a large single-center study reported by Buckley and colleagues,[27] 77 SCID patients were analyzed after HLA-haploidentical HCT. In this study, a survival rate of 77% was reported, with follow-up after transplantation ranging from 3 months to 16 years. All patients in this study underwent transplants without conditioning. Furthermore, the proportion of patients with B– SCID was very low, in contrast to the European study, in which this proportion was about 35%. An important prognostic factor for survival was noted to be age at transplantation; within the whole group of treated patients, infants who underwent transplant before the age of 3 to 5 months had a survival rate of 95% as compared with a survival rate of 76% in patients beyond that age.

In a previous multicenter EBMT study analyzing prognostic factors for long-term survival, normalization of T-cell immunity at 12 months was identified as a strong favorable indicator, whereas ineffective reconstitution, which may be because of poorly controlled GVHD or other complications, was found to be associated with a substantial mortality.[29]

The basis for improved survival after HLA-haploidentical HCT during more recent periods includes several factors, such as earlier diagnosis resulting in fewer sick patients at the time of transplantation, more effective prevention and treatment of disease-related and transplantation-induced complications (notably infections and GVHD), and effective prevention of graft failure by using conditioning prior to transplantation in patients at risk for this complication.

Efficient prevention of GVHD has been related in particular to the use of highly purified, GCSF-mobilized $CD34^+$ precursor cells from peripheral blood, which are obtainable in high numbers with minimal contamination by T cells.[10] In addition to de novo GVHD caused by imperfect T-cell depletion of grafts, another cause for this complication has been a primary engraftment of transplacentally acquired maternal T cells, which is a common phenomenon in SCID.[24,31] In the study by Buckley and colleagues[27] discussed earlier, 27 of 28 cases with GVHD were noted to have circulating maternal T cells before transplantation. In the authors' own experience of HLA-haploidentical HCT in a cohort of 137 SCID patients, 31 of 59 patients with maternal T-cell engraftment developed GVHD to variable degrees, whereas among the other 78 patients without maternal T cells, only 7 cases developed this complication (Friedrich W, unpublished data, 2009).

HCT WITHOUT AND WITH CONDITIONING

Cytoreductive conditioning in SCID patients, for which most commonly a combination of busulfan and cyclophosphamide is used, has been found to offer several advantages, including, in particular, an improved prevention of graft failure and a high chance of sustained, complete immune reconstitution. In the authors' experience of HLA-haploidentical HCT in SCID, they have observed better overall survival rates in patients who received preparative cytoreductive conditioning compared with those who did not, as demonstrated in **Fig. 3**. Causes of death in the latter group were manifold but included a significant proportion of earlier patients showing complete graft failures. There are, however, obvious disadvantages with this approach, most importantly potentially acute and long-term toxic side effects. In particular, in infants suffering from persistent viral disease or other poorly controllable complications, the risks of conditioning may outweigh its potential benefits. As already mentioned, conditioning does not alter the kinetics of immune reconstitution. Also, the use of highly purified $CD34^+$ cells at comparatively high numbers does not influence the slow pattern of T-cell reconstitution, whether conditioning is used or not.[10] As outlined later in this article, based on studies in long-term surviving patients, some concern has been raised regarding the stability of thymic functions in nonconditioned patients. Nevertheless, the decision to use or not to use conditioning requires careful consideration in each individual case, taking into account potential advantages and disadvantages.

LONG-TERM OUTCOME AND COMPLICATIONS AFTER HLA-HAPLOIDENTICAL HCT

Recently a single-center study analyzing long-term outcome of HCT in a large cohort of SCID patients was reported, assessing the occurrence of clinical events and the quality of life as well as quality and stability of immune functions.[32] Patients were

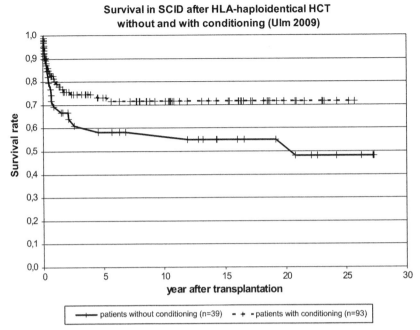

Fig. 3. Overall survival in SCID patients who underwent transplant either without or with preparative cytoreductive conditioning from HLA-haploidentical donors since 1982 at the University of Ulm.

observed from 2 to 34 years (medium 14 years) after transplantation, and the study included 51 cases with HLA-haploidentical donors, 22 cases with matched sibling donors, and 15 cases with other HLA-matched family donors. The investigators observed one or more significant late clinical events in about 50% of patients. These included persistent chronic GVHD (in 6 of 51 cases after haploid identical HCT); autoimmune and inflammatory manifestations (in 12 cases within the whole cohort of 90 cases) that included autoimmune hemolytic anemia in 6 cases and chronic inflammatory disease in 3 cases, requiring immunosuppressive treatment over periods of 1.5 to 17 years; opportunistic and nonopportunistic infections, including chronic human papilloma virus (HPV) infections; and prolonged nutritional support. Except HPV infections, these complications were commonly associated with chronic GVHD and its treatment. The rate of infectious complications tended to decrease with increasing time after transplantation, with the exception of severe HPV infection. This infection developed in 23 cases between 4 and 19 years after transplantation and was severe in 9 cases (as defined by the persistence of multiple lesions [>30] for more than 2 years and by poor therapeutic responsiveness) and milder in the others, resolving in 11 of 14 cases. As previously reported by the same group, severe HPV infections were restricted to B+ SCID patients with *yc and Jak3* deficiency, leading to the speculation that the continued deficiency in nonlymphoid cells of yc-dependent cytokine signaling, which may play a crucial part in local resistance of keratinocytes, is relevant for the cause of this complication.[33]

An important finding in the study was that T-cell immune reconstitution had failed to normalize in a significant proportion of patients, even after prolonged follow-up. At 1 and 2 years, about 25% of patients had a low CD4 T-cell number, and this percentage

Table 1
Late immune reconstitution in SCID after HLA-haploidentical HCT (Ulm 2009)

			No Conditioning							
UPN	SCID Variant	Time After BMT (y)	CD3+ Cells/μl	CD4+ Cells/μl	CD8+ Cells/μl	CD4/CD45RA+ Cells/μl	PHA(SI)	Donor B-cell Chimerism	Donor Myeloid Chimerism	IgG Subst
14	B+ (nd)	24	1420	470	820	280	110	No	No	No
15	B+ (yc)	25	1500	650	680	348	540	No	No	Yes
16	B− (Artemis)	26	2150	860	1270	140	140	No	No	Yes
17	B+ (yc)	24	2700	1400	1180	600	290	No	No	Yes
22	B+ (yc)	23	1200	560	430	150	650	No	No	Yes
39	B+ (yc)	17[a]	900	150	863	33	42	No	No	Yes
53	B− (Artemis)	18	1100	840	220	420	470	No	No	Yes
87	B+ (yc)	10[a]	2300	550	1600	30	60	No	No	Yes
88	B+ (yc)	21	1400	600	700	90	120	No	No	Yes
137	B+ (yc)	14	1300	500	610	330	480	Yes	Yes	No
188	B+ (yc)	14	500	140	300	60	115	No	No	Yes
201	B+ (yc)	13	1538	413	844	54	312	No	No	Yes
246	B+ (Jak3)	14	2570	700	1800	200	473	No	No	Yes
247	B+ (Jak3)	14	3600	800	2600	30	120	No	No	Yes
250	B+ (Jak3)	14	1520	1012	418	597	893	No	No	Yes
281	B+ (Jak3)	12	3040	960	1820	633	411	No	No	Yes
282	B− (Artemis)	12	710	520	160	155	140	No	No	Yes

With Conditioning

UPN	SCID Variant	Time after BMT (y)	CD3+ Cells/μl	CD4+ Cells/μl	CD8+ Cells /μl	CD4/CD45RA+ Cells/μl	PHA (SI)	Donor B-cell Chimerism	Donor Myeloid Chimerism	IgG Subst
26	ADA	21	2300	570	430	520	550	Yes	Yes	No
36	ADA	19	1470	710	550	380	650	Yes	Yes	No
74	B+ (IL7R)	18	1480	1000	400	390	170	Yes	Yes	No
77	Reticular dysgenesis	17	1930	760	740	400	140	Yes	Yes	No
81	B− (RAG)	21	1200	660	255	323	270	No	No	Yes
84	B+ (γc)	11	1390	562	600	300	690	Yes	Yes	No
101	B+ (Jak3)	17	2160	970	1300	600	260	Yes	Yes	No
128	B− (Artemis)	14	3700	2210	1220	780	760	Yes	Yes	No
172	B+ (γc)	15	2210	1500	490	1190	430	Yes	Yes	No
180	B+ (nd)	15	2170	890	1020	450	430	Yes	Yes	No
197	B− (RAG)	17	1840	1060	680	690	540	Yes	Yes	No
223	B− (RAG)	16	600	400	175	152	349	Yes	No	No
241	B+ autosomal	11	500	400	100	16	63	No	No	No
249	B+ (γc)	14	1500	1095	358	613	396	Yes	Yes	No
271	B+ (IL7R)	13	1600	814	682	850	495	Yes	Yes	No
310	B+ autosomal	12	1935	816	956	481	220	Yes	Yes	No

Abbreviations: nd, not determined; PHA, phytohemagglutinin; SI, stimulatory indices; Subst, substitution; UPN, unit patient number.
[a] Both patients died from late complications.

remained in the same range at follow-up between 5 and 15 years, confirming previous observations showing that CD4$^+$ T-cell numbers at 1 and 2 years after HCT were highly predictive of outcome and of late immune T-cell reconstitution.[29] The analysis also revealed that in patients with donor-derived myeloid cells, associated with previous myelosuppressive conditioning, CD4$^+$ T-cell counts tended to be higher at all evaluation times compared with values in patients without donor-derived myeloid cells.

In SCID patients with persisting subnormal reconstitution of T-cell immunity, repeat CD34$^+$ cell infusions without conditioning from the same donors have been attempted to improve graft function. This experience has failed to provide clear evidence for an advantage or efficiency of boost transplants, in particular if given late after initial transplantation.[34]

ADA deficiency is a systemic metabolic disease that may cause other complications beside SCID, including neurologic abnormalities. Late outcome after transplantation was reported in 12 long-term surviving ADA-deficient patients, 6 of whom had undergone HLA-nonidentical transplantation.[35] The analysis revealed that HCT commonly fails to control late central nervous system complications, because 6 of 12 patients showed marked late neurologic abnormalities, including mental retardation, motor dysfunction, and sensorineural hearing deficit. The study failed to reveal a correlation of these abnormalities with the transplant approach used. In another study addressing neurologic outcome in ADA-deficient patients, which included 16 patients and a control group that underwent transplant for nonmetabolic SCID, the authors reported striking behavioral abnormalities in ADA-deficient patients, but, in contrast to the above, no motor function abnormalities.[36]

STABILITY OF T-CELL IMMUNITY AND OF THYMIC FUNCTION

As already discussed, HLA-haploidentical transplantation without conditioning usually results in split chimerism, with donor cell development limited to T cells. Although T-cell lymphopoiesis clearly reflects thymic engraftment of progenitor cells, it remains presently unclear if the thymus is colonized immediately after transplantation during a limited time window when donor precursor progenitor cells are present in the circulation or, alternatively, if transient marrow engraftment takes place, allowing pre–T-cells to emigrate from the marrow to enter the thymus. Because longitudinal studies, with rare exceptions, fail to provide evidence for sustained progenitor cell marrow engraftment, at least based on conventional technologies failing to detect donor cells less than 1%, this latter scenario, in any case, would be operative only temporarily. Based on animal models, a periodical re-colonization of the thymus by precursor cells from the marrow is required to maintain sustained thymopoiesis because stem cells with self-replicating potential are absent in the normal thymus.[37] The possible consequences of the specific situation in SCID patients who undergo transplant without conditioning and in whom periodical re-colonization of the thymus likely does not occur has been addressed in several recent studies that evaluated long-term immune reconstitution and the stability of T-cell lymphopoiesis.[12,13,38,39] In one study,[13] 32 SCID patients surviving longer than 10 years were analyzed (**Table 1**). All patients had received HLA-haploidentical HCT, 17 cases without and 16 cases with myeloablative conditioning. Several findings emerged from this study. Most patients had sustained normal numbers and functions of circulating T cells, including distribution of CD4$^+$ and CD8$^+$ T-cell subsets. In 5 of the 32 patients, however, T cells were decreased to numbers less than 1000 per µl, of whom 3 patients had diminished phytohemagglutinin responses (stimulatory indices <100). Two of the cases with diminished T-cell immunity had died from late complications; 1 from complicating vari-cella, the other from chronic encephalopathy. Importantly, these 5 patients had never achieved completely normal T-cell immunity after transplantation. There was also a broad range in the number of CD45RA-expressing naive CD4$^+$ cells (see **Table 1**). The number of these cells tended to be lower in patients who underwent transplant without conditioning (mean, 244 per μL; range, 30–600 per μL) in comparison to patients with conditioning (mean, 508 per μL; range, 16–1190 per μL). The only patient in the latter group with a low naive T-cell number had shown only transient myeloid engraftment, similar to 1 other patient, despite conditioning. Patients who underwent transplant without conditioning, with the exception of 1 case, revealed no evidence of myeloid engraftment and lacked donor B-cell engraftment. Lower numbers of naive T cells were associated with diminished total T-cell numbers and/or functions in the 5 patients mentioned earlier, whereas 3 patients with low naive T-cell numbers showed otherwise normal T-cell immunity. Previous determinations of naive T cells in these 3 cases had revealed higher numbers.

Several groups also reported evidence for diminished thymic output in a proportion of long-term surviving SCID patients. In a study by Sarzotti-Kelsoe and colleagues,[38] 10 of 41 patients surviving longer than 10 years after T-cell depleted, haploidentical transplantation without conditioning were noted to lack thymic output of naive T cells, which in this study was based on measurements of TREC as an indicator of recent thymic emigration. Cavazzana-Calvo and colleagues[12] studied 32 SCID patients who survived long-term after transplantation performed either without or with myeloa-blation. In this study, persistent normal thymopoiesis, as defined by normal propor-tions of naive CD4$^+$ T cells carrying TREC, was strongly correlated with conditioning and donor myeloid cell engraftment. In nonconditioned patients, sus-tained thymic function was more common in patients with γc deficiency compared with patients with *RAG* and Artemis deficiency. There was no correlation between thymic function and age at transplantation, and younger age did not provide an advan-tage with regard to sustained thymic activity. Importantly, the long-term clinical outcome of patients in this study was found not to differ, regardless of the presence or absence of TREC+ T cells.

At present, the relevance of these findings, indicating limited long-term thymopoie-sis in a significant proportion of long-term surviving SCID patients, mostly trans-planted without myeloablative conditioning and lacking myeloid engraftment, remains open and requires longer observation. Whether the observation of persistent normal thymopoiesis in patients with myeloid chimerism favors the general use of myeloablation before HCT in SCID patients remains to be determined.

SUMMARY

Curative treatment of SCID by HCT remains a challenge, in particular in infants pre-senting with serious, poorly controllable complications, as is commonly the case in this disorder. In the absence of a matched family donor, HLA-haploidentical transplan-tation from parental donors represents a uniformly and readily available treatment option, offering a high chance to be successful. Concerning outcomes of HCT in SCID, other important parameters beside survival need to be taken into consideration, in particular, the stability and robustness of the graft and its function as well as poten-tial late complications related either to the disease or to the treatment. At present, strategies in performing haploidentical HCT are not uniform, in particular regarding the indication, intensity, and mode of preparative conditioning. To further advance and to arrive at consistent, solidly founded recommendations, coordinated strategies in the application of the treatment and systematic analysis of outcomes will remain important.

REFERENCES

1. Reisner Y, Kapoor N, Kirckpatrick D, et al. Transplantation for acute leukemia with HLA-A and B nonidentical parental bone marrow fractionated with soybean agglutinin and sheep red blood cells. Lancet 1981;2:327–31.
2. Reisner Y, Kapoor N, Kirkpatrich D, et al. Transplantation for severe combined immunodeficiency with HLA-A, B, D, DR incompatible parental marrow cells fractionated with soybean agglutinin and sheep red blood cells. Blood 1983;61: 341–8.
3. Friedrich W, Goldmann SF, Vetter U, et al. Immunoreconstitution in severe combined immunodeficiency after transplantation of HLA haploidentical, T-cell-depleted bone marrow. Lancet 1984;1(8380):761–4.
4. Friedrich W, Goldmann SF, Ebell W, et al. Severe combined immunodeficiency: treatment by bone marrow transplantation in 15 infants using HLA-haploidentical donors. Eur J Pediatr 1985;144:125–30.
5. Buckley RH, Schiff SE, Sampson HA, et al. Development of immunity in human severe primary T-cell deficiency following haploidentical bone marrow stem cell transplantation. J Immunol 1986;136:2398–407.
6. Cowan MJ, Wara DW, Weintrub PS, et al. Haploidentical bone marrow transplantation for severe combined immunodeficiency disease using soybean agglutinin-negative, T-depleted marrow grafts. J Clin Immunol 1985;5:370–6.
7. Fischer A, Durandy A, De Villarty JP, et al. HLA-haploidentical bone marrow transplantation for severe combined immunodeficiency using E-rosette fractionation and cyclosporine. Blood 1986;67:444–9.
8. Morgan G, Linen DC, Knott LT, et al. Successful haploidentical mismatched bone marrow transplantation in severe combined immunodeficiency: T-cell removal using CAMPATH-1 monoclonal antibody and E-rosetting. Br J Haematol 1986; 62:421–30.
9. O'Reilly RJ, Keever CA, Small TN, et al. The use of HLA-non-identical T-cell-depleted marrow transplants for correction of severe combined immunodeficiency disease. Immunodefic Rev 1989;1:273–309.
10. O'Reilly RJ, Small TN, Friedrich W. Hematopoietic cell transplant for immunodeficiency diseases. In: Thomas ED, Blume KG, Forman SJ, editors. Hematopoietic cell transplantation. 2nd edition. Malden (MA): Blackwell Science; 2004. p. 1430–42.
11. Tjonnfjord GE, Steen R, Veiby OP, et al. Evidence for engraftment of donor-type multipotent CD34+ cells in a patient with selective T-lymphocyte reconstitution after bone marrow transplantation. Blood 1994;84:3584–9.
12. Cavazzana-Calvo M, Carlier F, Le Deist F, et al. Long-term T-cell reconstitution after hematopoietic stem-cell transplantation in primary T-cell–immunodeficient patients is associated with myeloid chimerism and possibly the primary disease phenotype. Blood 2007;109:4576–80.
13. Friedrich W, Hoenig M, Mueller SM, et al. Long-term follow-up in patients with severe combined immunodeficiency treated by bone marrow transplantation. Immunol Res 2007;80:6621–8.
14. Krengler W, Schmidlin H, Cavadini G, et al. On the relevance of TCR rearrangement circles as molecular markers for thymic output during experimental graft-versus-host disease. J Immunol 2004;172:7359–67.

15. Knobloch C, Friedrich W. T cell receptor diversity in severe combined immunodeficiency following HLA-haploidentical bone marrow transplantation. Bone Marrow Transplant 1991;8(5):383–7.

16. Sarzotti M, Patel DD, Li X, et al. T cell repertoire development in humans with SCID after nonablative allogeneic marrow transplantation. J Immunol 2003; 170(5):2711–8.

17. Müller SM, Kohn T, Schulz A, et al. Similar pattern of thymic-dependent T-cell reconstitution in infants with severe combined immunodeficiency after human leukocyte antigen (HLA)-identical and HLA-nonidentical stem cell transplantation. Blood 2000;96(13):4344–9.

18. Schulz AS, Classen CF, Mihatsch WA, et al. HLA-haploidentical blood progenitor cell transplantation in osteopetrosis. Blood 2002;99(9):3458–60.

19. Friedrich W, Schütz C, Schulz A, et al. Results and long-term outcome in 39 patients with Wiskott-Aldrich syndrome transplanted from HLA-matched and mismatched donors. Immunol Res 2009;44(1–3):18–24.

20. White H, Thrasher A, Veys P, et al. Intrinsic defects of B cell function in X-linked severe combined immunodeficiency. Eur J Immunol 2000;30(3):732–7.

21. Cabatingan MS, Schmidt MR, Sen R, et al. Naive B lymphocytes undergo homeostatic proliferation in response to B cell deficit. J Immunol 2002;169(12): 6795–805.

22. van Zelm MC, Szczepanski T, van der Burg M, et al. Replication history of B lymphocytes reveals homeostatic proliferation and extensive antigen-induced B cell expansion. J Exp Med 2007;204(3):645–55.

23. Prockop SE, Petrie H. Regulation of thymus size by competition for stromal niches among early T cell progenitors. J Immunol 2004;173:1604–11.

24. Mueller SM, Ege M, Pottharst A, et al. Transplacentally acquired maternal T lymphocytes in severe combined immunodeficiency: a study of 121 patients. Blood 2001;98(6):1847–51.

25. Antoine C, Muller S, Cant A, et al. Long-term survival after transplantation of haematopoietic stem cells for immunodeficiencies: report of the European experience 1968–1999. Lancet 2003;361:553–60.

26. Bertrand Y, Landais P, Friedrich W, et al. Influence of severe combine immunodeficiency phenotype on the outcome of HLA non-identical, T cell depleted bone marrow transplantation: a retrospective European survey from the European group for bone marrow transplantation and the European society for immunodeficiency. J Pediatr 1999;134:740–8.

27. Buckley RH, Schiff SE, Schiff RI, et al. Hematopoietic stem-cell transplantation for the treatment of severe combined immunodeficiency. N Engl J Med 1999;340: 508–16.

28. Fischer A, Landais P, Friedrich W, et al. European experience of bone marrow transplantation for severe combined immunodeficiency. Lancet 1990;2:850–4.

29. Haddad E, Landais P, Friedrich W, et al. Long-term immune reconstitution and outcome after HLA-nonidentical T-cell-depleted bone marrow transplantation for severe combined immunodeficiency: a European retrospective study of 116 patients. Blood 1998;91:3646–53.

30. Bertrand Y, Mueller SM, Casanova JL, et al. Reticular dysgenesis: HLA non-identical bone marrow transplants in a series of 10 patients. Bone Marrow Transplant 2002;29(9):759–62.

31. Pollack MS, Kirkpatrick D, Kapoor N, et al. Identification by HLA typing of intrauterine-derived maternal T-cells in four patients with severe combined immunodeficiency. N Engl J Med 1982;307:662–6.

32. Neven B, Leroy S, Decaluwe H, et al. Long-term outcome after hematopoietic stem cell transplantation of a single-center cohort of 90 patients with severe combined immunodeficiency. Blood 2009;113(17):4114–24.
33. Laffort C, Le Deist F, Favre M, et al. Severe cutaneous papillomavirus disease after haemopoietic stem-cell transplantation in patients with severe combined immune deficiency caused by common gamma cytokine receptor subunit or JAK-3 deficiency. Lancet 2004;363(9426):2051.
34. Booth C, Ribeil JA, Audat F, et al. CD34 stem cell top-ups without conditioning after initial haematopoietic stem cell transplantation for correction of incomplete haematopoietic and immunological recovery in severe congenital immunodeficiencies. Br J Haematol 2006;135(4):533–7.
35. Hoenig M, Albert MH, Schulz A, et al. Patients with adenosine deaminase deficiency surviving after hematopoietic stem cell transplantation are at high risk of CNS complications. Blood 2007;109(8):3595–602.
36. Rogers MH, Lwin R, Fairbanks L, et al. Cognitive and behavioral abnormalities in adenosine deaminase deficient severe combined immunodeficiency. J Pediatr 2001;139(1):44–50.
37. Frey JR, Ernst B, Surh CD, et al. Thymus-grafted SCID mice show transient thymopoiesis and limited depletion of V beta 11+ T cells. J Exp Med 1992;175(4):1067–71.
38. Sarzotti-Kelsoe M, Win CM, Parrott RE, et al. Thymic output, T-cell diversity, and T-cell function in long-term human SCID chimeras. Blood 2009;114(7):1445–53.
39. Mazzolari E, Forino C, Guerci S, et al. Long-term immune reconstitution and clinical outcome after stem cell transplantation for severe T-cell immunodeficiency. J Allergy Clin Immunol 2007;120(4):892–9.

Haploidentical Bone Marrow Transplantation in Primary Immune Deficiency: Stem Cell Selection and Manipulation

David Hagin, MD, Yair Reisner, PhD*

KEYWORDS

• Immunodeficiency • Stem cell transplantation • T cell depletion

Primary immunodeficiency (PID) describes a group of inherited disorders character-ized by impairment of innate or adaptive immunity. Although rare, PID commonly leads to lethal complications mainly as a result of severe and recurrent infections. In the last 50 years there has been enormous progress in understanding and identifying the genetic variability causing PID, with more than 150 different primary immune defi-ciency syndromes known today.[1–3] Despite this variability in etiology, especially for severe cases of immune deficiency, hematopoietic stem cell transplantation (HSCT) remains the major curative treatment to correct the immunodeficiency and reverse the predicted poor prognosis. The first HSCT for treatment of severe combined immu-nodeficiency was performed in 1968 using a bone marrow donation from an human leukocyte antigen (HLA) identical sister to correct the immune function of an infant with severe combined immunodeficiencies (SCID).[4] However, because of the lethal complication of graft versus host disease (GVHD), the procedure could be employed only in patients who had an HLA identical donor.[5] It was 12 years later that successful stem cell selection, using differential agglutination with soybean agglutinin (SBA) and subsequent T cell depletion (TCD) with sheep red blood cells (SRBC), made it possible to perform lifesaving stem cell transplantations using a haploidentical stem cell donor, without causing lethal GVHD.[6]

A version of this article was previously published in the *Immunology and Allergy Clinics of North America*, 30:1.
Department of Immunology, Weizmann Institute of Science, PO Box 26, Rehovot 76100, Israel
* Corresponding author.
E-mail address: yair.reisner@weizmann.ac.il

T CELL DEPLETED STEM CELL TRANSPLANTATION

Stem cell transplantation offers a curative treatment for many patients with a severe form of immune deficiency, as well as malignant and nonmalignant hematologic disorders. As an identical, related, stem cell donor is available only in a small minority of cases (15%–20%),[7] alternative donors are needed. The 2 alternative options are allogeneic stem cell transplantation from an unrelated identical donor and haploidentical related donor (in which the donor and recipient share only 1 of 2 possible HLA haplotypes). For the first option, despite the world registry network, the odds of finding a matched unrelated donor in the registries varies with the patient's race and ranges from approximately 60% to 80% for whites to less than 10% for ethnic minorities.[8,9] Another major disadvantage is the time required to identify a donor from a potential panel; the severely immune compromised patient may succumb to severe infectious complications during this time. Furthermore, with the development of molecular analysis, close matching has become more accurate in an attempt to reduce the risk of GVHD but, at the same time, the chance of finding a suitable matched donor reduces even more. For these reasons, allogeneic identical stem cell transplantation is not available for most treatment candidates. On the other hand, virtually all patients have a readily available haploidentical family member. Using a full haplotype mismatched related donor offers several significant advantages:

1. Immediate donor availability
2. Immediate access to donor-derived cellular therapies if required after transplantation, including repeated transplantation from the same donor or from the other haploidentical parental donor in case of graft failure
3. Ability to select the donor of choice out of several available relatives by their clinical status and natural killer (NK) alloreactivity.

However, the use of haploidentical donors has presented a major challenge in the past 4 decades, because of life-threatening GVHD. Following a lead originally attributed to Delta Uphoff,[10] the possibility that fetal liver at the appropriate time in development, lacking post-thymic immunocompetent cells, could be used as a source of stem cells without producing GVHD was studied.[11,12] Later, similar results were achieved using splenocytes from neonatally thymectomized mice to protect lethally irradiated mice without causing GVHD.[11]

Further work in the late 1970s using specific anti-T cell antibodies in mice[10,11] or antilymphocyte antibodies in rats[13] demonstrated that TCD can effectively enable radioprotection without GVHD. Furthermore, as many as 0.3% of mature T cells in the donor graft can cause a high incidence of lethal GVHD.[13] In parallel with this work, we have demonstrated that the lectin SBA can effectively separate hemapoietic stem cells from T cells, to enable successful bone marrow transplantation in lethally irradiated mice from fully disparate donors. This procedure was established based on the earlier observation that the peanut agglutinin (PNA) and SBA, which are exposed on hematopoietic stem cells (HSCs), are masked by sialic acid in the maturation process in the thymus medulla (**Fig. 1**).[14,15]

It was then clear that the key to successful haploidentical stem cell transplantation is dependent on a highly T cell depleted stem cell graft.

Based on the initial work on rodents with SBA[16,17] we further tested our ability to purify bone marrow stem cells from mature T cells in primates. Although a modification of the separation protocol was needed, a successful TCD was achieved[18] and an allogeneic T cell depleted stem cell transplantation was fully engrafted without causing GVHD.[19]

Model for changes in lectin receptors on murine lymphocyte
surfaces during differentiation and maturation

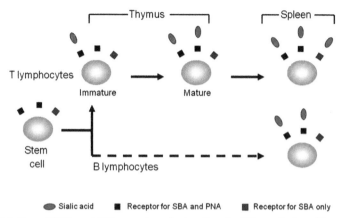

Fig. 1. Sialylation of PNA and SBA receptors during thymic differentiation. (*From* Reisner Y. Changes in lectin receptors during lymphocyte differentiation: application to bone marrow transplantation. Lectins Biol Biochem Clin Biochem 1983;3:681; with permission.)

In 1980, following further adaptation to human bone marrow to attain more than 3 log TCD, this approach finally enabled us to perform an allogeneic haploidentical bone marrow transplantation on a 10-month-old girl with acute leukemia.[6] Eight weeks after transplantation of a haploidentical paternal graft, the girl showed complete recovery of the stem cell graft with T cells and other marrow cells of the donor type, without any evidence of GVHD in the absence of GVHD prophylaxis. In parallel, this method was used successfully in 1980 for the treatment of the first SCID patient with his mother's bone marrow.[20]

The era of T cell depleted stem cell transplantations had begun.

METHODS OF TCD

Three major TCD methods have been used successfully for the treatment of PID patients.

Stem Cells Fractionation by Lectins

Lectins are sugar-binding proteins that are highly specific for their carbohydrate moieties. Stem cell fractionation using lectins is based on the principle that cell subpopulations expressing different lectin receptors can be separated by differential agglutination. Of the different lectins used for cell separation and identification, plant lectin SBA was shown to be useful in the separation of bone marrow cells and depletion of mature T cells.[18] After several modifications, an efficient and rapid technique was developed for the large-scale removal of T lymphocytes from human bone marrow. The method achieved a highly purified cell population rich in blast cells and all myeloid precursors but depleted of T lymphocytes. Briefly, there are 4 main steps in this process[6]: (1) selective removal of red blood cells (RBCs) by gravity sedimentation; (2) agglutination with SBA and differential sedimentation of the agglutinated (SBA$^+$) cells; (3) removal of E-rosette forming T cells from the SBA$^-$ cell fraction by centrifugation over Ficoll (RBCs form around human T cells on incubation); (4)

repetition of the E-rosetting step using neuraminidase-treated sheep RBCs to eliminate residual T cells in the SBA$^-$E$^-$ fraction. The cells collected at the end of the process (SBA$^-$E$^-$E$_N^-$) were used for transplantation.

Following the successful transplantation of a haploidentical stem cell graft in a patient with acute leukemia as described earlier,[6] this method was used in the treatment of patients with SCID using a haploidentical stem cell parental graft.[20–22]

Although the initial reports were limited because of the small number of recipients and short duration of follow-up, several significant issues were demonstrated. First, although more than 1 stem cell donation was needed in some of the patients, durable engraftment was achieved. Each of the patients developed mixed chimerism with T cells that were exclusively of donor type, and non-T populations that were either of mixed or host origin. Second, full reconstitution of cell-mediated immunity and partial reconstitution of humoral immunity was achieved. Despite the capability of engrafted paternal lymphocytes for a strong alloreactive response, reactivity against host cells in vitro was diminished. Third, no significant GVHD developed.

A modification of the method described is the use of E-rosetting with neuraminidase-treated SRBCs without prior lectin separation. Although the degree of TCD was less than that described earlier, requiring posttransplant immunosuppressive treatment to prevent GVHD, it was hoped that the presence of more donor T cells in the graft might enable better engraftment and faster immune reconstitution.[23]

TCD Using Anti-T Cells Monoclonal Antibodies

Shortly after the development of lectin-based cell separation, another method using monoclonal antibodies was examined. The first antibody used was the anti-CD3 monoclonal antibody OKT3. Although engraftment was achieved, significant acute GVHD (aGVHD) could not be prevented.[24,25] This could be explained by insufficient ex vivo TCD and by the inability of this murine antibody to activate human complement and continuously inactivate donor T cells after transplantation.

In 1983 a new monoclonal antibody was presented by Hale and colleagues.[26] The antibody, a rat monoclonal anti-CD52 designated CAMPATH 1(alemtuzumab in the humanized form), has been proved to fix human complement and efficiently eliminate lymphocytes (>99% depletion) when incubated with complement-containing autologous plasma, while sparing the colony-forming cells in the bone marrow. Comparison between the 2 methods for TCD showed a similar degree of reduction in bone marrow T cells (99.8% for SBA vs 99.4% for Campath 1).[27] Soon after, Campath 1 became widely used for T cell depletion in allogeneic bone marrow transplantation for the treatment of malignant diseases and a significant reduction in the occurrence and degree of GVHD relative to untreated bone marrow was reported, although most of these preliminary studies described patients who received transplants from HLA-matched donors[28–30] and with posttransplant immune suppression. Since then, anti-CD52 antibodies has been used for prevention of graft rejection[31] in organ transplantation and as an antineoplastic drug.[32]

Positive Selection of Hematopoietic CD34+ Stem Cells

In the late 1990s, following a successful positive selection of CD34+ stem cells,[33–35] this approach afforded a third option for TCD. The most commonly used methods, Isolex or the Milteney CliniMACS system, based on magnetic beads attached to an anti-CD34 antibody, enable marked purification of CD34+ stem cells.[36] This procedure can be performed with or without additional negative depletion of CD3+ cells. In particular, in this method peripheral blood can be used as a source of stem cells affording up to 4 log TCD.

The following paragraphs summarize the efficacy of TCD HSCT in relation to overall survival, GVHD prevention, and recovery after transplantation and immune reconstitution. As most of the larger retrospective studies regarding HSCT in PID compare TCD haploidentical HSCT to unmanipulated identical HSCT (either related or unrelated), without distinguishing between the method used for T cell depletion, most of the data presented focuses on the differences between TCD HSCT and unfractionated HSCT. Data regarding the effect of the method used for TCD on posttransplantation outcome is presented where available.

LONG-TERM SURVIVAL AFTER TCD HSCT

A review of the literature regarding the long-term results of T cell depleted stem cell transplantation reveals an unexpected variability in the outcome and survival of patients treated. Some of the disparity could result from the nature of the primary disease but other variables should be considered, such as supportive care, the degree of TCD, pretreatment conditioning regimen (CR) and posttransplantation prophylaxis.

Survival in SCID Patients

When considering the information on the overall survival of TCD HSCT in SCID patients, a careful analysis of the data should be made. Although the overall survival in the European Group for Blood and Marrow Transplantation multicenter study, which was published in 1998, showed a poor prognosis of 52% long-term survival,[37] almost at the same time 2 other studies published by Buckley and colleagues[38] and Small and colleagues[39] in North America reported a long-term survival rate of near 80% (**Fig. 2**A). However, there are some significant differences between the groups. The method used for TCD in the North American studies was SBA and E-rosetting; the depletion in the European study comprised several methods including E-rosetting ± albumin gradient separation, SBA and E-rosetting or monoclonal antibodies with complement lysis. The difference in the degree of TCD might be associated with the disparity presented. In addition, the CR and the posttransplantation prophylactic treatment were different between the groups. In consideration of the marked sensitivity of SCID patients even to mild conditioning, in the early studies during the 1980s the North American groups preferred to avoid using conditioning and largely resorted to repeated transplantation. Moreover, no GVHD prophylaxis was used. On the other hand, in the European study conditioning and posttransplantation prophylaxis were given in 73% and 33% of the cases, respectively. Two other areas of uncertainty are the phenotypical composition of the SCID population involved (as discussed later) and the quality of supportive care used. The quality of supportive care is supported by a more recent analysis from the European group (based on data gathered in the SCETIDE (Stem Cell Transplantation for Immunodeficiencies) registry and includes the largest cohort of patients described) demonstrating significant improvement in long-term survival with time (**Fig. 2**B)[40] (reaching near 80% in transplantation performed after 1996, in accordance with the data presented by the North American groups). In 1996, CD34+ positive selection[40] began to be used as a method for TCD. Better TCD and improvement in the diagnosis and treatment of infectious complications can explain improved survival.

There is no doubt that related HLA identical stem cell transplantations result in the highest survival with more than a 90% long-term survival rate.[41] This survival rate can be further improved, even with haploidentical TCD HSCT, when performed in the neonatal period.[42] However, for most patients,[39] the haploidentical stem cell graft is

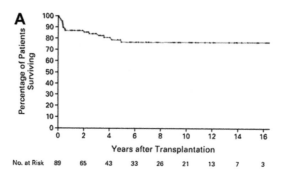

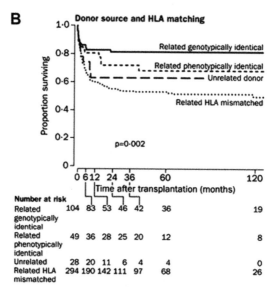

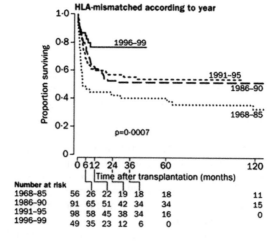

more than a reasonable alternative in the absence of an HLA identical family member, even compared with unmanipulated, matched, unrelated donor graft with ~80% survival rate.[37]

Despite the favorable results of TCD HSCT, there is much diversity in the outcome of SCID patients based on the disease phenotype and genetic cause. To simplify matters, based on the existence of B lymphocytes, SCID can be separated into 2 main groups: the first is the autosomal recessive (AR) inherited, characterized by the absence of T and B lymphocytes but by the presence of normal NK cells (T−B−NK+ SCID); the second is either X-linked or AR, characterized by the absence of T cells and NK cells but by the presence of nonfunctional B cells (T−B+NK− SCID). In general, the results of haploidentical TCD HSCT are significantly better for patients with T−B+NK− SCID (60% survival) than for T−B−NK+ SCID (35%).[43] Although with time, and younger age at transplantation and the use of conditioning treatment, these results improved, the outcome of B− SCID transplantations are still less favorable with overall survival near 50%.[41,43] Similar disparity was not found with an identical related stem cell donor.[40] It is traditionally believed that existing NK cells are responsible for graft rejection, causing a low rate of engraftment and poor prognosis.

ADA SCID represents another group of patients in which the efficacy of TCD HSCT is difficult to evaluate. In a retrospective study, data from 87 patients demonstrated a 1-year survival of 88%, 67%, and 29% to 43% with related identical donor, unrelated identical donor, and haploidentical donor, respectively.[40] However, when evaluating patients who received a highly T cell depleted haploidentical stem cell graft, without any pretransplantation treatment, the long-term survival rate approximates 75%, almost the same as in other B+ SCID.[44]

Survival in Non-SCID PID Patients

Despite supportive management, premature mortality mostly as a result of infectious complications, has led to the use of HSCT as a curative treatment. Although a heterogeneous group of diseases, combined analysis of the available data predicts an unfavorable outcome for TCD haploidentical HSCT compared with matched related HSCT (71% vs 42% 3-year survival),[40] without evidence for improvement over time.

Of the non-SCID PIDs treated with HSCT, patients with Wiskott-Aldrich syndrome (WAS) are the largest group. A recent analysis of 96 patients treated with HSCT for WAS showed inferior results for haploidentical HSCT relative to mostly unmanipulated identical HSCT, either related or unrelated (55%, 88% and 71%, respectively).[45]

The data suggest that when considering the treatment of choice for non-SCID PID, as the threat of imminent death does not exist, a search for a fully matched stem cell donor should be conducted, as long as the procedure is performed at a young age.[46]

Fig. 2. Long-term survival rate after T cell depleted haploidentical SCT. (*A*) Kaplan-Meier survival curve for 89 patients with severe combined immunodeficiency who received stem cell transplants; 12 received transplants from related identical donors. *From* Buckley RH, Schiff SE, Schiff RI, et al. Hematopoietic stem-cell transplantation for the treatment of severe combined immunodeficiency. N Engl J Med 1999;340(7):510; with permission. (*B*) Cumulative probability of survival in SCID patients, according to donor source (related or unrelated donor) and HLA matching, and year of transplantation. (*From* Antoine C, Müller S, Cant A, et al. Long-term survival and transplantation of haemopoietic stem cells for immunodeficiencies: report of the European experience 1968–99. Lancet 2003;361(9357):556; with permission.)

Method of T Cell Depletion and Survival

Because of the lack of data comparing the efficacy of the different methods for TCD, it is almost impossible to conclude which is the preferred method for T cell depletion. One study has demonstrated reduced engraftment and survival in T−B−NK+ SCID patients when monoclonal antibodies were used for T cell depletion.[43] Similarly, although not analyzed for statistical significance, a slightly reduced survival was implicated when comparing the long-term sequelae of anti-CD52 depletion and CD34+ positive selection (19/27 vs 19/22).[36] As these studies reflect separation procedures which, in part, were performed more than 10 years ago, it is more than reasonable to assume that improvement in separation techniques will render this difference insignificant.

GVHD AND TCD HSCT

TCD was developed as a method to prevent GVHD when using haploidentical stem cell grafts. The prevention of GVHD is of great importance as retrospective analysis has shown it is a significant risk factor for reduced survival when appearing either in the early form of aGVHD or when present 6 months after transplantation in the form of cGVHD.[37,40]

In addition, as was recently suggested, GVHD might impair thymic function and affect long-term T cell immune reconstitution.[47,48] Despite the initial results which showed near complete prevention of GVHD, data presented in larger studies describe a higher incidence of GVHD than previously expected. However, the incidence and severity of GVHD was significantly lower than that observed with unmanipulated stem cell grafts.

Acute GVHD

In several studies of SCID patients, different rates of acute GVHD were reported. For TCD haploidentical HSCT the incidence rate was 34% at the Duke University group (grades I–III),[2] and between 40% and 22% in the European group (grade II or higher) with improvement over the years.[40] These results are comparable and somewhat better than those achieved with identical related HSCT (30.8%–40%[2,41]), but significantly superior in incidence and severity compared with patients receiving transplants from unmanipulated, matched, unrelated donor (73.1% incidence, 3/41 patients died as a consequence of aGVHD, the most common cause of death).[41]

No GVHD prophylaxis was used in the Duke series, but patients in the European group who received haploidentical TCD HSCT were treated with at least 2 months of cyclosporin A. Considering the mild degree of the GVHD that developed, and the small reduction (if any) in the incidence of GVHD in patients receiving prophylactic treatment, careful evaluation of the risks of chemoprophylactic treatment should be made, as it is possible that more vigorous T cell depletion by itself would achieve similar results.

Most of the cases of GVHD after haploidentical TCD HSCT occurred when there was persistence of transplacentally transferred maternal T cells,[2] a phenomenon that was seen in up to 40% of SCID patients.[49]

There is general lack of data regarding the prevalence and severity of acute GVHD after HSCT for non-SCID patients. The European study describes aGVHD as a poor prognostic factor independent of the origin of the donor.[40] In a WAS study the incidence of significant aGVHD (grades II–IV) was affected by the origin of the donor with an incidence of 16% for HLA identical sibling donors, 30% for other related donors, and 56% for unrelated donor transplant, although in the last 2 groups, not all of the grafts were T depleted.[46]

Chronic GVHD

In SCID patients chronic GVHD is an infrequent complication. In several series of T cell depleted haploidentical HSCT, there was a low incidence (<2%) of low-grade chronic GVHD (cGVHD).[2,36,41] In a more recent study describing a long-term follow-up of up to 34 years after HSCT, the incidence of cGVHD when using haploidentical HSCT was 10%. At least in some of these patients the disease was of higher grade and disseminated.[50] These frequencies are significantly lower than those described for matched unrelated donors (23%).[41]

Method of TCD and GVHD

It is reasonable to assume that better TCD will result in lower incidence and severity of GVHD; however, in the absence of well-controlled comparative studies, this point cannot be easily demonstrated.

Several issues should be mentioned about GVHD. GVHD should be considered as a double risk for the patient: the clinical risk of severe and lethal disease and the long-term immunologic risk of thymic dysfunction and reduced thymopoiesis. Posttransplantation prophylaxis could be considered as a measure for prevention of GVHD, but the possible risk of thymic damage without an obvious benefit of the preventive treatment as described earlier, requires a careful and thoughtful decision making when choosing the appropriate treatment for the patient.

ENGRAFTMENT AND IMMUNE RECONSTITUTION FOLLOWING TCD HSCT
Engraftment

In the first series of TCD HSCT in SCID patients the problem of early graft rejection, which could be corrected by a second transplant from the other parent, was observed. In the initial work of Reisner and colleagues[20] from 1983, all 3 patients who underwent TCD HSCT required repeat stem cell grafts as a result of early graft rejection. Several subsequent studies in which the rate of early graft rejection reached up to 30% and necessitated repeated transplantation confirmed these results.[2,38,41] This observation and the fear of increased mortality during the prolonged time of severe immune deficiency led to the use of somewhat reduced TCD, together with GVHD prophylaxis in the hope of achieving better graft engraftment.[23] The overall rate of 30% graft rejection is significantly higher than that observed when using a matched unrelated HSC donor.[41] In particular, NK+ SCID might lead to a higher rate of early graft rejection in the absence of conditioning treatment, unless prior maternal engraftment is present and the mother is the HSC donor.[7] However, although the main concern in early graft rejection is the prolonged period of vulnerability to infections, even with a higher incidence of graft rejection, requiring more than 1 transplant, overall survival was not inferior to that observed in other studies.[2]

T Cell Recovery

Twenty years ago T cell recovery was evaluated through the development of normal T cell counts and proliferative responses to phytohemagglutinin antigen, recall antigens such as purified protein derivative, and tetanus or allogeneic stimulators. In recent years attention has focused on long-lasting thymic activity that results in continuous production and development of a diverse T cell repertoire.

One method for evaluating T cell reconstitution and thymic function is the measurement of T cell receptor (TCR) rearrangement excisional circles (TRECs), which are found only in progenitor T cells undergoing TCR rearrangement and, for this reason, represent recently released naive T cells.[51]

In addition, based on differential T cell phenotypes, it has been shown that after HSCT, T cells may develop from 2 independent sources.[52,53] The first is mature memory donor T cells contained in the graft, expressing the surface marker CD45RO. These cells can undergo substantial and rapid expansion; mediate protective immunity early after transplantation but at the same time may induce GVHD. The second source is naive T cells, expressing the surface marker CD45RA, generated from thymic engrafted stem cells. The appearance of CD4+CD45RA+ T cells after transplantation represents thymic-derived naive T cells.

It is to be expected that a different pattern of T cell reconstitution will follow unmanipulated HSCT and TCD HSCT. The unmanipulated graft consists of progenitor cells and mature T cells. Therefore, T cell reconstitution is bimodal, with early expansion of mature T cells followed by a second wave of naive T cells resulting in neothymopoiesis. Although early T cell expansion supports rapid elevation of the lymphocyte count, it is unclear whether this T cell population provides sufficient immunity against infection, as these cells proliferate from a limited number of precursors and carry a TCR repertoire of limited diversity.[54]

Highly diverse naive T cells (CD45RA+) usually appear 3 to 6 months after transplantation and continue to increase during the first 2 years following transplantation. The initial time interval between transplantation and the appearance of naive T cells most likely reflects the time required for the complex process of intrathymic lymphoid maturation, and remains similarly independent of the donor type or stem cell manipulation.[55–58] One exception is unmanipulated, matched, unrelated donor graft, which in several studies in non-PID patients was thought to result in delayed immune reconstitution as a result of a higher incidence and severity of GVHD.[56,59]

Of several factors that were suspected of inhibiting T cell reconstitution, GVHD was found to be of great importance. It is thought that GVHD induces injury to host thymic and other lymphoid organs required for T cell reconstitution,[60] as reflected by the decreased TRECs number[56,59] and increased morbidity and mortality.[50,61] Prevention of GVHD in HSCT from other than an identical HSC donor is, therefore, of high priority and requires a more careful evaluation of the methods used for TCD.

Over the years, longer follow-up data have caused concern regarding the long-term results of T cell reconstitution following HSCT for PID. Patel and colleagues[57] and Sarzotti and colleagues[62] showed that despite satisfactory early T cell reconstitution, a rapid decline in thymic function follows HSCT in SCID patients. TRECs levels have declined to undetectable levels over a period of 14 years compared with approximately 80 years in a normal control patient, representing rapid thymic exhaustion. As most of the patients in these studies were transplanted with TCD haploidentical HSC donor, T cell depletion may be the cause of the apparent decline in thymopoiesis. However, other studies did not find similar results, and were able to demonstrate a positive correlation between continuous measurable TRECs level and the development of myeloid chimerism in the transplanted patient.[63,64] It has been suggested that early T cell reconstitution does not require marrow engraftment of donor CD34+ cells.[58] Therefore, it is possible that the lack of marrow engraftment is responsible for the late loss of thymic function in the absence of a continuous supply of marrow progenitor cells.[58,65] Although long-lasting thymic function was shown to correlate with myeloid donor chimerism,[60,61] which, in most cases, can be achieved only with myeloablative CR, patients in the studies describing thymic exhaustion did not receive any CR before transplantation.[57,59] The data may cause an uneasy dilemma for the patient and caregiver having to choose between an aggressive CR, which might result in reduced survival in the short-term, and long-term thymic exhaustion which might result in significant morbidity and mortality in the long-term. However, according to the available data (for some patients >18 years after TCD HSCT), the decline in thymic function was not associated with recurrent infection.[38,57,62]

B Cell Recovery

In general, B cell function in SCID patients does not develop as well as T cells following HSCT, and a substantial proportion of patients require immunoglobulin replacement therapy to prevent infections, even when using a related identical HSC graft in the absence of donor stem cell engraftment.[38,47]

Several factors have been shown to be associated with B cell recovery. T cell reconstitution 6 months after bone marrow transplant correlates with improved B cell function.[37] T−B−SCID was associated with a lower rate of B cell recovery, especially when no CR was given.[37,43] When evaluating B cell function in T−B+ SCID patients, engraftment of donor B cells offered the best chance for B cell recovery. However, chimerism was achieved only in a minority of the patients independent of HSC origin or nonmyeloablative CR.[66] Some SCID patients with normal B cells enjoy long-lasting functional host B cell function following the development of competent donor T cells.[47,66]

Of the different methods used for TCD, a comparison between CD34+ positive selection and anti-CD52 depletion showed an advantage for the anti-CD52–treated stem cells, as represented by a higher rate of normal IgG levels, a higher rate of class-switched memory B cells and a trend toward more complete B lymphocyte donor chimerism.[36] The findings could be explained by the hypothesis that positive stem cells selection (in contrast to T cell depletion) might result in removal of key stromal cells[67] or alloreactive NK cells from the graft and reduce engraftment.

Dependence on immunoglobulin replacement therapy tends to resolve in some patients over the years, independent of chimerism and SCID diagnosis.[50]

METHODS TO ENHANCE RECOVERY FOLLOWING TCD HSCT

The delayed T cell reconstitution following TCD HSCT is a major clinical problem as it is a period of profound immune deficiency during which the patient is exposed to lethal infectious complication. Several modalities have been suggested in an attempt to shorten the period of risk.

Haploidentical TCD HSCT in the neonatal period improved overall survival rate (95%) and might shorten the period between HSCT and normal T cell function.[42] Early CD34+ stem cell boost as a means to correct incomplete immune recovery was found to be beneficial when performed in the first year following transplantation.[68] Recently, several experimental methods using cell therapy have been suggested as a possible method of accelerating immune reconstitution, including treatment with nonalloreactive T cells, specific antiviral effector T cells and, hopefully in the future, ex vivo expanded T cell precursors to achieve rapid thymic seeding.[48,69]

One of the most encouraging results presented in recent years is the study of Dvorak and colleagues[70] describing a megadose CD34+ cell graft in a SCID patient. Administration of a megadose of CD34+ HSC has been reported to induce tolerance and enhance engraftment.[71] In accordance with this, a megadose of haploidentical CD34+ cells, together with a fixed number of CD3+ cells, without myeloablative chemotherapy, has been shown to result in a high rate of engraftment (73%), accelerated recovery of CD4 counts (1.2 months for CD4 >200) and a favorable overall survival rate of 87% despite relatively older age (median 5.7 months) and significant infections at the time of transplantation. However, there was a relatively high rate of grade II aGVHD (58%) and B cell function failed to develop in most patients.[70] Despite the small number of patients treated (15), the data are highly convincing and validate the haploidentical TCD HSC graft as the appropriate source for donor graft in the absence of an identical related donor.

SUMMARY

Several primary immune deficiency diseases can be cured by allogeneic HSCT. In the more severe form of otherwise lethal SCID disease, with the exception of experimental gene therapy, HSCT is the only curative treatment. It is well established that HSCT from an identical related donor offers the best survival outcome, lowest GVHD rate, and to some extent improved immune reconstitution. However, as a matched sibling donor is available for only a few patients, and because SCID is a medical emergency, a T cell depleted haploidentical stem cell donation from a close relative (mostly parents) has emerged as an alternative option.

Most of the data available for the assessment of TCD HSCT in PID patient is difficult to analyze as in many cases it involves multicenter studies, different cell preparations, and variable pre- and posttransplantation treatment. This is the result of several factors including the rarity of diseases, evolution of separation techniques, supportive treatments, CRs, progressive understanding of the different types of PIDs, and the clinical status of the patients which mandates a different approach from one patient to another. However, several issues are relevant when considering TCD HSCT.

With improved survival rates over the years,[38,40,70] TCD haploidentical HSCT is a reasonable alternative in the absence of an identical related donor. This is the case for SCID patients with T−B+ phenotype, but haploidentical TCD carries a much less favorable outcome when performed in T−B− SCID patients and in several other non-SCID PIDs compared with matched unrelated donor.[43,45]

GVHD and early immune reconstitution after TCD HSCT are 2 complicated issues that deserve specific consideration. Both have a significant effect on overall survival and, in a way, the 2 are directly linked to each other. GVHD is a significant risk factor for increased morbidity and mortality and impaired immune reconstitution.[40,47,50,56,60] Efforts have been made to reduce the incidence and severity of GVHD. However, posttransplant GVHD prophylaxis with immunosuppressive agents can be related to increased mortality and morbidity and perhaps delayed immune reconstitution. Given the low grade of GVHD following 3 log T cell depletion, it is difficult to justify the use of such treatments.[38] On the other hand, methods used to enhance engraftment and recovery, including myeloablative treatment and administration of grafts containing larger amounts of T cells, can aggravate GVHD, either through a direct effect of the transplanted T cells or, theoretically, through chemotherapy-mediated thymic injury and inferior tolerance induction. The authors, therefore, believe that the data support the compelling use of highly depleted stem cell grafts as a means of preventing GVHD, together with conservative patient support while waiting for immune reconstitution to develop. This suggestion is based, in part, on the observation that between 1980 and 1996 the North American groups, using largely an extensive T cell depletion with SBA and E-rosetting, attained better survival compared with that described by the European study, in which many patients received less rigorously deleted bone marrow and were therefore also treated by posttransplant GVHD prophylaxis. Furthermore, results in the European study following 1996, at which time T cell depletion was enhanced using positive selection of CD34 cells, reached the same survival rate as reported in the North American study.

Long-term immune reconstitution following TCD HSCT has remained a problem especially when considering humoral immunity. As B cell reconstitution was shown to be associated with B cell engraftment,[66] the use of myeloablative treatment to achieve the desirable donor chimerism could be considered. However, as such protocols were shown to be associated with increased early mortality and long-term clinical effects (especially in several types of SCID patients who are highly sensitive to irradiation and chemotherapy because of the basic genetic defect) and immunologic effects (possible thymic injury), it is difficult to justify such treatments over the more cautious approach avoiding the use of conditioning.

One approach to replace conventional conditioning could be the use of alloreactive NK cells, shown in mouse models to empty bone marrow niches[72] and thereby may enable engraftment of long-term HSCs, important for the establishment of long-lasting B and T cell reconstitution.

Over the years T cell depletion has become a synonym for haploidentical stem cell graft. However, because GVHD is an obvious problem when using an unmanipulated identical unrelated donor as a source for HSCT,[41] the use of T cell depleted stem cell graft should be considered, especially in situations in which haploidentical HSCT was shown to carry a less favorable outcome.

Finally, the encouraging results of a megadose of CD34+ haploidentical stem cell graft presented recently[60] makes this new approach highly compelling and attractive for use in other lethal PID conditions and with different stem cell donors. In particular, this approach could be used in conjunction with other tolerizing cells, such as anti–third-party CTLs[73,74] or immature dendritic cells,[75] in patients known to exhibit immune rejection.

Furthermore, early posttransplant T cell reconstitution might be enhanced by adoptive transfer of nonalloreactive T cells depleted of graft versus host reactivity ex vivo. In addition, recent results in leukemia patients suggest that combining effector donor T cells with donor natural T regulatory cells can effectively enhance immune reconstitution without GVHD (Martelli and colleagues, unpublished results, 2009).

TCD haploidentical HSCT has been shown to be a lifesaving procedure for SCID patients in the absence of an identical related donor. However, the multiplicity of reported studies and the diversity of PID diseases and methods used for treatment, stress the need for prospective studies in more homogeneous patient populations to evaluate the effect of the method used, the source of cells, and the extent of T cell depletion on the posttransplantation outcome.

REFERENCES

1. Geha RS, Notarangelo LD, Casanova JL, et al. The International Union of Immunological Societies (IUIS) primary immunodeficiency diseases (PID) classification committee. J Allergy Clin Immunol 2007;120(4):776.
2. Buckley RH. Molecular defects in human severe combined immunodeficiency and approaches to immune reconstitution. Annu Rev Immunol 2004;22:625–55.
3. Fischer A. Primary immunodeficiency diseases: an experimental model for molecular medicine. Lancet 2001;357(9271):1863–9.
4. Gatti R, Meuwissen H, Allen H, et al. Immunological reconstitution of sex-linked lymphopenic immunological deficiency. Lancet 1968;2(7583):1366.
5. Bortin M, Rimm A. Severe combined immunodeficiency disease. Characterization of the disease and results of transplantation. JAMA 1977;238(7):591–600.

6. Reisner Y, Kapoor N, Kirkpatrick D, et al. Transplantation for acute leukaemia with HLA-A and B nonidentical parental marrow cells fractionated with soybean agglutinin and sheep red blood cells. Lancet 1981;2(8242):327–31.

7. Griffith LM, Cowan MJ, Kohn DB, et al. Allogeneic hematopoietic cell transplantation for primary immune deficiency diseases: current status and critical needs. J Allergy Clin Immunol 2008;122(6):1087–96.

8. Zuckerman T, Rowe JM. Alternative donor transplantation in acute myeloid leukemia: which source and when? Curr Opin Hematol 2007;14:152–61.

9. Tiercy JM, Bujan-Lose M, Chapuis B, et al. Bone marrow transplantation with unrelated donors: what is the probability of identifying an HLA-A/B/Cw/DRB 1/B 3/B 5/DQB 1-matched donor? Bone Marrow Transplant (Basingstoke) 2000; 26(4):437–41.

10. Uphoff D. Preclusion of secondary phase of irradiation syndrome by inoculation of fetal hematopoietic tissue following lethal total-body x-irradiation. J Natl Cancer Inst 1958;20:625.

11. Yunis E, Good R, Smith J, et al. Protection of lethally irradiated mice by spleen cells from neonatally thymectomized mice. Proc Natl Acad Sci U S A 1974; 71(6):2544.

12. Bortin M, Saltzstein E. Graft-versus-host inhibition: fetal liver and thymus cells to minimize secondary disease. Transplantation 1969;8(5):712.

13. Korngold B, Sprent J. Lethal graft-versus-host disease after bone marrow transplantation across minor histocompatibility barriers in mice. Prevention by removing mature T cells from marrow. J Exp Med 1978;148(6):1687–98.

14. Reisner Y, Linker-Israeli M, Sharon N. Separation of mouse thymocytes into two subpopulations by the use of peanut agglutinin. Cell Immunol 1976;25(1): 129–34.

15. Reisner Y, Ravid A, Sharon N. Use of soybean agglutinin for the separation of mouse B and T lymphocytes. Biochem Biophys Res Commun 1976;72(4): 1585–91.

16. Reisner Y, Itzicovitch L, Meshorer A, et al. Hemopoietic stem cell transplantation using mouse bone marrow and spleen cells fractionated by lectins. Proc Natl Acad Sci U S A 1978;75(6):2933–6.

17. Reisner Y, Ikehara S, Hodes MZ, et al. Allogeneic hemopoietic stem cell transplantation using mouse spleen cells fractionated by lectins: in vitro study of cell fractions. Proc Natl Acad Sci U S A 1980;77(2):1164–8.

18. Reisner Y, Kapoor N, O'Reilly R, et al. Allogeneic bone marrow transplantation using stem cells fractionated by lectins: VI, in vitro analysis of human and monkey bone marrow cells fractionated by sheep red blood cells and soybean agglutinin. Lancet 1980;2(8208–8209):1320–4.

19. Reisner Y, Kapoor N, Good R, et al. Allogeneic bone marrow transplantation in mouse, monkey and man using lectin-separated grafts. In: Slavin S, editor. Tolerance in bone marrow and organ transplantation. Amsterdam (NY): Elsevier Science Publishing Co; 1984. p. 293.

20. Reisner Y, Kapoor N, Kirkpatrick D, et al. Transplantation for severe combined immunodeficiency with HLA-A, B, D, DR incompatible parental marrow cells fractionated by soybean agglutinin and sheep red blood cells. Blood 1983; 61(2):341.

21. O'Reilly R, Kapoor N, Kirkpatrick D, et al. Transplantation for severe combined immunodeficiency using histoincompatible parental marrow fractionated by soybean agglutinin and sheep red blood cells: experience in six consecutive cases. Transplant Proc 1983;15(1):1431.

22. Friedrich W, Goldmann SF, Vetter U, et al. Immunoreconstitution in severe combined immunodeficiency after transplantation of HLA-haploidentical, T-cell-depleted bone marrow. Lancet 1984;1(8380):761–4.

23. Fischer A, Durandy A, De Villartay J, et al. HLA-haploidentical bone marrow transplantation for severe combined immunodeficiency using E rosette fractionation and cyclosporine. Blood 1986;67(2):444.

24. Filipovich AH, McGlave PB, Ramsay NK, et al. Pretreatment of donor bone marrow with monoclonal antibody OKT3 for prevention of acute graft-versus-host disease in allogeneic histocompatible bone-marrow transplantation. Lancet 1982;1(8284):1266–9.

25. Hayward AR, Murphy S, Githens J, et al. Failure of a pan-reactive anti-T cell antibody, OKT 3, to prevent graft versus host disease in severe combined immunodeficiency. J Pediatr 1982;100(4):665–8.

26. Hale G, Bright S, Chumbley G, et al. Removal of T cells from bone marrow for transplantation: a monoclonal antilymphocyte antibody that fixes human complement. Blood 1983;62(4):873.

27. Frame JN, Collins NH, Cartagena T, et al. T cell depletion of human bone marrow. Comparison of Campath-1 plus complement, anti-T cell ricin A chain immunotoxin, and soybean agglutinin alone or in combination with sheep erythrocytes or immunomagnetic beads. Transplantation 1989;47(6):984–8.

28. Waldmann H, Hale G, Cividalli G, et al. Elimination of graft-versus-host disease by in-vitro depletion of alloreactive lymphocytes with a monoclonal rat anti-human lymphocyte antibody(CAMPATH-1). Lancet 1984;2(8401):483–5.

29. Apperley J, Jones L, Hale G, et al. Bone marrow transplantation for patients with chronic myeloid leukaemia: T-cell depletion with Campath-1 reduces the incidence of graft-versus-host disease but may increase the risk of leukaemic relapse. Bone Marrow Transplant 1986;1(1):53.

30. Hale G, Cobbold S, Waldmann H. T cell depletion with CAMPATH-1 in allogeneic bone marrow transplantation. Transplantation 1988;45(4):753.

31. Hale G, Zhang MJ, Bunjes D, et al. Improving the outcome of bone marrow transplantation by using CD52 monoclonal antibodies to prevent graft-versus-host disease and graft rejection. Blood 1998;92(12):4581.

32. Waldmann H, Hale G. CAMPATH: from concept to clinic. Philos Trans R Soc Lond B Biol Sci 2005;360(1461):1707.

33. Civin CI, Strauss LC, Fackler MJ, et al. Positive stem cell selection-basic science. Prog Clin Biol Res 1990;333:387–401 [discussion: 402].

34. Sutherland DR, Stewart AK, Keating A. CD34 antigen: molecular features and potential clinical applications. Stem Cells 1993;11(Suppl 3):50–7.

35. Shpall EJ, Gee A, Cagnoni PJ, et al. Stem cell isolation. Curr Opin Hematol 1995; 2(6):452–9.

36. Slatter MA, Brigham K, Dickinson AM, et al. Long-term immune reconstitution after anti-CD52-treated or anti-CD34-treated hematopoietic stem cell transplantation for severe T-lymphocyte immunodeficiency. J Allergy Clin Immunol 2008;121: 361–7.

37. Haddad E, Landais P, Friedrich W, et al. Long-term immune reconstitution and outcome after HLA-nonidentical T-cell-depleted bone marrow transplantation for severe combined immunodeficiency: a European retrospective study of 116 patients. Blood 1998;91(10):3646.

38. Buckley RH, Schiff SE, Schiff RI, et al. Hematopoietic stem-cell transplantation for the treatment of severe combined immunodeficiency. N Engl J Med 1999;340(7): 508–16.

39. Small TN, Friedrich W, O'Reilly RJ. Hematopoietic cell transplantation for immuno-deficiency diseases. In: Appelbaun FR, Forman SJ, Negrin S, et al, editors. Thomas' hematopoietic cell transplantation. 4th edition. Blackwell Publishing Ltd; 2009. p. 1105–24.
40. Antoine C, Müller S, Cant A, et al. Long-term survival and transplantation of hae-mopoietic stem cells for immunodeficiencies: report of the European experience 1968–99. Lancet 2003;361(9357):553–60.
41. Grunebaum E, Mazzolari E, Porta F, et al. Bone marrow transplantation for severe combined immune deficiency. JAMA 2006;295(5):508–18.
42. Myers LA, Patel DD, Puck JM, et al. Hematopoietic stem cell transplantation for severe combined immunodeficiency in the neonatal period leads to supe-rior thymic output and improved survival. Blood 2002;99(3):872.
43. Bertrand Y, Landais P, Friedrich W, et al. Influence of severe combined immuno-deficiency phenotype on the outcome of HLA non-identical, T-cell-depleted bone marrow transplantation: a retrospective European survey from the European Group for Bone Marrow Transplantation and the European Society for Immunode-ficiency. J Pediatr 1999;134(6):740.
44. Booth C, Hershfield M, Notarangelo L, et al. Management options for adenosine deaminase deficiency. Proceedings of the EBMT satellite workshop (Hamburg, March 2006). Clin Immunol 2007;123(2):139–47.
45. Ozsahin H, Cavazzana-Calvo M, Notarangelo LD, et al. Long-term outcome following hematopoietic stem-cell transplantation in Wiskott-Aldrich syndrome: collaborative study of the European Society for Immunodeficiencies and Euro-pean Group for Blood and Marrow Transplantation. Blood 2008;111(1):439.
46. Filipovich AH, Stone JV, Tomany SC, et al. Impact of donor type on outcome of bone marrow transplantation for Wiskott-Aldrich syndrome: collaborative study of the International Bone Marrow Transplant Registry and the National Marrow Donor Program. Blood 2001;97(6):1598.
47. Cowan MJ, Neven B, Cavazanna-Calvo M, et al. Hematopoietic stem cell trans-plantation for severe combined immunodeficiency diseases. Biol Blood Marrow Transplant 2008;14(1S):73–80.
48. Cavazzana-Calvo M, André-Schmutz I, Dal Cortivo L, et al. Immune reconstitution after haematopoietic stem cell transplantation: obstacles and anticipated prog-ress. Curr Opin Immunol 2009;21:544–8.
49. Scaradavou A, Carrier C, Mollen N, et al. Detection of maternal DNA in placental/umbilical cord blood by locus-specific amplification of the noninherited maternal HLA gene. Blood 1996;88(4):1494.
50. Neven B, Leroy S, Decaluwe H, et al. Long-term outcome after hematopoietic stem cell transplantation of a single-center cohort of 90 patients with severe combined immunodeficiency. Blood 2009;113(17):4114.
51. Douek DC, McFarland RD, Keiser PH, et al. Changes in thymic function with age and during the treatment of HIV infection. Nature 1998;396(6712):690–5.
52. Mackall C, Granger L, Sheard M, et al. T-cell regeneration after bone marrow transplantation: differential CD45 isoform expression on thymic-derived versus thymic-independent progeny. Blood 1993;82(8):2585.
53. Dumont-Girard F, Roux E, van Lier RA, et al. Reconstitution of the T-cell compart-ment after bone marrow transplantation: restoration of the repertoire by thymic emigrants. Blood 1998;92(11):4464.
54. Roux E, Helg C, Dumont-Girard F, et al. Analysis of T-cell repopulation after allo-geneic bone marrow transplantation: significant differences between recipients of T-cell depleted and unmanipulated grafts. Blood 1996;87(9):3984.

55. Small T, Papadopoulos E, Boulad F, et al. Comparison of immune reconstitution after unrelated and related T-cell-depleted bone marrow transplantation: effect of patient age and donor leukocyte infusions. Blood 1999;93(2):467.

56. Weinberg K, Blazar BR, Wagner JE, et al. Factors affecting thymic function after allogeneic hematopoietic stem cell transplantation. Blood 2001;97(5):1458.

57. Patel DD, Gooding ME, Parrott RE, et al. Thymic function after hematopoietic stem-cell transplantation for the treatment of severe combined immunodeficiency. N Engl J Med 2000;342(18):1325–32.

58. Muller SM, Kohn T, Schulz AS, et al. Similar pattern of thymic-dependent T-cell reconstitution in infants with severe combined immunodeficiency after human leukocyte antigen (HLA)-identical and HLA-nonidentical stem cell transplantation. Blood 2000;96(13):4344.

59. Lewin SR, Heller G, Zhang L, et al. Direct evidence for new T-cell generation by patients after either T-cell-depleted or unmodified allogeneic hematopoietic stem cell transplantations. Blood 2002;100(6):2235.

60. Dulude G, Roy DC, Perreault C. The effect of graft-versus-host disease on T cell production and homeostasis. J Exp Med 1999;189(8):1329–42.

61. Hazenberg MD, Otto SA, de Pauw ES, et al. T-cell receptor excision circle and T-cell dynamics after allogeneic stem cell transplantation are related to clinical events. Blood 2002;99(9):3449.

62. Sarzotti M, Patel DD, Li X, et al. T cell repertoire development in humans with SCID after nonablative allogeneic marrow transplantation 1. J Immunol 2003; 170(5):2711–8.

63. Borghans JA, Bredius RG, Hazenberg MD, et al. Early determinants of long-term T-cell reconstitution after hematopoietic stem cell transplantation for severe combined immunodeficiency. Blood 2006;108(2):763.

64. Cavazzana-Calvo M, Carlier F, Le Deist F, et al. Long-term T-cell reconstitution after hematopoietic stem-cell transplantation in primary T-cell-immunodeficient patients is associated with myeloid chimerism and possibly the primary disease phenotype. Blood 2007;109(10):4575.

65. Frey J, Ernst B, Surh C, et al. Thymus-grafted SCID mice show transient thymo-poiesis and limited depletion of V beta 11 T cells. J Exp Med 1992;175(4): 1067–71.

66. Haddad E, Deist FL, Aucouturier P, et al. Long-term chimerism and B-cell function after bone marrow transplantation in patients with severe combined immunodeficiency with B cells: a single-center study of 22 patients. Blood 1999;94(8): 2923.

67. Slatter M, Bhattacharya A, Flood T, et al. Polysaccharide antibody responses are impaired post bone marrow transplantation for severe combined immunodeficiency, but not other primary immunodeficiencies. Bone Marrow Transplant 2003;32(2):225–9.

68. Booth C, Ribeil JA, Audat F, et al. CD34 stem cell top-ups without conditioning after initial haematopoietic stem cell transplantation for correction of incomplete haematopoietic and immunological recovery in severe congenital immunodeficiencies. Br J Haematol 2006;135(4):533–7.

69. André-Schmutz I, Six E, Bonhomme D, et al. Shortening the immunodeficient period after hematopoietic stem cell transplantation. Immunol Res 2009;44(1):54–60.

70. Dvorak CC, Hung GY, Horn B, et al. Megadose CD34 cell grafts improve recovery of T cell engraftment but not B cell immunity in patients with severe combined immunodeficiency disease undergoing haplocompatible nonmyeloablative transplantation. Biol Blood Marrow Transplant 2008;14(10):1125–33.

71. Rachamim N, Gan J, Segall H, et al. Tolerance induction by "megadose" hematopoietic transplants: donor-type human CD34 stem cells induce potent specific reduction of host anti-donor cytotoxic T lymphocyte precursors in mixed lymphocyte culture. Transplantation 1998;65(10):1386–93.

72. Ruggeri L, Capanni M, Urbani E, et al. Effectiveness of donor natural killer cell alloreactivity in mismatched hematopoietic transplants. Science 2002; 295(5562):2097.

73. Bachar-Lustig E, Reich-Zeliger S, Reisner Y. Anti-third-party veto CTLs overcome rejection of hematopoietic allografts: synergism with rapamycin and BM cell dose. Blood 2003;102(6):1943.

74. Edelshtein Y, Ophir E, Bachar-Lustig E, et al. Ex-vivo acquisition of central memory phenotype is critical for tolerance induction by donor anti-3rd party CD8 T cells in allogeneic bone marrow transplantation. Blood (ASH Annual Meeting Abstracts) 2008;112:2323.

75. Yu P, Xiong S, He Q, et al. Induction of allogeneic mixed chimerism by immature dendritic cells and bone marrow transplantation leads to prolonged tolerance to major histocompatibility complex disparate allografts. Immunology 2009;127(4): 500–11.

Bone Marrow Transplantation Using HLA-Matched Unrelated Donors for Patients Suffering from Severe Combined Immunodeficiency

Eyal Grunebaum, MD, Chaim M. Roifman, MD, FRCPC, FCACB*

KEYWORDS

• Immunodeficiency • Transplantation • Unrelated • Long-term

Severe combined immunodeficiency (SCID) is a heterogeneous group of inherited diseases characterized by significantly impaired T-cell immunity that leads to death in infancy. The diagnosis of SCID relies on distinct clinical manifestations and laboratory features, and ideally is confirmed by the identification of mutations in genes known to be critical for T lineage development and function. Complete cure can be attained in the majority of patients suffering from SCID by using allogeneic bone marrow transplantation (BMT). The best outcome is achieved by family-related genotypically HLA-identical donors (RID). Among populations with high consanguinity marriage, RID account for the majority of transplants for SCID[1]; however, in most European and North American populations, RID are found for only 15% to 25% of the patients.[2,3] BMT using phenotypically HLA-matched family-related donors (PMD) have resulted in a relatively high success rate[4]; however, PMD are not frequently found.[2] The lack of RID or PMD for more than 75% of SCID patients led many groups to search for alternative sources, such as parents who are often HLA-haploidentical donors (HID) or HLA-matched unrelated donors (MUD).

A version of this article was previously published in the *Immunology and Allergy Clinics of North America*, 30:1.
Division of Immunology and Allergy, Department of Pediatrics, The Hospital for Sick Children, 555 University Avenue, Toronto, Ontario M5G 1X8, Canada
* Corresponding author.
E-mail address: chaim.roifman@sickkids.ca

The first attempt to treat SCID with unmodified MUD transplant was performed in 1973. A patient diagnosed with SCID, whose similarly affected sister died previously after receiving a transplant from her HLA-haploidentical parent, underwent BMT from a partially MUD found among 800 normal individuals registered in Denmark. The patient achieved durable engraftment with complete hematopoietic and immunologic reconstitution, but suffered from skin and oral mucosa chronic graft versus host disease (GvHD).[5]

Difficulties finding HLA-matched unrelated donors and the lack of adequate means to control GvHD, together with the increased availability of T-cell depleted HID BMT in the early 1980s resulted in limited use of MUD BMT for SCID. However, it soon became apparent that with some exceptions,[6] the success rate of HID BMT consistently hovered around 50% at best, regardless of the T-cell depletion method[1,2,7–13] (D. Kohn, Los Angeles, California, personal communication, 2006; L. Notarangelo, Brescia, Italy, personal communication, 2006).

During the late 1980s, several events including the disappointment from HID BMT for SCID, the surge in the number of bone marrow donor registries (**Fig. 1**), and the development of efficient medications to control GvHD, such as cyclosporine A (CsA), prompted Dr Roifman to systematically explore the systematic use of MUD BMT for SCID in their center. Therefore, in 1987, Dr Roifman created a protocol for MUD BMT in SCID. The protocol included strict patient isolation in private HEPA-filtered rooms from diagnosis until discharge, intensive pretransplant antimicrobial management with intravenous immunoglobulins (to maintain IgG≥6 g/L), *Pneumocystis jiroveci* pneumonia prophylaxis, close Herpes virus group surveillance, and nutritional support. Pretransplant conditioning consisted of oral or intravenous busulfan in 16 doses over 4 days (total amount ranging from 16 to 20 mg/kg), in accordance with busulfan blood levels, followed by a 4-day course of cyclophosphamide. Patients received 3 to 5 × 10^8 nucleated cells per kilogram body weight from bone marrow that was unmodified except for volume reduction and plasma removal in blood group mismatch. The amount of nucleated bone marrow harvested from the adult donors was often greater than that required for the infant SCID, therefore excess bone marrow was frozen as backup for graft failure. Patients also received aggressive GvHD prophylaxis and treatment, detailed later in this article, as well as granulocyte-macrophage colony stimulating factor or granulocyte colony stimulating factor from the day

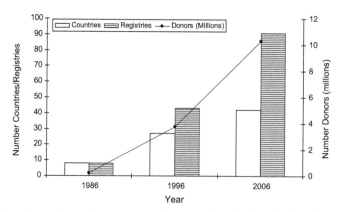

Fig. 1. Increase in registered bone marrow donors and registries. Number of countries that have bone marrow registries, number of registries, and number of donors (in millions) registered in 1986, 1996, and 2006.

of transplant (or day +5 in some cases). This protocol led to improved engraftment and patient survival, which was summarized in 2000 by Dalal and colleagues.[14] Among the first 15 patients with SCID and CID in the authors' center who underwent BMT from HLA-matched or 1 non-DR antigen mismatched unrelated donors, survival was 73.3% with a mean follow-up of 47.4 months (range 18–101 months). All patients had leukocytes engraftment, which were demonstrated to be 100% donor by restriction length fragment polymorphism. Deaths were directly attributed to GvHD disease in 2 patients, while the third patient died of *Streptococcus viridans* sepsis and bone marrow aplasia 1 year after transplant, presumably also due to GvHD.

Other centers using MUD BMT for SCID also achieved excellent engraftment, with survival ranging from 71.5% to 83.3%.[13,15,16] These reports suffered from drawbacks such as the small number of patients in each study, which represented only single centers and lacked long-term evaluation of immune reconstitution. Therefore, in 2004 the authors initiated a study comparing the outcome of 94 patients with SCID who received BMT from 1990 until 2004 at the Hospital for Sick Children, Toronto, Canada and Brescia, Italy. Of importance, this study contained the largest group of patients with SCID to have undergone MUD BMT. The study also provided a unique opportunity for direct and detailed comparison of 40 patients transplanted using HLA-mismatched related donors (MMRD), mostly HID, with 41 patients transplanted with MUD.[3] The clinical presentation, age of diagnosis, molecular diagnosis, and gender, as well as maintenance prior to and after BMT were similar in both centers and among both transplant groups (**Table 1**). Of note is that among 9 patients initially considered as clinically unstable, 4 could be stabilized and only a few required "rush" BMT. The latter emphasizes that while the diagnosis and initial treatment of SCID is a medical emergency, once patients have been stabilized, the BMT itself should be performed with the best available donor.

The median time from diagnosis to MUD BMT in the authors' study was only 4 months, which is shorter than previously reported, probably because of the expansion and improvement of bone marrow registries. Still, the median time from diagnosis to MMRD BMT was only 2 months. However, 30% of the MMRD recipients lost the graft

Table 1
Comparison between pretransplant features of SCID patients who received MMRD or MUD BMT

	MUD (N = 41)	MMRD (N = 40)	P
Males/females	28/13	29/11	0.78
Diagnosis before 3 mo of age	11	14	0.43
Diagnosis between 3 and 12 mo of age	27	25	0.75
Diagnosis after 12 mo of age	3	1	0.32
Failure to thrive	13	8	0.17
Lung disease	14	19	0.16
Diarrhea	5	9	0.17
Rash	6	8	0.36
Candida	6	7	0.48
Unstable clinical condition	4	5	0.48
No clinical abnormalities	8	6	0.40
T−B+NK− immune phenotype	14	16	0.29
T−B−NK+ immune phenotype	12	15	0.20

and required repeat BMT (see later discussion), therefore the actual median time from diagnosis to the final MMRD BMT increased to 3 months, eliminating some of the potential disadvantage of MUD.

Most importantly, long-term survival was significantly better after MUD BMT than after MMRD BMT (80.5% compared with 52.5%, respectively), as demonstrated in **Fig. 2**. The survival after MUD BMT was similar in Toronto and Brescia, suggesting that the outcome was not specific to one center. In addition, there was no difference in outcome whether BMT was performed between 1990 and 1997 or between 1998 and 2004, suggesting lack of effect by change of antimicrobial or supportive management over the years. Survival of patients with B− SCID phenotype, associated previously with poor prognosis,[17] was not different to that in B+ SCID, nor did the specific molecular defect causing SCID affect survival. Moreover, as described later by the authors[18] and by others,[19] patients with Omenn syndrome or residual T cells (T+) SCID also had excellent outcome after MUD BMT, which is discussed in an article elsewhere in this issue.

Engraftment of hematopoietic cell lineages was robust after MUD BMT (**Fig. 3**), with all patients demonstrating 100% donor leukocyte engraftment by 1 month after transplant. Graft failure was observed in only 3 of the 41 (7.3%) patients who received MUD BMT. The authors repeated BMT in 2 of these patients using frozen bone marrow from the unrelated donors following conditioning with cyclophosphamide and total lymphoid irradiation. Both patients achieved complete donor engraftment, which persists 10 and 8 years after transplant, respectively. In marked contrast, a significantly ($P = .009$) higher frequency of donor graft failure was observed after MMRD BMT (**Fig. 4**), with 12 patients (30%) requiring a second transplant. Repeated MMRD BMT led to donor engraftment in only 4 patients. Two patients underwent a third MMRD BMT, one of which was successful. Increased frequency of graft failures after MMRD BMT in patients with SCID were also reported by other centers. Three of 16 patients in Florida also required repeat transplant, with only 1 of them surviving,[11] while 8 of 24 patients in San Francisco required more than 1 MMRD transplant.[7] Graft failure was particularly common when myeloablative conditioning was withheld or significantly altered, although some patients in the authors' study, as well as in other reports, failed to engraft after MMRD despite myeloablation, possibly because the T-cell depletion and ex vivo manipulation can also affect hematopoietic progenitors.

The ultimate purpose of BMT for SCID is to fully restore immune function and return patients to normal unrestricted lives indefinitely. Therefore, the authors were

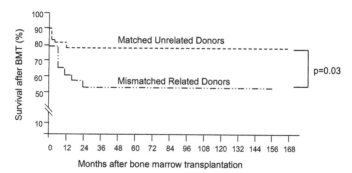

Fig. 2. Survival of patients with SCID who received BMT from MUD or MMRD. Percentage of patients surviving after MUD or MMRD BMT. For patients who received multiple transplants, survival was calculated from the date of the last transplant.

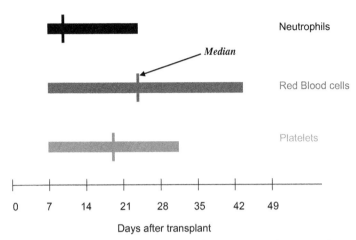

Fig. 3. Engraftment of hematopoietic lineages after MUD BMT for SCID. The numbers of days required to achieve engraftment of neutrophils (absolute neutrophil count >500/μL), red blood cells (last red blood cells transfusion), and platelets (platelets >20,000/μL) after MUD BMT for patients with SCID at the Hospital for Sick Children, Toronto, Canada.

particularly interested in long-term immune reconstitution, 2 or more years after BMT, when most patients had stopped immune suppressive medications. Again, better results were achieved with MUD BMT compared with MMRD BMT, with complete donor lymphocyte engraftment in 88.5% and 66%, respectively. Lymphocyte subsets, in vitro responses of T lymphocytes to mitogens and T-cell receptor excision circles, which represent new thymic emigrants, were normal in all but one of the patients tested after MUD BMT. Similar results were also found after MMRD BMT. In contrast, normal distribution of T-cell receptor variable beta-chain expression was demonstrated in 18 (94.7%) of 19 MUD BMT patients, compared with only 11 (61.1%) of 18 MMRD BMT patients (**Fig. 5**). The latter findings are in agreement with other reports detailing immune dysfunction following MMRD for SCID. Among 11 patients in the Netherlands that received HID BMT for SCID, 4 were considered to have poor long-term T-cell immune reconstitution.[20] The abnormal T-cell immune reconstitution might

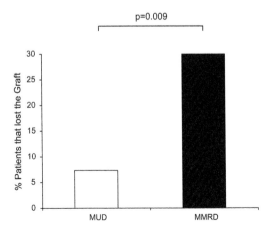

Fig. 4. Graft loss after MUD or MMRD BMT for SCID. Percentage of patients with SCID that lost donor lymphocyte engraftment after MUD or MMRD BMT.

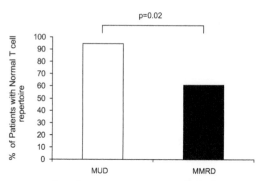

Fig. 5. T-cell receptor repertoire after MUD or MMRD BMT for SCID. Percentage of patients with SCID that achieved normal T-cell repertoire, as determined by T-cell receptor variable beta chain expression, after MUD or MMRD BMT.

be related to the rigorous depletion of donor T cells required for HID BMT. Of importance, the authors continue to monitor the patients every year, and have observed normal immune function in all patients even 20 years after MUD BMT (**Table 2**).

Patients with SCID are particularly prone to respiratory track infections. Indeed, lower respiratory tract infections and pneumonitis, most frequently caused by viral or fungal infections, occurred in 14 SCID patients after MMRD BMT and was the cause of death in 12 patients (**Fig. 6**). In contrast, only 3 SCID patients who received MUD BMT experienced pneumonitis, which was the cause of death in only one patient. Other infections were also infrequent among MUD BMT recipients, possibly because of the rapid and robust immune reconstitution described earlier. Of note, veno-occlusive disease of the liver, which has been reported in some patients with SCID undergoing BMT,[13,21] was not detected in any of the authors' patients despite their use of myeloablative conditioning, possibly because myeloablation is administered when the patients were clinically stable. Mucositis and hemorrhagic cystitis, commonly seen with the use of busulfan and cyclophosphamide, similarly have been rare and relatively mild among SCID patients undergoing MUD BMT.

The use of MUD was expected to be associated with significant GvHD; Therefore, all the authors' patients received GvHD prophylaxis, which consisted of intravenous CsA and methylprednisolone (MPO). CsA (3 mg/kg/d) was initially given from the day before transplant although currently the authors begin CsA as early as 3 days before transplant. CsA doses were adjusted to maintain a trough level of 150 to 200 µg/L.

Table 2
Long-term immune reconstitution after MUD BMT at the Hospital for Sick Children, Toronto, Canada

	No. of Patients Tested	Percent of Patients with Normal Results
Complete donor lymph engraftment	32	100%
T-cell numbers	22	100%
T-cell mitogenic responses	20	100%
Antibody production	21	100%
T-cell receptor excision circles	15	100%
T-cell receptor V-beta diversity	13	100%

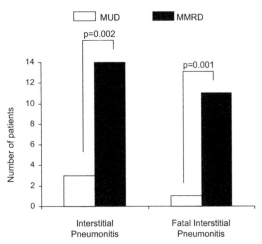

Fig. 6. Pneumonitis after MUD or MMRD BMT for SCID. Number of patients with SCID that suffered interstitial pneumonitis and died of interstitial pneumonitis after MUD or MMRD BMT.

MPO (2 mg/kg/d) was given from the day of the transplant divided into 2 doses. The authors tried adding methotrexate, 10 mg/m^2 on days 3, 6, 11, and 18 in a few SCID patients, as suggested by other investigators[22]; however, the lack of clear benefit and the frequent need to omit several doses of methotrexate because of liver abnormalities led to the removal of methotrexate from the protocol. Despite the aggressive GvHD prophylaxis, acute GvHD did develop in 73.1% of the 41 SCID patients who received MUD BMT in Toronto and Brescia. Although acute GvHD was transient and limited to the skin in most SCID patients after MUD BMT, it was the major cause of death in these patients. Therefore, the authors were particularly aggressive in treating acute GvHD and have treated patients who developed grade II or higher acute GvHD with high-dose steroid pulses. Among the 16 SCID patients in the authors' center that developed acute GvHD after MUD BMT, 13 had grade II or higher acute GvHD.[23] These patients were treated with high-dose MPO for 3 days, each followed by gradual dose reduction. Ten of these 13 patients received a pulse of 30 mg/kg/d, whereas 3 patients were given lower doses (10–20 mg/kg/d). Of note, 2 of the 3 patients who received the lower doses of MPO pulse as well as 2 of the patients who had low-grade GvHD and were not pulsed developed chronic GvHD, whereas none of the patients who received high-dose MPO pulse therapy developed chronic GvHD ($P = .015$). Pulse therapy was given to patients at a mean of 13.5 days after BMT (range, 7–35 days) and a mean of 0.6 days after the first symptoms of acute GvHD were apparent (range, 0–7 days). This treatment was effective in reversing 12 of 14 episodes of grade II or higher acute GvHD (one patient received 2 steroid pulses). Episodes of acute GvHD involving multiple organs including skin, liver, and gut were less likely to fully respond to MPO pulse therapy. The 2 patients who failed to respond to pulse therapy also failed other acute GvHD medications and eventually succumbed to GvHD. Patients usually tolerated the MPO pulse regimen without significant adverse effects. An increase in blood pressure (as determined by the need to add antihypertension medications to keep systolic blood pressure≤95th percentile) was the most common side effect. The increased blood pressure may have also contributed to the development of hypertrophic cardiomyopathy, which reversed after discontinuation of MPO.[24] Most patients, however, already had hypertension before the pulse therapy due to the use of standard dose steroids and CsA. Other adverse effects included hyperglycemia, which was evident in 12.5% of patients. Four patients who received MPO had gastrointestinal bleeding, which was likely related to acute gut GvHD. Of importance, 2 SCID patients who received anti T-cell specific antibodies for acute GvHD developed Epstein-Barr virus–associated posttransplant lymphoproliferative disease and lymphoma, which was fatal in one patient, emphasizing again that high-dose steroids may be the best treatment for SCID patients failing GvHD prophylaxis.

The authors' aggressive treatment of acute GvHD may have also been the reason for the good outcome, that is, although the frequency of acute GvHD after MUD BMT was significantly higher than after MMRD BMT ($P = .009$), the frequency of grade III and IV GvHD after MUD BMT was not different than after MMRD BMT (**Fig. 7**). GvHD after the first few months of transplant, which often involved the skin and mucous membranes, was diagnosed in 8 of 35 patients after MUD BMT, a frequency that was not significantly different to that found among MMRD BMT recipients ($P = .06$). After MUD BMT, one patient developed fatal GvHD of the liver, and another had bone marrow failure that may have been associated with chronic GvHD. Chronic GvHD was the cause of death in one child after MMRD BMT. GvHD tended to surface when immune suppressive medications were changed from intravenous to oral or when prednisone doses were tapered rapidly (>5 mg/wk), particularly if they were not monitored closely by physicians experienced with such patients; the authors therefore tend to reduce immune suppression very gradually (not more than 25% of the total dose on alternate days) over extended periods (not more frequent than once every 2 weeks), which often continues for 6 to 12 months.

Other immune-mediated disorders that occurred during the 2 years after MUD BMT included autoimmune hematopoietic cytopenia (6 patients) and myocarditis (2 patients), while polymyositis and bronchiolitis obliterans were each diagnosed in one patient. Hematopoietic cytopenia was documented in 5 SCID patients after MMRD BMT. In contrast to the high frequency of complications shortly after transplant, late complications after MUD BMT were rare. Three patients had chronic GvHD that persisted for up to 7 years after MUD BMT, which resolved in 2. One of these patients died 6 years after transplant from an unknown cause. Significant neurologic defects after MUD BMT were found in 2 SCID patients, one who already suffered from neurologic abnormalities before transplant and the other who had a defect in the DNA Ligase IV gene, which is known to cause such abnormalities.[25]

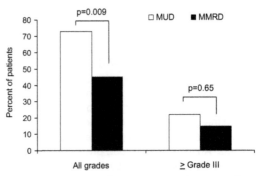

Fig. 7. Acute graft versus host disease after MUD or MMRD BMT for SCID. Percentage of patients with SCID that suffered acute graft versus host disease or grade III and higher acute graft versus host disease after MUD or MMRD BMT.

The low frequency of late complications that the authors observed after MUD BMT is in stark contrast to a recent report.[26] Among 90 patients who were 2 or more years after BMT (57% after MMRD, 24.5% after RID, 16.5% after PMD, and 2% after MUD), 10 patients had persistent chronic GvHD and 12 patients displayed other immune-mediated complications. Three patients died of chronic GvHD and related infectious complications, while 5 died of other immune-mediated disorders. A detailed description of 20 long-term survivors after MMRD BMT in Brescia[10] similarly revealed immune-mediated complications in 5 patients (25%). There were also 5 patients (25%) who suffered from neurologic abnormalities.[10] In contrast, among the 10 long-term survivors after MUD BMT in Brescia, only one patient had immune-mediated complications and none had neurologic abnormalities.

The data described clearly show that MUD BMT is an excellent alternative source of hematopoietic stem cells for patients with SCID. Therefore, in the authors' center, for SCID patients who do not have an RID or PMD and are clinically stable or can be stabilized through intensive care, a search for a MUD is initiated. For the few patients who cannot be stabilized, the option of HID would be offered. For patients for whom the authors failed to find a MUD, particularly if they are from populations not well represented in donor registries, HID does remain an option, although it is expected that the percentage of such patients will decrease with the expansion of bone marrow registries and cord blood banks. In addition, advances in HLA analysis and better management of GvHD are expected to further improve outcome of MUD BMT for SCID.

In conclusion, the close to 80% long-term survival, excellent immune reconstitution, and normal quality of life that the authors' and other groups have demonstrated after MUD BMT suggest that in the absence of RID or PMD, MUD BMT should be offered to patients suffering from SCID.

ACKNOWLEDGMENTS

The Audrey and Donald Campbell, The Jeffery Modell Foundation, and The Canadian Immunodeficiency Society for their support of Dr Roifman and data collection at the Hospital for Sick Children, Toronto, Canada. Brenda Reid, Advanced Practice Nurse in the division of Immunology, Hospital for Sick Children, Toronto, Canada. The dedicated team of physicians, nurses, pharmacists, dieticians and social workers at the Blood and Marrow Transplant Unit, and the post-BMT outpatient clinic for SCID, Hospital for Sick Children, Toronto, Canada.

REFERENCES

1. Al-Ghonaium A. Stem cell transplantation for primary immunodeficiencies: King Faisal Specialist Hospital experience from 1993 to 2006. Bone Marrow Transplant 2008;42(Suppl 1):S53–6.
2. Antoine C, Müller S, Cant A, et al. European Group for Blood and Marrow Transplantation; European Society for Immunodeficiency. Long-term survival and transplantation of haemopoietic stem cells for immunodeficiencies: report of the European experience 1968–99. Lancet 2003;361(9357):553–60.
3. Grunebaum E, Mazzolari E, Porta F, et al. Bone marrow transplantation for severe combined immune deficiency. JAMA 2006;295(5):508–18.
4. Caillat-Zucman S, Le Deist F, Haddad E, et al. Impact of HLA matching on outcome of hematopoietic stem cell transplantation in children with inherited diseases: a single-center comparative analysis of genoidentical, haploidentical or unrelated donors. Bone Marrow Transplant 2004;33(11):1089–95.

5. O'Reilly RJ, Dupont B, Pahwa S, et al. Reconstitution in severe combined immunodeficiency by transplantation of marrow from an unrelated donor. N Engl J Med 1977;297(24):1311–8.

6. Buckley RH, Schiff SE, Schiff RI, et al. Hematopoietic stem-cell transplantation for the treatment of severe combined immunodeficiency. N Engl J Med 1999;340(7): 508–16.

7. Dror Y, Gallagher R, Wara DW, et al. Immune reconstitution in severe combined immunodeficiency disease after lectin-treated, T-cell-depleted haplocompatible bone marrow transplantation. Blood 1993;81(8):2021–30.

8. Fischer A, Landais P, Friedrich W, et al. European experience of bone-marrow transplantation for severe combined immunodeficiency. Lancet 1990; 336(8719):850–4.

9. Gennery AR, Dickinson AM, Brigham K, et al. CAMPATH-1M T-cell depleted BMT for SCID: long-term follow-up of 19 children treated 1987-98 in a single center. Cytotherapy 2001;3(3):221–32.

10. Mazzolari E, Forino C, Guerci S, et al. Long-term immune reconstitution and clinical outcome after stem cell transplantation for severe T-cell immunodeficiency. J Allergy Clin Immunol 2007;120(4):892–9.

11. Petrovic A, Dorsey M, Miotke J, et al. Hematopoietic stem cell transplantation for pediatric patients with primary immunodeficiency diseases at All Children's Hospital/University of South Florida. Immunol Res 2009;44(1–3):169–78.

12. Roifman CM, Grunebaum E, Dalal I, et al. Matched unrelated bone marrow transplant for severe combined immunodeficiency. Immunol Res 2007;38(1–3): 191–200.

13. Tsuji Y, Imai K, Kajiwara M, et al. Hematopoietic stem cell transplantation for 30 patients with primary immunodeficiency diseases: 20 years experience of a single team. Bone Marrow Transplant 2006;37(5):469–77.

14. Dalal I, Reid B, Doyle J, et al. Matched unrelated bone marrow transplantation for combined immunodeficiency. Bone Marrow Transplant 2000;25(6):613–21.

15. Filipovich AH, Shapiro RS, Ramsay NK, et al. Unrelated donor bone marrow transplantation for correction of lethal congenital immunodeficiencies. Blood 1992;80(1):270–6.

16. Rao K, Amrolia PJ, Jones A, et al. Improved survival after unrelated donor bone marrow transplantation in children with primary immunodeficiency using a reduced-intensity conditioning regimen. Blood 2005;105(2):879–85.

17. Bertrand Y, Landais P, Friedrich W, et al. Influence of severe combined immunodeficiency phenotype on the outcome of HLA non-identical, T-cell-depleted bone marrow transplantation: a retrospective European survey from the European group for bone marrow transplantation and the European society for immunodeficiency. J Pediatr 1999;134(6):740–8.

18. Roifman CM, Somech R, Grunebaum E. Matched unrelated bone marrow transplant for T+ combined immunodeficiency. Bone Marrow Transplant 2008;41(11):947–52.

19. Mazzolari E, Moshous D, Forino C, et al. Hematopoietic stem cell transplantation in Omenn syndrome: a single-center experience. Bone Marrow Transplant 2005; 36(2):107–14.

20. Borghans JA, Bredius RG, Hazenberg MD, et al. Early determinants of long-term T-cell reconstitution after hematopoietic stem cell transplantation for severe combined immunodeficiency. Blood 2006;108(2):763–9.

21. Bhattacharya A, Slatter MA, Chapman CE, et al. Single centre experience of umbilical cord stem cell transplantation for primary immunodeficiency. Bone Marrow Transplant 2005;36(4):295–9.

22. Storb R, Deeg HJ, Whitehead J, et al. Methotrexate and cyclosporine compared with cyclosporine alone for prophylaxis of acute graft versus host disease after marrow transplantation for leukemia. N Engl J Med 1986;314(12):729–35.
23. Somech R, Kavadas FD, Atkinson A, et al. High-dose methylprednisolone is effective in the management of acute graft-versus-host disease in severe combined immune deficiency. J Allergy Clin Immunol 2008;122(6):1215–6.
24. Bulley SR, Benson L, Grunebaum E, et al. Cardiac chamber hypertrophy following hematopoietic stem cell transplantation for primary immunodeficiency. Biol Blood Marrow Transplant 2008;14(2):229–35.
25. Grunebaum E, Bates A, Roifman CM. Omenn syndrome is associated with mutations in DNA ligase IV. J Allergy Clin Immunol 2008;122(6):1219–20.
26. Neven B, Leroy S, Decaluwe H, et al. Long-term outcome after hematopoietic stem cell transplantation of a single-center cohort of 90 patients with severe combined immunodeficiency. Blood 2009;113(17):4114–24.

Purified Hematopoietic Stem Cell Transplantation: The Next Generation of Blood and Immune Replacement

Agnieszka Czechowicz, PhD*, Irving L. Weissman, MD

KEYWORDS

- Hematopoeitic stem cell transplantation
- Nonmalignant hematolymphoid disorders
- Nonmyeloablative conditioning • Immune tolerance
- Autoimmune diseases

Severe combined immunodeficiency (SCID), systemic lupus erythematosus (SLE), and type 1 diabetes share one commonality: these diverse disorders can all be attributed to faulty immune effector cells largely caused by genetic mutations that alter hematopoietic cell-intrinsic function. These defective immune cells inherit their genetic deficiencies from hematopoietic stem cells (HSCs) as they differentiate. Thus, each of these unique diseases should be theoretically curable through the same strategy: replacement of patients' HSCs carrying the problematic mutation with normal HSCs from disease-free donors, thereby generating entire new, healthy hematolymphoid systems. Replacement of disease-causing stem cells with healthy ones has been achieved clinically via hematopoietic cell transplantation (HCT) for the last 40 years,

This investigation was supported by National Institutes of Health grants R01CA086065 and R01HL058770 (to I.L.W.). A.C. is supported by the Medical Scientist Training Program at Stanford University School of Medicine, as well as a grant from The Paul and Daisy Soros Fellowships for New Americans. The program is not responsible for the views expressed.
Affiliations that might be perceived to have biased this work are as follows: I.L.W. cofounded and consulted for Systemix, is a cofounder and director of Stem Cells, Inc, and cofounded and is a former director of Cellerant, Inc. A.C. declares no financial or commercial conflict of interest.
A version of this article was previously published in the *Immunology and Allergy Clinics of North America*, 30:2.
Institute of Stem Cell Biology and Regenerative Medicine, Stanford University School of Medicine, Lorry I. Lokey Stem Cell Research Building, G3165, 265, Campus Drive, Stanford, CA 94305-5323, USA
* Corresponding author.
E-mail address: aneeshka@stanford.edu

as a treatment modality for a variety of cancers and immunodeficiencies with moderate, but increasing success. This modality has traditionally included transplantation of mixed hematopoietic populations that include HSCs and other cells, such as T cells. This article explores and delineates the potential expansion of this technique to treat a variety of inherited diseases of immune function, the current barriers in HCT and pure HSC transplantation, and the up-and-coming strategies to combat these obstacles.

ADVANTAGES OF PURIFIED ALLOGENEIC HEMATOPOIETIC STEM CELL TRANSPLANTATION

HSCs are the only cells within the body that at a clonal level have the ability to self-renew for life as well as give rise to all the different distinct mature effectors cells that comprise the blood and immune system.[1] These 2 properties give HSCs the sole responsibility for the proper lifelong maintenance of hematopoietic homeostasis. However, genetic abnormalities within HSCs can result in diseases such as immunodeficiency, autoimmunity, hemoglobinopathies, or hematologic malignancies, as these defects are passed down from the HSCs to their mature cell progeny, which then generate the diseased blood or immune system.

The first successful hematopoietic cell transplant involving reconstitution of an infant immunologic deficiency was accomplished by Good and colleagues in 1968.[2] Since then, HCT has been employed as an effective strategy to treat a multitude of hematolymphoid diseases. This procedure, more commonly known as allogeneic bone marrow transplantation, replaces mutant HSCs with functional ones from donor bone marrow grafts, which thereafter give rise to a complete normal hematolymphoid system that if stably engrafted persists for life.[3] Although allogeneic HCT can be an effective cure for most hematopoietic-intrinsic blood or immune diseases, it is rarely performed clinically except for life-threatening diseases and in near-death scenarios because of the toxicity of the procedure. Under current practices, allogeneic HCT has a transplant mortality rate of approximately 10% to 20%, far too high to justify its routine use in most nonmalignant settings.[4]

One of the most frequent and dangerous complications associated with allogeneic HCT is graft versus host disease (GvHD).[5] GvHD is a complex, immunologically mediated, host-directed, inflammatory response that is attributed to transplanted donor cells genetically disparate to their host. During GvHD, grafted mature T cells, having undergone tolerization on donor rather than host thymic epithelium, upon infusion into the host result in a violent immunologic response and particularly react against host lymphoid organs, skin, liver, and gut.[6,7] Although the likelihood and severity of GvHD can be minimized by transplantation from donors that are a close histocompatible match,[8] the risks and effects of GvHD remain unacceptably high and dramatically limit HCT.

Based on presentation of symptoms, GvHD has historically been classified into 2 distinct classes: acute and chronic. Acute GvHD is rapid, occurring within 100 days of HCT and presenting as a syndrome of dermatitis, enteritis, and/or hepatitis.[7] Chronic GvHD occurs at later time points and differs drastically from acute GvHD, often consisting of an autoimmune-like syndrome combining impairment of multiple organs or organ systems.[7] To these 2 commonly studied subsets of GvHD is added a third important subtype, subclinical but immunosuppressive GvHD (see later discussion).[9] Although T cells have been shown to play a dominant role in these severe complications of HCT, the exact molecular and cellular mechanisms underlying each subtype remain largely unknown.[10]

Despite a lack of complete understanding of the pathogenesis of GvHD, one potential solution to prevent its occurrence is to transplant purified HSCs. Often the terms hematopoietic stem cell transplantation (HSCT) and HCT/bone marrow transplantation (BMT) are used interchangeably in the literature, but in reality the clinical methodology differs dramatically. Although the efficacy of BMT relies on the activity of HSC, bone marrow is composed of a heterogeneous mixture of cells, including stem, multipotent progenitors, and mature blood cells, all of which are transferred to the patient in BMT. In contrast, HSCT refers to transfer of a highly purified population of strictly HSCs obtained from the donor bone marrow. The inclusion of cell populations other than HSCs and their resulting effects are what differentiate HCT/BMT from HSCT.

HSCs are defined as cells that can give rise to long-term multilineage reconstitution, as demonstrated when they are transferred into a hematolymphoid-depleted, irradiated host. Separation based on expression of discrete phenotypic cell surface markers and verification of their functionality in this manner led to identification and isolation of human[11] and murine HSCs.[1] HSCs are exceedingly rare cells, making up less than 0.1% of a bone marrow graft. Based on the efforts of multiple scientific groups, the HSC population has been prospectively isolated and refined to purity. All long-term HSC activity in adult mouse bone marrow is believed to be contained within a population marked by the composite phenotype of c-Kit$^+$, Thy-1.1^{lo}, lineage marker$^{-/lo}$, Sca-1$^+$, Slamf1$^+$, Flk2$^-$, and CD34$^-$.[1,12–16] Similarly, the phenotypic profile of human HSCs was validated to consist of CD34$^+$ and Thy-1$^+$, in addition to lacking CD38$^-$, CD45RA$^-$, and mature lineage markers.[11,17,18] Cells with these specific phenotypes are capable of giving rise to lifelong hematopoiesis on transplantation at the single mouse-cell level into congenic myeloablated mice,[17,19–21] and at the 10 human-cell level in xenogeneic models with myeloablated immunodeficient mice.[18] Validation of in vivo human HSC activity with cells of this phenotype was confirmed in several phase 1 clinical trials, which showed autologous HSC-rescued blood formation in myeloablated recipients and provided sustained, prolonged hematopoiesis.[22–24]

Isolation of HSCs based on the cell surface markers listed above can be accomplished by combining magnetic bead selection and fluorescence activated cells sorting (FACS) methods, yielding purified HSCs that are depleted of other polluting hematopoietic populations such as T cells.[1] Prospective isolation of HSCs in this manner is the only effective way to completely purge grafts of contaminating, unwanted populations from clinically transplantable HSC populations. In the case of autologous transplantation to treat malignancy, human HSCs purified in this manner provide long-term hematolymphoid repopulating activity and are free of contaminating resident or metastasized cancer cells.[22] However, in allogeneic transplantation for malignancies, HSC purification eliminates T cells that may function against the cancer and be responsible for the beneficial graft versus tumor (GvT) effect.[25]

In allogeneic HCT for nonmalignant diseases, purification of HSCs can be profoundly beneficial and can lead to significantly diminished procedure-related toxicity. Purified HSCT decreases the adverse outcomes of HCT/BMT; because removal of T cells from allografts completely eliminates GvHD.[26] Purification of HSCs from a graft eliminates the possibility of cotransplantation of host-reactive mature donor T cells, which are often contained within a graft and are primarily responsible for both acute and chronic GvHD.[10] In addition to the gross lesions associated with transplantation of T cells, low doses of T cells within a graft also contribute to underappreciated subclinical GvHD. In HCT, delays in immune reconstitution can be observed even in the setting where GvHD is not readily recognized, attributable to subclinical GvHD. Even after transplantation of grafts containing minimal contaminating T cells, donor T cells attack host lymphoid tissue and destroy tissue architecture, leaving the recipient vulnerable to opportunistic infections. Transplantation of purified HSCs eliminates subclinical GvHD and results in significantly accelerated immune reconstitution,[9] further increasing transplantation safety. As such, the complications and toxicities of BMT and HSCT are distinct, and further advocate for the transplantation of purified hematopoietic stem cells especially in nonmalignant settings.

APPLICATION OF HSCT: CURING A VARIETY OF NONMALIGNANT HEMATOLYMPHOID DISEASES

Toxicity associated with HCT has dramatically restricted its current practice to life-threatening disorders such as hematologic malignancies and bone marrow failure states, where few other therapeutic options exist. However, HCT has other important potential applications beyond its current uses if HCT-associated toxicity could be eliminated. HCT has been shown to effectively reverse nonmalignant genetic hematologic disorders such as sickle cell anemia and β-thalassemia, as well as primary immune deficiencies,[27] if sufficient hematopoietic chimerism is achieved. In addition, early experimentation in rodents revealed that marrow transplantation could not only protect against irradiation death and prevent hematopoietic failure, but in the process could induce immune tolerance, resulting in the creation of hematopoietic chimeras that would accept skin grafts from the donor or host strain.[28] These and subsequent studies opened the opportunity to expand this technique as a therapeutic modality for a variety of immunologic diseases, and provided a potential alternative to lifelong administration of immunosuppressive drugs following organ transplantation—the aims of transplant biologists and clinicians now for over half a century.[29–32]

This phenomenon of permanent transplant tolerance is attributable to the elimination of donor-reactive T cells, primarily through negative selection in the thymus of developing T cells with donor-reactive antigen receptors. Transplantation of donor HSCs results in new immune cell generation on a chimeric microenvironment, leading to deletion of reactive immune effector cells against both host (via the thymic medullary epithelium) and donor (via donor derived thymic dendritic cells).[6,33] Recent studies illustrate that allotransplantation of purified HSCs either before or concurrent with transplantation of matched donor heart tissue precludes injury and subsequent rejection of donor organs.[34] Due to cotransplantation of either tissue organs and/or tissue stem cells with HSCs, long-term immune tolerance to donor tissues by the host can be achieved and the need for hazardous lifelong immunosuppression eliminated, as best illustrated in recent trials of kidney/bone marrow transplant patients.[30,35] The use of HSCT in this manner may significantly abrogate complications of solid organ transplantation, extending organ longevity and decreasing infection susceptibility. Future cotransplantation of HSCs and solid organ tissue generated in vitro from the same embryonic or induced pluripotent stem cell may be possible, expanding the pool of transplant candidates.

The concept of induced immune tolerance by HSCT can additionally be extended to the treatment of autoimmune diseases. HCT and HSCT have been demonstrated to have utility in blocking disease pathogenesis of a wide variety of autoimmune disorders such as diabetes mellitus type 1,[36] multiple sclerosis,[37] and SLE.[38,39] These autoimmune diseases are complex, multifactorial diseases often containing an environmental component; however, they also bear a genetic element and involve HSCs predisposed to generating self-reactive T-cell and/or B-cell clones that can react against and attack host tissues.[40] Transplantation of the disease can be achieved by transplantation of HSCs from donors predisposed to or bearing the disorder into otherwise healthy recipients.[41] Conversely, allogeneic transplantation of normal donor HSCs into diseased recipients generates tolerance and prevents attack of otherwise reactive tissues.

Cure of these diseases can be achieved by elimination of the host's reactive T cells, and subsequent generation of a new nonself-reactive T-cell compartment from the disease-resistant donor. Current transplantation procedures eliminate host immune cells and thus at least initially suppress the autoimmune disease, regardless of whether autologous or allogeneic HCT is performed. However, in these autoimmune disorders the HSCs are defective and predisposed to generating self-reactive immune cells, thus autologous transplantation as illustrated in mouse models of type 1 diabetes, allergic encephalomyelitis, and SLE is not curative. As such, syngeneic transplantation of purified HSCs in a mouse model of spontaneous autoimmune diabetes mellitus provides no long-term survival benefit.[41] Conversely, transplanted allogeneic HSCs are predisposed to generating nonself-reacting immune cells, and indeed in the same model completely prevent diabetes development throughout life.[41] Clinical data regarding autologous transplantation for autoimmune diseases is variable. In such settings, a naïve immune system is transplanted and, depending on environmental factors, may not always result in rapid re-creation of the diseased state. Some patients show excellent and long-lived clinical remission of disease, whereas others enjoy initial symptomatic benefit with subsequent relapse.[42]

Autologous transplantation reintroduces the host's defective HSCs, and therefore may not result in long-term cure. As the molecular basis for various monogenic hematolymphoid diseases is determined, gene therapy may become a realistic strategy to correct autologous HSCs before transplantation. On transplantation, these few modified HSCs could reconstitute a complete, corrected hematolymphoid system that persists for life. This strategy would be instrumental in the treatment of immune diseases, in addition to genetic and acquired nonmalignant blood diseases, such as sickle cell anemia for which currently allogeneic HCT is occasionally performed. In addition, gene therapy for HSCs may play a pivotal role in generating HSCs that produce immune cells predisposed to attacking tumors. However, to date gene therapy is individual specific, and is limited by the current inability to achieve reliable and rapid gene transduction with vectors that do not by insertional mutagenesis induce diseases such LMO2-activated acute lymphocytic leukemia.[43]

Furthermore, transplantation of HSCs generating mature cells resistant to infectious agents may prove an effective strategy to combat a magnitude of viral agents. Case reports of human immunodeficiency virus (HIV)-infected patients transplanted with HSCs from donors resistant to the disease resulted in at least preliminary cure of these patients. In these select scenarios, transplanted donor HSCs generated donor T cells bearing CCR5 defects, making them impenetrable to HIV.[44] Long-term outcome of these studies is unknown and the feasibility of such treatments using currently available transplantation strategies is questionable. However, these studies illustrate a potential new therapeutic use of HCT if other hurdles such as supply of resistant-matched donor cells are overcome.[45]

HCT has been repeatedly confirmed to be the singular curative therapy for this plethora of blood and immune diseases. To date, however, HCT has not been routinely applied in these manners to treat the hundreds of thousands of patients who suffer from these ailments, primarily because of concerns regarding the morbidity and mortality of allografting procedures. With elimination of GvHD by transplantation of purified HSCs that are debulked of reactive T cells, therapy of this nature may become a mainstream reality.

BARRIERS TO EXPANSION OF HSCT

Continued improvements in the control of regimen-related toxicities are necessary to expand the applications of HCT. Current HCT methods hold exorbitant risk to the patient in terms of the transplant procedure–related morbidity and mortality, providing a major impediment to extrapolation of these practices to a multitude of conditions.

Although GvHD may be eliminated by transplantation of purified HSCs, much toxicity of HCT is also attributable to the conditioning regimens necessary to enable HSC engraftment. Current conditioning methods include irradiation and cytotoxic drugs such as high-dose chemotherapy, which can cause infertility, secondary malignancies, endocrine dysfunction, and organ damage.[46] Whereas in the malignant settings this conditioning serves the dual purpose of tumor eradication as well as preparation of the host, in the nonmalignant disease setting these regimens lead to inexcusable, nonbeneficial toxicity. Despite the ability of BMT/HSCT to cure many nonmalignant diseases, they have seldom been employed in the treatment of nonlife-threatening yet debilitating diseases, largely due to these associated risks. This situation necessitates the need for more specific and less toxic methods to allow efficient HSC engraftment.

Stable, robust chimerism is necessary in the treatment of these diseases, with disorders such as sickle cell anemia requiring approximately 20% chimerism to ameliorate the side effects of the disease.[47,48] In the absence of myeloablative therapy, this can be difficult to achieve.[49] In addition, engraftment of purified HSCs in the absence of other facilitator populations in the bone marrow poses an even larger engraftment challenge. Various facilitator populations that augment HSC engraftment, including in mice CD8 T cells or CD8+ TCR− dendritic cells, have been identified in bone marrow; however, many of these cells may also contribute to GvHD and therefore their transplantation should be avoided.[50] Moreover, the identification and subsequent purification of non–T-cell facilitator populations in humans has not been executed, further limiting our ability to enhance the engraftment of HSC.

Historical clinical data have shown that T-cell depletion results in increased graft failure.[51,52] T-cell depletion is a major impediment to transplantation of purified HSCs, thwarting the current practice and consequently exposing patients to GvHD. Various "nonmyeloablative" protocols have been developed to permit engraftment of donor cells with attenuated conditioning regimens[53]; however, although these protocols are not completely myeloablative they are still nonspecific, ablate the bone marrow, and have severe regimen-related toxicities, instigating the need for better preparative regimens.

However, transplanting HSCs without traditional conditioning has been difficult.[54] Traditional myeloablative conditioning is thought to play a role in immune suppression as well as creating space for transplanted donor HSCs.[55] HSCs are thought to reside in specialized microenvironments in the bone marrow that can serve as fixed tissue niches for HSCs, thereby regulating HSC numbers and behavior. Although the precise identities of the niche cells are still largely unknown and controversial, there is a large amount of data indicating that HSC niches exist and are critical to HSC maintenance.[56]

HSCs require specific and special growth factors and cytokines to preserve their unique state. How they receive these signals has been a growing field of research and controversy. In 1978 Schofield[55] proposed that an HSC site-specific niche must exist to provide these signals and in this way oversee HSC numbers, by regulating an HSC's decision to undergo self-renewal, differentiation, or apoptosis. In a setting of finite numbers of such niches, transplantation of HSCs in excess of these spaces would be predicted to be futile; initial experimentation performed by Micklem and colleagues[57] supports this hypothesis. Others have since argued that space is not an important factor to donor HSC engraftment, and have shown that in unirradiated recipients, transplantation of whole donor bone marrow readily displaces endogenous host marrow. Rather than by specialized sites, the argument can be made that HSC number is regulated by availability of diffusible factors and thus conditioning need not be done to ensure HSC engraftment.[58–60] However, these experiments were performed with whole bone marrow, and the conclusions about broad HSC behavior and purified HSC engraftment ability must be taken into consideration in this context.

Using purified HSC transplants, the authors have recently shown that in normal and immunodeficient mice, at any one point only a small number of HSC niches are readily available for transplanted donor HSCs, and transplants without conditioning lead to very low donor HSC chimerism (0.5%).[61] Regardless of the number of HSCs transplanted, once the available HSC niches are saturated additional engraftment cannot be obtained.[62] Of importance, only HSCs can saturate these niches and cotransplantation of 1000 fold-excess of progenitors does not affect HSC engraftment, arguing that HSCs occupy discrete niches from their downstream progeny.[62] These data mimic those observed by clinical transplanters who, even in the absence of immune barriers, observe similar very low levels of donor HSC chimerism on transplantation of hematopoietic cells enriched for human HSCs into immunodeficient patients not receiving conditioning.[63] The low level of HSC engraftment in these patients is sufficient to restore immune function transiently through proliferation and expansion of immune progenitors; however, over time these few engrafted HSCs encounter exhaustion and loss of the graft is occasionally observed, thereby necessitating ways to increase initial HSC engraftment even in the immunodeficiency setting.[64]

Taken together, these studies suggest that in the absence of conditioning or facilitator populations, in both humans and mice donor HSC engraftment is limited by the availability of appropriate niches. Endogenous HSCs occupy appropriate, otherwise transplantable HSC niches, and therefore one strategy to enhance donor HSC engraftment may be to deplete host HSCs. The development of reagents that specifically displace host HSCs, rather than myeloablative conditioning techniques currently in use, could lead to safer transplantation-based therapies for hematological and nonhematological disorders.

UP-AND-COMING STRATEGIES TO IMPROVE HSCT

HSCs are migratory cells.[65] Under homeostatic conditions they can be found in blood circulation in addition to bone marrow, albeit at very low but physiologically relevant frequency.[66] Recent studies have shown that HSCs enter the blood stream via division-independent egress from the bone marrow, leaving behind empty HSC niches available for transplantation, and explaining why low levels of engraftment are observed in nonconditioned settings.[66] HSCs continually egress from the marrow and enter the blood, suggesting that additional HSC niches may become available over time. Concordantly, saturation of engrafted HSC niches is transient and indeed, repeat rounds of HSCT transplantation lead to additional donor HSC chimerism.[61,66] This strategy may be one important path through which donor HSC engraftment can be increased with ease.

The natural vacancy of HSC niches admittedly is very slow, and therefore one proposed strategy to increase the competition between the donor and host HSCs is to augment the vacancy of the HSC niches through mobilizing endogenous host HSCs out of their marrow microenvironments and into circulation. This goal may be accomplished with reagents such as AMD3100, which cause significant mobilization without noteworthy proliferation.[67] Limited murine studies have shown such drugs to function as effective nontoxic conditioning therapeutics.[68] However, even in the setting of HSC mobilization, transplanted donor HSCs must still compete with displaced host HSCs for HSC space. Therefore, alternative strategies to enhance engraftment by eliminating endogenous competing HSCs are desired.

HSCs rely on a variety of signals for survival and maintenance of their stem cell state. Specifically, HSCs have been shown to require continual c-kit ligand (SCF) for survival, and inhibition of this signal results in apoptosis.[69] The authors have recently shown that ACK2, an antagonistic monoclonal antibody to the murine c-kit receptor[70] in immunodeficient mice, eliminates murine HSCs and creates vacant HSC niches available for transplantation.[62] Donor HSC engraftment efficiency is significantly increased with such conditioning, without any toxic side effects other than transient graying (as c-kit is additionally present on melanocytes). Transplantation of high doses of HSCs or multiple rounds of ACK2 followed by HSCs result in very high levels of mixed chimerism (>90%).[62] Translation of such strategies, targeting human HSCs, may result in nonmyeloablative regimens that promote donor HSC engraftment with minimal toxicity, thereby significantly decreasing the morbidity and mortality currently experienced with present conditioning regimens.

Such novel conditioning strategies may be effective at obtaining high levels of HSC engraftment. However, conditioning methods including irradiation and cytotoxic agents not only play a role in the creation of incoming space for HSC, but additionally act as immune suppressants and play a role in immune-mediated HSC resistance. In immunodeficient patients, such novel "space-creating" strategies in conjunction with purification of HSCs may be sufficient to eliminate entirely the current toxicities associated with HCT. However, in immunocompetent settings additional reagents will need to be explored to inhibit the host's immune system, thereby preventing rejection of the incoming transplanted cells. T lymphocytes and natural killer (NK) cells classically are considered the primary immune mediators of allogeneic HSC resistance.[71] When transplant pairs are fully matched at the major histocompatibility complex (MHC) loci, T-cell immunity predominates. However, if MHC disparities exist, as in, for example, haploidentical transplantations, NK cells also play an important role. Thus, reagents to eliminate the engraftment barrier must deplete or significantly impair the function of both types of lymphoid cells. Monoclonal antibodies may play a significant future role, as they may be used to transiently deplete host T cells and host NK cells before donor cell infusion. Multiple immunosuppressive monoclonal antibodies to human lymphocytes currently exist, including anti-CD2, -CD52, -CD3, -CD4, and -CD8, facilitating the generation of purely antibody-based nontoxic conditioning.

REVOLUTIONIZING HCT

Almost 60 years has passed since the early dismal but promising transplants performed by Thomas and colleagues,[72] and since then we have learned much about the biology of blood and immune transplantation. Yet today we still face many of the same hurdles faced by our predecessors, namely, the competing challenges of (1) complications arising from GvHD syndrome and (2) toxicities associated with preparative regimens necessary for cell engraftment.

Recent data suggest we may be bordering on developing therapies that overcome these obstacles. By combining these strategies, we may be at the tipping point of changing the practice and therefore application of HCT. If the strategies outlined in this article, or others in their stead, are employed successfully, we may witness a new exciting wave of HCT, and an expansion of the use of HCT from primarily for patients with rapidly lethal diseases to those with a variety of other hematolymphoid diseases for which HCT is currently unacceptable.

From the beginning of clinical HCT, immunodeficiency has been a good initial disease target because it allows for separation of the immune transplant barrier from the other transplantation obstacles, affording scientists and clinicians the ability to sequentially optimize individual treatment components. In this manner, SCID will likely be the first disease treated with the modalities outlined herein before they are extended to other applications. Moving forward, purified HSCT and novel conditioning strategies should allow for better treatment of SCID, obtaining higher donor engraftment without GvHD. Addition of antibody-based immunodepletion will subsequently allow for the combating of nonmalignant blood diseases. Thereafter, transplant tolerance may be achievable using such strategies as cotransplantation of HSCs and tissues/organs, and similarly, autoimmunity may be treated. The final goal is to treat patients whose organs have already been destroyed during autoimmune attacks, such as insulin-dependent type 1 diabetics lacking islet cells and, as has been shown in mice, concurrently transplant them with new organs as well as HSCs that impede rejection of the organ graft, prevent subsequent autoimmunity, and do not lead to GvHD.[41] Such dreams may become a reality in the distant future; meanwhile the incremental successes in any of these realms will allow for the gradual expansion of HCT as a therapeutic option for thousands of patients suffering from the diverse diseases of the blood and immune system.

ACKNOWLEDGMENTS

The authors thank D. Bhattacharya and M. Howard for insightful review of the manuscript.

REFERENCES

1. Spangrude GJ, Heimfeld S, Weissman IL. Purification and characterization of mouse hematopoietic stem cells. Science 1988;241(4861):58–62.
2. Gatti RA, Meuwissen HJ, Allen HD, et al. Immunological reconstitution of sex-linked lymphopenic immunological deficiency. Lancet 1968;2(7583):1366–9.
3. McCulloch EA, Till JE. The radiation sensitivity of normal mouse bone marrow cells, determined by quantitative marrow transplantation into irradiated mice. Radiat Res 1960;13:115–25.
4. Michlitsch JG, Walters MC. Recent advances in bone marrow transplantation in hemoglobinopathies. Curr Mol Med 2008;8(7):675–89.
5. Barnes DW, Loutit JF, Micklem HS. "Secondary disease" of radiation chimeras: a syndrome due to lymphoid aplasia. Ann N Y Acad Sci 1962;99:374–85.
6. Keever CA, Flomenberg N, Brochstein J, et al. Tolerance of engrafted donor T cells following bone marrow transplantation for severe combined immunodeficiency. Clin Immunol Immunopathol 1988;48(3):261–76.
7. Ferrara JL, Deeg HJ. Graft-versus-host disease. N Engl J Med 1991;324(10): 667–74.
8. Schierman LW, Nordskog AW. Influence of the B bloodgroup-histocompatibility locus in chickens on a graft-versus-host reaction. Nature 1963;197:511–2.
9. Tsao GJ, Allen JA, Logronio KA, et al. Purified hematopoietic stem cell allografts reconstitute immunity superior to bone marrow. Proc Natl Acad Sci U S A 2009; 106(9):3288–93.

10. Sprent J, Miller JF. Fate of H2-activated T lymphocytes in syngeneic hosts. II. Residence in recirculating lymphocyte pool and capacity to migrate to allografts. Cell Immunol 1976;21(2):303–13.

11. Baum CM, Weissman IL, Tsukamoto AS, et al. Isolation of a candidate human hematopoietic stem-cell population. Proc Natl Acad Sci U S A 1992;89(7): 2804–8.

12. Kiel MJ, Yilmaz OH, Iwashita T, et al. SLAM family receptors distinguish hematopoietic stem and progenitor cells and reveal endothelial niches for stem cells. Cell 2005;121(7):1109–21.

13. Whitlock CA, Tidmarsh GF, Muller-Sieburg C, et al. Bone marrow stromal cell lines with lymphopoietic activity express high levels of a pre-B neoplasia-associated molecule. Cell 1987;48(6):1009–21.

14. Christensen JL, Weissman IL. Flk-2 is a marker in hematopoietic stem cell differentiation: a simple method to isolate long-term stem cells. Proc Natl Acad Sci U S A 2001;98(25):14541–6.

15. Matsuoka S, Ebihara Y, Xu M, et al. CD34 expression on long-term repopulating hematopoietic stem cells changes during developmental stages. Blood 2001; 97(2):419–25.

16. Adolfsson J, Borge OJ, Bryder D, et al. Upregulation of Flt3 expression within the bone marrow Lin(−)Sca1(+)c-kit(+) stem cell compartment is accompanied by loss of self-renewal capacity. Immunity 2001;15(4):659–69.

17. Osawa M, Hanada K, Hamada H, et al. Long-term lymphohematopoietic reconstitution by a single CD34-low/negative hematopoietic stem cell. Science 1996; 273(5272):242–5.

18. Majeti R, Park CY, Weissman IL. Identification of a hierarchy of multipotent hematopoietic progenitors in human cord blood. Cell Stem Cell 2007;1(6): 635–45.

19. Matsuzaki Y, Kinjo K, Mulligan RC, et al. Unexpectedly efficient homing capacity of purified murine hematopoietic stem cells. Immunity 2004;20(1):87–93.

20. Wagers AJ, Christensen JL, Weissman IL. Cell fate determination from stem cells. Gene Ther 2002;9(10):606–12.

21. Camargo FD, Chambers SM, Drew E, et al. Hematopoietic stem cells do not engraft with absolute efficiencies. Blood 2006;107(2):501–7.

22. Negrin RS, Atkinson K, Leemhuis T, et al. Transplantation of highly purified CD34+Thy-1+ hematopoietic stem cells in patients with metastatic breast cancer. Biol Blood Marrow Transplant 2000;6(3):262–71.

23. Vose JM, Bierman PJ, Lynch JC, et al. Transplantation of highly purified CD34+Thy-1+ hematopoietic stem cells in patients with recurrent indolent non-Hodgkin's lymphoma. Biol Blood Marrow Transplant 2001;7(12):680–7.

24. Michallet M, Philip T, Philip I, et al. Transplantation with selected autologous peripheral blood CD34+Thy1+ hematopoietic stem cells (HSCs) in multiple myeloma: impact of HSC dose on engraftment, safety, and immune reconstitution. Exp Hematol 2000;28(7):858–70.

25. Ito M, Shizuru JA. Graft-vs.-lymphoma effect in an allogeneic hematopoietic stem cell transplantation model. Biol Blood Marrow Transplant 1999;5(6):357–68.

26. Shizuru JA, Jerabek L, Edwards CT, et al. Transplantation of purified hematopoietic stem cells: requirements for overcoming the barriers of allogeneic engraftment. Biol Blood Marrow Transplant 1996;2(1):3–14.

27. Barth E, Malorgio C, Tamaro P. Allogeneic bone marrow transplantation in hematologic disorders of childhood: new trends and controversies. Haematologica 2000;85(11 Suppl):2–8.

28. Main JM, Prehn RT. Successful skin homografts after the administration of high dosage X radiation and homologous bone marrow. J Natl Cancer Inst 1955; 15(4):1023–9.
29. Starzl TE, Demetris AJ, Murase N, et al. Cell migration, chimerism, and graft acceptance. Lancet 1992;339(8809):1579–82.
30. Scandling JD, Busque S, Dejbakhsh-Jones S, et al. Tolerance and chimerism after renal and hematopoietic-cell transplantation. N Engl J Med 2008;358(4): 362–8.
31. Millan MT, Shizuru JA, Hoffmann P, et al. Mixed chimerism and immunosuppressive drug withdrawal after HLA-mismatched kidney and hematopoietic progenitor transplantation. Transplantation 2002;73(9):1386–91.
32. Alexander SI, Smith N, Hu M, et al. Chimerism and tolerance in a recipient of a deceased-donor liver transplant. N Engl J Med 2008;358(4):369–74.
33. Shizuru JA, Weissman IL, Kernoff R, et al. Purified hematopoietic stem cell grafts induce tolerance to alloantigens and can mediate positive and negative T cell selection. Proc Natl Acad Sci U S A 2000;97(17):9555–60.
34. Gandy KL, Weissman IL. Tolerance of allogeneic heart grafts in mice simultaneously reconstituted with purified allogeneic hematopoietic stem cells. Transplantation 1998;65(3):295–304.
35. Kawai T, Cosimi AB, Spitzer TR, et al. HLA-mismatched renal transplantation without maintenance immunosuppression. N Engl J Med 2008;358(4):353–61.
36. Nikolic B, Takeuchi Y, Leykin I, et al. Mixed hematopoietic chimerism allows cure of autoimmune diabetes through allogeneic tolerance and reversal of autoimmunity. Diabetes 2004;53(2):376–83.
37. van Gelder M, Kinwel-Bohre EP, van Bekkum DW. Treatment of experimental allergic encephalomyelitis in rats with total body irradiation and syngeneic BMT. Bone Marrow Transplant 1993;11(3):233–41.
38. Traynor AE, Schroeder J, Rosa RM, et al. Treatment of severe systemic lupus erythematosus with high-dose chemotherapy and haemopoietic stem-cell transplantation: a phase I study. Lancet 2000;356(9231):701–7.
39. Smith-Berdan S, Gille D, Weissman IL, et al. Reversal of autoimmune disease in lupus-prone New Zealand black/New Zealand white mice by nonmyeloablative transplantation of purified allogeneic hematopoietic stem cells. Blood 2007; 110(4):1370–8.
40. Todd JA, Bell JI, McDevitt HO. HLA-DQ beta gene contributes to susceptibility and resistance to insulin-dependent diabetes mellitus. Nature 1987;329(6140): 599–604.
41. Beilhack GF, Scheffold YC, Weissman IL, et al. Purified allogeneic hematopoietic stem cell transplantation blocks diabetes pathogenesis in NOD mice. Diabetes 2003;52(1):59–68.
42. Krauss AC, Kamani NR. Hematopoietic stem cell transplantation for pediatric autoimmune disease: where we stand and where we need to go. Bone Marrow Transplant 2009;44(3):137–43.
43. McCormack MP, Rabbitts TH. Activation of the T-cell oncogene LMO2 after gene therapy for X-linked severe combined immunodeficiency. N Engl J Med 2004; 350(9):913–22.
44. Hutter G, Nowak D, Mossner M, et al. Long-term control of HIV by CCR5 Delta32/ Delta32 stem-cell transplantation. N Engl J Med 2009;360(7):692–8.
45. van Griensven J, De Clercq E, Debyser Z. Hematopoietic stem cell-based gene therapy against HIV infection: promises and caveats. AIDS Rev 2005;7(1): 44–55.

46. Ferry C, Socie G. Busulfan-cyclophosphamide versus total body irradiation-cyclophosphamide as preparative regimen before allogeneic hematopoietic stem cell transplantation for acute myeloid leukemia: what have we learned? Exp Hematol 2003;31(12):1182–6.

47. Walters MC, Patience M, Leisenring W, et al. Stable mixed hematopoietic chimerism after bone marrow transplantation for sickle cell anemia. Biol Blood Marrow Transplant 2001;7(12):665–73.

48. Iannone R, Luznik L, Engstrom LW, et al. Effects of mixed hematopoietic chimerism in a mouse model of bone marrow transplantation for sickle cell anemia. Blood 2001;97(12):3960–5.

49. Storb R, Yu C, Sandmaier BM, et al. Mixed hematopoietic chimerism after marrow allografts. Transplantation in the ambulatory care setting. Ann N Y Acad Sci 1999; 872:372–5 [discussion: 375–6].

50. Gandy KL, Domen J, Aguila H, et al. CD8+TCR+ and CD8+TCR– cells in whole bone marrow facilitate the engraftment of hematopoietic stem cells across allogeneic barriers. Immunity 1999;11(5):579–90.

51. Kernan NA, Bordignon C, Heller G, et al. Graft failure after T-cell-depleted human leukocyte antigen identical marrow transplants for leukemia: I. Analysis of risk factors and results of secondary transplants. Blood 1989;74(6):2227–36.

52. Marmont AM, Horowitz MM, Gale RP, et al. T-cell depletion of HLA-identical transplants in leukemia. Blood 1991;78(8):2120–30.

53. Maloney DG, Sandmaier BM, Mackinnon S, et al. Non-myeloablative transplantation. Hematology Am Soc Hematol Educ Program 2002;392–421.

54. Tomita Y, Sachs DH, Sykes M. Myelosuppressive conditioning is required to achieve engraftment of pluripotent stem cells contained in moderate doses of syngeneic bone marrow. Blood 1994;83(4):939–48.

55. Schofield R. The relationship between the spleen colony-forming cell and the haemopoietic stem cell. Blood Cells 1978;4(1–2):7–25.

56. Morrison SJ, Spradling AC. Stem cells and niches: mechanisms that promote stem cell maintenance throughout life. Cell 2008;132(4):598–611.

57. Micklem HS, Clarke CM, Evans EP, et al. Fate of chromosome-marked mouse bone marrow cells transfused into normal syngeneic recipients. Transplantation 1968;6(2):299–302.

58. Saxe DF, Boggs SS, Boggs DR. Transplantation of chromosomally marked syngeneic marrow cells into mice not subjected to hematopoietic stem cell depletion. Exp Hematol 1984;12(4):277–83.

59. Stewart FM, Crittenden RB, Lowry PA, et al. Long-term engraftment of normal and post-5-fluorouracil murine marrow into normal nonmyeloablated mice. Blood 1993;81(10):2566–71.

60. Wu DD, Keating A. Hematopoietic stem cells engraft in untreated transplant recipients. Exp Hematol 1993;21(2):251–6.

61. Bhattacharya D, Rossi DJ, Bryder D, et al. Purified hematopoietic stem cell engraftment of rare niches corrects severe lymphoid deficiencies without host conditioning. J Exp Med 2006;203(1):73–85.

62. Czechowicz A, Kraft D, Weissman IL, et al. Efficient transplantation via antibody-based clearance of hematopoietic stem cell niches. Science 2007;318(5854): 1296–9.

63. Muller SM, Kohn T, Schulz AS, et al. Similar pattern of thymic-dependent T-cell reconstitution in infants with severe combined immunodeficiency after human leukocyte antigen (HLA)-identical and HLA-nonidentical stem cell transplantation. Blood 2000;96(13):4344–9.

64. Cavazzana-Calvo M, Carlier F, Le Deist F, et al. Long-term T-cell reconstitution after hematopoietic stem-cell transplantation in primary T-cell-immunodeficient patients is associated with myeloid chimerism and possibly the primary disease phenotype. Blood 2007;109(10):4575–81.
65. Wright DE, Wagers AJ, Gulati AP, et al. Physiological migration of hematopoietic stem and progenitor cells. Science 2001;294(5548):1933–6.
66. Bhattacharya D, Czechowicz A, Ooi AG, et al. Niche recycling through division-independent egress of hematopoietic stem cells. J Exp Med 2009;206(12): 2837–50.
67. Broxmeyer HE, Orschell CM, Clapp DW, et al. Rapid mobilization of murine and human hematopoietic stem and progenitor cells with AMD3100, a CXCR4 antagonist. J Exp Med 2005;201(8):1307–18.
68. Chen J, Larochelle A, Fricker S, et al. Mobilization as a preparative regimen for hematopoietic stem cell transplantation. Blood 2006;107(9):3764–71.
69. Domen J, Weissman IL. Hematopoietic stem cells need two signals to prevent apoptosis; BCL-2 can provide one of these, Kitl/c-Kit signaling the other. J Exp Med 2000;192(12):1707–18.
70. Ogawa M, Matsuzaki Y, Nishikawa S, et al. Expression and function of c-kit in hemopoietic progenitor cells. J Exp Med 1991;174(1):63–71.
71. Murphy WJ, Kumar V, Bennett M. Acute rejection of murine bone marrow allografts by natural killer cells and T cells. Differences in kinetics and target antigens recognized. J Exp Med 1987;166(5):1499–509.
72. Thomas ED, Lochte HL Jr, Lu WC, et al. Intravenous infusion of bone marrow in patients receiving radiation and chemotherapy. N Engl J Med 1957;257(11): 491–6.

Gene Therapy for Primary Immunodeficiencies

Alain Fischer, MD, PhD[a,b,c,*], S. Hacein-Bey-Abina, PharmD, PhD[a,b,d,e],
M. Cavazzana-Calvo, MD, PhD[a,b,d,e]

KEYWORDS

- Severe combined immunodeficiencies • Gene therapy
- Hematopoietic stem cells • Retrovirus • Lentivirus
- Wiskott Aldrich • Chronic granulomatous disease • Clinical trial

The concept of gene therapy emerged as a way of correcting monogenic inherited diseases by introducing a normal copy of the mutated gene into at least some of the patients' cells.[1] Although this concept has turned out to be quite complicated to implement, it is in the field of primary immunodeficiencies (PIDs) that proof of feasibility has been undoubtedly achieved. There is now a strong rationale in support of gene therapy for at least some PIDs, as discussed later in this article.

RATIONALE

Many PIDs are lethal diseases. In the absence of treatment, severe combined immunodeficiencies (SCIDs) cause death within the first year of life. Many other combined deficiencies of adaptive immunity (such as Wiskott Aldrich syndrome [WAS] and diseases causing hemophagocytic lymphohistiocytosis [HLH]) can also be fatal in young infants. Allogeneic hematopoietic stem cell transplantation (HSCT) can cure many of these disorders by replacing the diseased hematopoietic lineages with normal

A version of this article was previously published in the *Immunology and Allergy Clinics of North America*, 30:2.

[a] Developpement Normal et Pathologique du Systeme Immunitaire, INSERM U 768, Hopital Necker, 149 rue de sevres, Paris 75015, France

[b] Paris-Descartes University, Hopital Necker, 149 rue de sevres, Paris 75015, France

[c] Unité d'Immunologie et Hématologie Pédiatrique, Assistance Publique, Hôpital Necker Enfants Malades, Hopital Necker, 149 rue de sevres, Paris 75015, France

[d] Department of Biotherapy, Hopital Necker-Enfants Malades, Assistance Publique-Hôpitaux de Paris (AP-HP), Université René Descartes, Hopital Necker, 149 rue de sevres, Paris 75015, France

[e] INSERM, Centre d'Investigation Clinique intégré en Biothérapies, Groupe Hospitalier Universitaire Ouest, AP-HP, Hopital Necker, 149 rue de sevres, Paris 75015, France

* Corresponding author. Developpement Normal et Pathologique du Systeme Immunitaire, INSERM U 768, Hopital Necker, 149 rue de sevres, Paris 75015, France.

E-mail address: alain.fischer@inserm.fr

ones.[2] These results prove that transplantation of normal hematopoietic stem cells or their progenitors can correct a large variety of PIDs of the adaptive and innate immune systems. However, HSCT is associated with several serious adverse events, including the toxicity of myeloablative chemotherapy and, above all, the consequences of the potential immune conflict between donor and recipient. The latter can result in either graft failure or, conversely, graft-versus-host disease, a cause of serious morbidity and mortality.[3] In the context of human leukocyte antigen (HLA) mismatch, the risk for immune conflict can be alleviated by removing donor T cells from the stem cell inoculum. However, this type of approach is still marred by the risk for graft failure and prolonged immunodeficiency before donor-derived immunity develops. Although advances in HSCT methodology may provide better solutions to these problems,[4] it is clearly legitimate to search for alternative, gene-based approaches.

Most PIDs display Mendelian inheritance, so that addition of a normal copy of the mutated gene can correct the deficiency provided that the right cells are targeted and transgene expression is appropriate. At present, the pathophysiological mechanisms of many PIDs have been worked out and provide further clues to the use of gene therapy.

Information on gene expression pattern and regulation is essential for assessing the therapeutic feasibility. For instance, the tightly regulated expression of CD40L (the protein that is deficient in X-linked hyper IgM syndrome) precludes gene therapy in its present form because such precise regulatory control cannot yet be mimicked. Indeed, continuous expression of CD40L led to the development of lymphoma when tested in CD40L-deficient mice.[5] Given that several of the genes mutated in PIDs encode proteins involved in cell survival/proliferation, their expression is expected to provide a significant growth advantage over non-corrected cells during differentiation (see later discussion). This key point was eventually verified in the first successful clinical trials.

While the pathophysiology of many PIDs was being deciphered, significant advances were also made in the development of vectors capable of efficiently trans-ducing mature lymphocytes and progenitor cells. These new vectors (γ retroviruses, lentiviruses, spumaviruses, and possibly retrotransposons) are all characterized by their ability to integrate into the host genome so that the therapeutic transgene is repli-cated during cell division and thus is stably transmitted to the progeny.[6] This property is mandatory for gene therapy in mitotic cells, such as immune cell precursors and mature lymphocytes. Initial attempts used the long terminal repeat (LTR) of retrovi-ruses as a promoter, whereas progress toward the use of internal promoters in conjunction with deletion of the LTR enhancer activity (the so-called self-inactivated LTR [SIN-LTR]) were made to promote safety (see later discussion).[7] Furthermore, the technical aspects of ex vivo gene transfer into hematopoietic progenitors have been improved over the years by using appropriate cytokine cocktails to put cells in cycle retrovirus (RV) or in G1 of the cell cycle lentivirus (LV) and thus facilitate vector integration. Use of fibronectin fragments also promotes cell infection by vectors. These developments made gene therapy a feasible option for some PIDs at least.[6]

GENE THERAPY FOR SEVERE COMBINED IMMUNODEFICIENCIES -X1

The most frequent SCID is SCID-X1; the condition is caused by a deficiency in the common γc cytokine receptor subunit, which causes a complete block in T-cell and Natural killer (NK)-cell development.[8] It was first thought that SCID-X1 was the most accurate model for assessing gene therapy because spontaneous reversion of the mutation in the γc-encoding IL2RG gene led to significant correction of the immune deficiency. This observation supported the hypothesis whereby transduced lymphocyte progenitors have a selective advantage over their non-transduced counterparts.[9] Furthermore, IL2RG is expressed by all hematopoietic cells and is not tightly regulated, thus reducing the risk for toxicity related to aberrant expression. It was thus expected that gene correction of a proportion of lymphoid progenitors would be enough to restore at least the T-cell compartment and that the effect would be long lasting (because T cells live for several decades).

Thus, following in vitro and in vivo preclinical tests in γc-deficient mice, clinical trials were designed. The vectors were based on the use of RV constructs in which IL2GR was placed under the transcriptional control of the LTR, with the use of either an amphotropic envelope[10] or the gibbon ape leukemia virus envelope.[11] Between 1999 and 2006, 20 subjects with archetypal SCID-X1 were treated in two trials in Paris and then London.[10–15] All the subjects lacked an HLA-identical donor. They received ex vivo transduced CD34 cells in the absence of any additional therapy. The outcome of these trials (in toxicity and then efficacy) can be summarized as follows. Five of the 20 subjects developed T-cell leukemia 2.5 to 5 years after gene therapy.[14,16,17] In four cases, chemotherapy was easily able to destroy abnormal clones so that these children are currently in remission and doing well. However, despite chemotherapy, the one remaining subject died from refractory leukemia.[17] The occurrence of these complications was serious enough to prompt discontinuation of the trials. Considerable efforts were made to understand the mechanism by which (with an unexpectedly high frequency) this complication had occurred. It was found that proliferative clones carried RV integrations within oncogenes loci.[14,17] One oncogene in particular (LMO-2) was targeted in four out five cases. Integration of the vector containing a functional LTR enhancer had led to uncontrolled expression activity of the oncogenes.[14,16,17] Secondary genomic modifications, such as loss of the p19Arf locus and NOTCH1-activating mutations, contributed to the clonal selection. It was then realized that the pattern of RV integration was, in contrast to previous hypotheses, semi-random with selective integration into gene loci (60% of all integrations) equally distributed between regulatory sequences 5' from the transcription start site and the gene itself (including the first few introns).[18] Furthermore, integrations were more frequent in genes being actively expressed in the target cells, as it is the case for several proto-oncogenes (including LMO-2) in hematopoietic progenitor cells.[14,16,17] It thus became clear that RV-mediated gene transfer could deregulate proto-oncogene expression through the LTRs enhancer activity. It is nevertheless likely that additional factors are involved, because none of the 14 subjects successfully treated with a similar gene-therapy approach for another SCID (adenosine deaminase [ADA] deficiency,[19] see later discussion) developed leukemic complications, despite the fact that a similar RV integrations pattern was found.[20,21] These observations suggest that either γc expression by lymphoid progenitors exerts some form of synergistic effect with oncogene deregulation (although there is no evidence of γc overexpression or active downstream signaling) or that an impairment in progenitor cell distribution caused by γc or ADA deficiency influences the risk for oncogene transactivation.

Indeed, progenitor cells differ in their sensitivity to transformation, perhaps because of gene expression or activation or the cell cycle patterns. These considerations are obviously of the utmost importance for further assessment of the risk associated with gene therapy. At present, there is a consensus that use of SIN vectors featuring an internal promoter with weak enhancer activity should reduce this risk. Although this is supported by in vitro experiments,[22] the available in vivo experimental models do not yet constitute a sufficiently predictive toxicity assay despite considerable experimental efforts.[23,24] Further safety measures include the presence of insulators in the vector (to prevent the transactivation of neighboring genes) and the potential addition of a suicide gene.[25,26] However, none of these modifications are likely to be absolute solutions and may carry disadvantages.

Lentiviral vectors based on HIV might be safer because they do not target 5' regulatory responses.[27] However, they still integrate into genes. Given the overall higher transduction efficiency of LV (as based on the number of integration sites in progenitor cells), LV and RV vectors do not greatly differ in oncogenicity.[28] Spumaviruses may also be of value because they integrate into genes less frequently than RVs and LVs do.[29] Nevertheless, significant issues in vector production must be solved before the effective use of spumaviruses can be envisaged.

The efficacy of γc gene transfer has been clearly demonstrated. Between 4 and 10.5 years after gene therapy, 17 of the 20 subjects are alive and display full or nearly full correction of the T-cell immunodeficiency[10,12,14]: T-cell subset counts, sustained detection of naive T cells (even in the subjects who had been treated for leukemia), a diversified T-cell repertoire, and T-cell–mediated immune functions. The γc gene transfer led to clear clinical benefits, because patients first recovered from ongoing infections with a poor prognosis and were then able to live in a normal environment without any evidence of particular susceptibilities to infection. The extent of correction of the NK-cell deficiency was not as impressive. Despite an early rise, NK-cell counts eventually dropped to low values. Remarkably, this was also observed in patients with non-myeloablated SCID-X1 who had undergone allogeneic HSCT. A partially persistent NK-cell deficiency does not appear to be harmful. This finding indicates that NK-cell population dynamics (cell development, expansion, and survival) differ significantly from those of T cells. The frequency of transduced B cells was low (<1%) and these cells were no longer detected in the blood 2 to 3 years after gene therapy. This observation emphasizes the lack of persistence of transduced progenitors in the bone marrow. In contrast, the sustained detection of naive T cells (even in patients having undergone chemotherapy for leukemia) strongly suggests the persistence of transduced (T) cell precursors that have perhaps localized in the thymus. Despite the apparent lack of persistent γc+ B cells, most patients do not require immunoglobulin substitution. Overall, these results constitute the first proof of principle of gene therapy and its sustained efficacy. As anticipated in this context, efficacy is based on the selective advantage provided by γc expression in lymphoid progenitors. These data pave the way for further use of gene therapy in patients with SCID-X1, as now scheduled in an international trial (in the United Kingdom, United States, and France) using SIN vectors. Similar attempts have been made to treat patients with atypical SCID-X1 (caused by hypomorphic mutations) or those who displayed limited T-cell reconstitution following HSCT. Effective CD34-cell transduction resulted in little or no improvement in T-cell production, probably as a consequence of thymic function loss.[30,31] This parameter must therefore also be taken into account when considering gene therapy in patients who are T-cell deficient after the first few years of life.

GENE THERAPY FOR ADENOSINE DEAMINASE DEFICIENCY

Adenosine deaminase deficiency is a rare, autosomal recessive PID characterized by a profound impairment in the generation of T, B, and NK lymphocytes. It is thus a particularly severe form of SCID, with early onset of infectious complications.[32] Adenosine deaminase deficiency results in a purine metabolism defect; the accumulation of adenosine, deoxyadenosine and their metabolites (notably deoxyadenosine triphosphate [dATP]) induces the premature death of lymphoid progenitor cells. It is a disease with broad consequences, because ADA deficiency also impairs (to a varying extent) bone, brain, lungs, liver functions and perhaps the epithelia. It is thus one of the SCIDs with the worst overall prognosis. Adenosine deaminase deficiency was the first PID in which gene therapy was tested. The initial approach was ex vivo ADA gene transfer into peripheral T cells that were obtained from patients undergoing enzyme substitution therapy. Although this approach failed to reconstitute immunity, it demonstrated the feasibility of gene transfer and the long-term viability (>10 years) of transduced CD8 T cells at least in one subject.[33] Adenosine deaminase deficiency was also the first PID in which researchers tested ex vivo ADA gene transfer mediated by an RV vector in CD34 progenitor cells from bone marrow and cord blood .[34,35] At that time, gene-transfer technology was not efficient enough to ensure sufficient progenitor cell transduction and correction of the PID. Nevertheless, long-term detection of a few transduced T cells was confirmed.[36,37] Concomitant enzyme substitution therapy also optimally reduced the transduced cells' selective advantage.

In the modern era of gene therapy, efficient ex vivo ADA gene transfer mediated by an RV vector in CD34 cells has been achieved. When combined with a partially myeloablative conditioning regimen (4 mg/kg busulfan), this protocol corrected the PID in 14 out of 20 patients treated once enzyme substitution had been withdrawn (or was not initiated).[19,38] Sustained correction has now been observed for up to 8 years, with clear-cut clinical benefits and no toxicity (see earlier discussion). Because of the administration of busulfan, it was found that transduced cells were detectable not only in T populations (all of which were transduced) but also in NK, B, and myeloid populations. The degree of T-cell correction in ADA deficiency does not appear to be as complete as in SCID-X1; this is probably a consequence of additional effects of ADA deficiency, such as damage to the thymic epithelium, that are not amenable to correction by ex vivo gene transfer into CD34 cells. In any case, the reproducible, sustained correction of the consequences of immunodeficiency in two SCIDs clearly proves the feasibility of this approach and suggests that, provided oncogene transactivation can be prevented, ex vivo gene transfer is an alternative to HSCT in the absence of available HLA-identical donors.

GENE THERAPY FOR OTHER SEVERE COMBINED IMMUNODEFICIENCIES AND OTHER SEVERE T-CELL IMMUNODEFICIENCIES

Fifteen distinct genetic defects have been found in association with SCID.[39] These conditions are all potential candidates for gene therapy, although the extreme rarity of some of them may hamper efforts to develop an appropriate vector up to the clinical phase. At the preclinical level, gene transfer efficacy has been shown for Rag-2, Artemis, JAK3, and ZAP70 deficiencies.[40–44] A clinical trial for the T- B- SCID condition caused by Artemis deficiency is being planned. An interesting strategy has been tested in a murine model of ZAP70 deficiency, with direct, intrathymic injection of the RV vector.[44] This treatment led to significant correction of the immunodeficiency, although it is not known whether this approach will enable the sufficiently long-term persistence of transduced progenitors. Furthermore, in humans, the accessibility of the T-cell–devoid thymus is questionable. For unknown reasons, it has not yet been possible to achieve reproducible, sustained correction of Rag-1 deficiency in mice without using a high vector multiplicity of infection to achieve integration of multiple copies per transduced cell, which is a setting with a high risk for insertional mutagenesis and oncogene transactivation.[45]

GENE THERAPY FOR WISKOTT ALDRICH SYNDROME

Wiskott Aldrich syndrome is an X-linked condition characterized by a multicell immunodeficiency that affects at least T and B lymphocytes and dendritic cells and by a thrombocytopenia. It is caused by loss-of-function mutations in the WAS protein (WASp) gene,[46] which is usually ubiquitously expressed within the hematopoietic system. When activated, WASp regulates the actin cytoskeleton. A WASp deficiency induces multiple defects in cell migration, activation, and survival. The severity of WAS depends on the type of mutation. Severe forms are life-threatening in childhood because of vulnerability to several pathogens associated with the onset of severe autoimmune manifestations, and in some cases, tumors. Following fully or partially myeloablative chemotherapy, allogeneic HSCT can cure WAS. The outcome for HSCT from HLA identical donors is good, whereas mortality is high in other settings. This is why several groups have considered WAS as a good candidate for gene therapy. RV and LV vectors are able to transduce WASp-deficient murine progenitor cells and correct (mild) WAS disease in mice.[47,48] Furthermore, in vitro experiments have shown that transduced human T cells and dendritic cells can be generated and recover normal functions.[49–51] Of particular interest is the LV vector in which the endogenous WASP promoter is being used to drive WASp expression at a physiologic level.[51] It is expected that transduced CD34 cells should have some degree of selective advantage over non-transduced cells, which facilitates clinical efficacy. The first clinical trial, based on a conventional RV vector with the WASP gene under the control of the LTR, has been initiated. After partially myeloablative conditioning, CD34 cells are ex vivo transduced and reinjected.[52] Although the preliminary data (after 2 to 3 years of follow-up) suggest that the manifestations of WAS have been effectively corrected, the safety concern is still to be addressed. Trials based on the use of a SIN LV vector with the endogenous WASP promoter are being planned. One possible concern for the long-term efficacy of gene therapy for WAS (and HSCT, in fact) stems from the observation that patients with WAS having undergone allogeneic HSCT are at a greater risk for relapse of autoimmune manifestations if autologous B cells persist post-HSCT.[53]

GENE THERAPY FOR OTHER PRIMARY IMMUNODEFICIENCIES OF THE ADAPTIVE IMMUNE SYSTEM

Hemophagocytic lymphohistiocytosis (HLH) is a condition generated by a group of genetic diseases (notably perforin, Munc13-4, Rab27a, Syntaxin11, Munc18-2, and SH2DIA deficiencies) in which cytotoxic lymphocyte function is impaired.[54] The condition is fatal in the absence of therapy and can be cured by allogeneic HSCT. Two gene-therapy strategies can be considered here: ex vivo gene transfer into peripheral CD8 T cells (to restore cytotoxic function) or CD34+ progenitor cells. The first scenario has some advantages: RV (LV)-mediated transfer into T cells is safe[55] and does not require prior myeloablation of the patients (in contrast to the HSCT approach). However, it might be difficult to tailor the efficacy of therapy in transduced CD8 T cells to be injected and the frequency of repeat injections. Relevant murine models might address these questions to some extent.

Similarly, immunoproliferative, entheropathy X-linked (IPEX) syndrome is a very severe condition that results in defective FOXP3 CD4+ CD25+ regulatory T cells. It is caused by loss-of-function mutations in the gene encoding FOXP3.[56] The syndrome is characterized by devastating, early-onset inflammation of the gut, which is often associated with diabetes, autoimmune cytopenia, and severe skin allergies. Hematopoietic stem-cell transplantation can cure IPEX, although reports of success are still scarce. Ex vivo transduction of CD4 T cells (leading to FOXP3 expression) would be an elegant and probably nontoxic approach for generating regulatory T cells able to control disease manifestations. There are, however, several questions to be solved before clinical applications can be envisaged (as is also the case for HLH): the number of cells to be injected, the control of FOXP3 expression, the injection frequency, and the quality of the in vivo function in the induced regulatory T cells.

B-cell immunodeficiencies could also be candidates for gene therapy. X-L agammaglobulinemia (XLA) has been considered as a model, because transduction of bone marrow progenitors with a vector carrying the BTK gene (which is mutated in XLA) could restore B-cell differentiation.[57] However, XLA is not as life threatening as the PIDs discussed earlier and so safety issues would have to be completely solved before clinical trials are initiated. In particular, BTK expression should be restricted to B cells (monocytes and mast cells) to avoid possible toxicity (over activation?) of cells in which BTK is not usually expressed, such as T lymphocytes.

GENE THERAPY FOR CHRONIC GRANULOMATOUS DISEASE

Chronic granulomatous disease (CGD) is an inherited (X-linked or autosomal recessive) condition characterized by defective killing of bacteria and fungi by neutrophils and monocytes/macrophages because of defective generation of reactive oxygen species in the phagosome membrane.[58] Life-threatening infections and chronic inflammation are the main consequences of this defect. Mutations in five genes encoding various components of nicotinamide adenine dinucleotide phosphate (NADPH) oxidase have been described in patients with CGD.

The most frequent form of CGD is X-linked and is caused by a lack of the gp91 phox protein. At present, patients with poor infection control are treated (with some success) with allogeneic HSCT. Hence, there is a rationale for a gene-therapy approach, although, unlike what was observed in SCID and is generally expected in WAS, expression of gp91 phox or the other defective proteins in myeloid precursor cells is not going to provide a selective advantage. Furthermore, the short life span of neutrophils (around 2 days) implies that a large number of stem cells will have to be transduced to ensure the long-term production of corrected neutrophils and monocytes. Thus, CGD is a tough candidate for gene therapy. The approach will require a combination of fully myeloablative conditioning and efficient transduction of stem cells (probably with LV vectors). This hypothesis was confirmed by the outcome of the first clinical trial of CGD gene therapy performed in the absence of myeloablation. Only low (<1%) levels of transduced neutrophils were transiently detected.[59] More recently, Grez and colleagues reported the apparently efficient correction of CGD in two adult subjects who had received myeloablative conditioning. Gene transfer of the gp91 phox-encoding gene was mediated by using an RV vector with a strong ability to induce gene expression in myeloid cells (spleen focus-forming virus [SFFV] LTR).[60] In both subjects, progressive accumulation of transduced neutrophils and monocytes in the blood was observed over the first few months post-injection. Restored NADPH oxidase activity was found on these cells. Clinical benefit was observed, because the subjects managed to clear concurrent chest *Aspergillus* infections. It was found that myelopoiesis was oligoclonal and driven by clones in which the vector had integrated near to three known oncogenes (Evi-1, PRD1M16, and STBP1). These oncogenes had been transactivated and thus provided the clones serendipitously with a selective advantage. Unfortunately, a myelodysplastic syndrome developed and was associated (in one subject) with extinction of transgene expression and a fatal outcome.[61] This observation also highlights the importance of the selective advantage that can be conferred by either transgene expression (in SCID, for example) or transactivation of an endogenous gene (leukemia in SCID-X1 and CGD). Further developments of gene therapy for CGD[62] will thus have to combine full myeloablative chemotherapy (to get rid of several non-transduced cells) and ex vivo gene transfer into HSCs by using a SIN LV vector. It was recently reported that the same approach gave stable transgene expression (more than 3 years, to date) in hematopoietic lineages in three subjects with adrenoleukodystrophy.[63] The transgene is expressed by about 10% to 15% of blood cells, which is a proportion that would be sufficient to clear CGD symptoms. Thus, the experience gathered in this non-PID model is encouraging for use of gene therapy for PIDs of the innate immune system, such as CGD and perhaps also leukocyte adhesion deficiency. The latter disease was reportedly cured in a murine model by using ex vivo β2 integrin gene transfer with a spumavirus vector.[64]

SUMMARY

The last decade has witnessed the effective advent of gene therapy as a treatment for two severe PIDs. Provided that safety issues can be mastered, today's technology opens the way to applying gene therapy to several life-threatening PIDs, including those in which transduction with the transgene does not provide a selective advantage. There will be several mandatory conditions: a carefully designed clinical research protocol, extensive monitoring of enrolled subjects, and real-time access to the results for the whole community to adjust practice worldwide and limit the occurrence of adverse events. Given the extensive requirements of these approaches, international collaborations are needed. Further progress can be expected. For example, PIDs caused by dominant mutations with negative effects, such as autoimmune lymphoproliferative syndrome or certain interferon γ, receptor deficiencies, could be treated by allele-specific oligonucleotide transfer, inducing degradation of the mutated allele.[65] Some mutations in complex genes with multiple exons might be treated by the exon-skipping methodology that is presently being tested in certain forms of Duchenne muscular dystrophy.[66]

Potentially, gene transfer could be targeted to a safe harbor in a genome area devoid of oncogenes.[67] An initial approach using bacterial integrases turned out to be cytotoxic but technology based on homologous recombination with engineered endonucleases (Zinc finger nucleases or meganucleases derived from the yeast Isce-1 endonuclease) might be useable.[68,69] The same approach could also be used for direct mutated gene repair by providing a template for homologous recombination.[69] This approach was effective for IL2RG in certain cell lines, although potential off-target action and the efficacy of homologous recombination in stem cells remain significant hurdles.

As was the case for HSCT, PIDs are at the forefront of development efforts in gene therapy. It is likely that during the next decade we shall see a significant shift toward gene therapy in the treatment of several PIDs.

ACKNOWLEDGMENTS

The authors are grateful to Malika Tiouri-Sifouane for her excellent secretarial assistance.

REFERENCES

1. Friedmann T, Roblin R. Gene therapy for human genetic disease? Science 1972; 175(25):949–55.
2. Antoine C, Muller S, Cant A, et al. Long-term survival and transplantation of hae-mopoietic stem cells for immunodeficiencies: report of the European experience 1968–99. Lancet 2003;361(9357):553–60.

3. Socie G, Blazar BR. Acute graft-versus-host disease: from the bench to the bedside. Blood 2009;114(20):4327–36.
4. Hagin D, Reisner Y. Haploidentical bone marrow transplantation in primary immune deficiency: stem cell selection and manipulation. Immunol Allergy Clin North Am 2010;30(1):45–62.
5. Brown MP, Topham DJ, Sangster MY, et al. Thymic lymphoproliferative disease after successful correction of CD40 ligand deficiency by gene transfer in mice. Nat Med 1998;4(11):1253–60.
6. Verma IM, Weitzman MD. Gene therapy: twenty-first century medicine. Annu Rev Biochem 2005;74:711–38.
7. Yu SF, von Ruden T, Kantoff PW, et al. Self-inactivating retroviral vectors designed for transfer of whole genes into mammalian cells. Proc Natl Acad Sci U S A 1986; 83(10):3194–8.
8. Leonard WJ. Cytokines and immunodeficiency diseases. Nat Rev Immunol 2001; 1:200–8.
9. Bousso P, Wahn V, Douagi I, et al. Diversity, functionality, and stability of the T cell repertoire derived in vivo from a single human T cell precursor. Proc Natl Acad Sci U S A 2000;97(1):274–8 [In Process Citation].
10. Cavazzana-Calvo M, Hacein-Bey S, De Saint Basile G, et al. Gene therapy of human severe combined immunodeficiency (SCID)-X1 disease. Science 2000; 288:669–72.
11. Gaspar HB, Parsley KL, Howe S, et al. Gene therapy of X-linked severe combined immunodeficiency by use of a pseudotyped gammaretroviral vector. Lancet 2004;364(9452):2181–7.
12. Hacein-Bey-Abina S, Le Deist F, Carlier F, et al. Sustained correction of X-linked severe combined immunodeficiency by ex vivo gene therapy. N Engl J Med 2002;346(16):1185–93.
13. Deichmann A, Hacein-Bey-Abina S, Schmidt M, et al. Vector integration is nonrandom and clustered and influences the fate of lymphopoiesis in SCID-X1 gene therapy. J Clin Invest 2007;117(8):2225–32.
14. Howe SJ, Mansour MR, Schwarzwaelder K, et al. Insertional mutagenesis combined with acquired somatic mutations causes leukemogenesis following gene therapy of SCID-X1 patients. J Clin Invest 2008;118(9):3143–50.
15. Schmidt M, Hacein-Bey-Abina S, Wissler M, et al. Clonal evidence for the transduction of CD34+ cells with lymphomyeloid differentiation potential and self-renewal capacity in the SCID-X1 gene therapy trial. Blood 2005;105(7): 2699–706.
16. Hacein-Bey-Abina S, Von Kalle C, Schmidt M, et al. LMO2-Associated clonal T cell proliferation in two patients after gene therapy for SCID-X1. Science 2003; 302(5644):415–9.
17. Hacein-Bey-Abina S, Garrigue A, Wang GP, et al. Insertional oncogenesis in 4 patients after retrovirus-mediated gene therapy of SCID-X1. J Clin Invest 2008; 118(9):3132–42.
18. Wu X, Li Y, Crise B, et al. Transcription start regions in the human genome are favored targets for MLV integration. Science 2003;300(5626):1749–51.
19. Aiuti A, Cattaneo F, Galimberti S, et al. Gene therapy for immunodeficiency due to adenosine deaminase deficiency. N Engl J Med 2009;360(5): 447–58.
20. Aiuti A, Cassani B, Andolfi G, et al. Multilineage hematopoietic reconstitution without clonal selection in ADA-SCID patients treated with stem cell gene therapy. J Clin Invest 2007;117(8):2233–40.

21. Cassani B, Montini E, Maruggi G, et al. Integration of retroviral vectors induces minor changes in the transcriptional activity of T cells from ADA-SCID patients treated with gene therapy. Blood 2009;114(17):3546–56.

22. Modlich U, Bohne J, Schmidt M, et al. Cell-culture assays reveal the importance of retroviral vector design for insertional genotoxicity. Blood 2006;108(8): 2545–53.

23. Shou Y, Ma Z, Lu T, et al. Unique risk factors for insertional mutagenesis in a mouse model of XSCID gene therapy. Proc Natl Acad Sci U S A 2006; 103(31):11730–5.

24. Montini E, Cesana D, Schmidt M, et al. Hematopoietic stem cell gene transfer in a tumor-prone mouse model uncovers low genotoxicity of lentiviral vector integration. Nat Biotechnol 2006;24(6):687–96.

25. Li CL, Xiong D, Stamatoyannopoulos G, et al. Genomic and functional assays demonstrate reduced gammaretroviral vector genotoxicity associated with use of the cHS4 chromatin insulator. Mol Ther 2009;17(4):716–24.

26. Baum C. I could die for you: new prospects for suicide in gene therapy. Mol Ther 2007;15(5):848–9.

27. Schroder AR, Shinn P, Chen H, et al. HIV-1 integration in the human genome favors active genes and local hotspots. Cell 2002;110(4):521–9.

28. Modlich U, Navarro S, Zychlinski D, et al. Insertional transformation of hematopoietic cells by self-inactivating lentiviral and gammaretroviral vectors. Mol Ther 2009;17(11):1919–28.

29. Trobridge GD, Miller DG, Jacobs MA, et al. Foamy virus vector integration sites in normal human cells. Proc Natl Acad Sci U S A 2006;103(5):1498–503.

30. Thrasher AJ, Hacein-Bey-Abina S, Gaspar HB, et al. Failure of SCID-X1 gene therapy in older patients. Blood 2005;105(11):4255–7.

31. Chinen J, Davis J, De Ravin SS, et al. Gene therapy improves immune function in preadolescents with X-linked severe combined immunodeficiency. Blood 2007; 110(1):67–73.

32. Blackburn MR, Kellems RE. Adenosine deaminase deficiency: metabolic basis of immune deficiency and pulmonary inflammation. Adv Immunol 2005;86:1–41.

33. Muul LM, Tuschong LM, Soenen SL, et al. Persistence and expression of the adenosine deaminase gene for 12 years and immune reaction to gene transfer components: long-term results of the first clinical gene therapy trial. Blood 2003;101(7):2563–9.

34. Bordignon C, Notarangelo LD, Nobili N, et al. Gene therapy in peripheral blood lymphocytes and bone marrow for ADA- immunodeficient patients. Science 1995;270(5235):470–5.

35. Kohn DB, Hershfield MS, Carbonaro D, et al. T lymphocytes with a normal ADA gene accumulate after transplantation of transduced autologous umbilical cord blood CD34+ cells in ADA-deficient SCID neonates. Nat Med 1998;4(7): 775–80.

36. Schmidt M, Carbonaro DA, Speckmann C, et al. Clonality analysis after retroviral-mediated gene transfer to CD34+ cells from the cord blood of ADA-deficient SCID neonates. Nat Med 2003;9(4):463–8.

37. Aiuti A, Slavin S, Aker M, et al. Correction of ADA-SCID by stem cell gene therapy combined with nonmyeloablative conditioning. Science 2002;296(5577):2410–3.

38. Gaspar HB, Aiuti A, Porta F, et al. How I treat ADA deficiency. Blood 2009; 114(17):3524–32.

39. Buckley RH. Molecular defects in human severe combined immunodeficiency and approaches to immune reconstitution. Annu Rev Immunol 2004;22:625–55.

40. Yates F, Malassis-Seris M, Stockholm D, et al. Gene therapy of RAG-2-/- mice: sustained correction of the immunodeficiency. Blood 2002;22:22.
41. Mostoslavsky G, Fabian AJ, Rooney S, et al. Complete correction of murine Artemis immunodeficiency by lentiviral vector-mediated gene transfer. Proc Natl Acad Sci U S A 2006;103(44):16406–11.
42. Benjelloun F, Garrigue A, Demerens-de Chappedelaine C, et al. Stable and functional lymphoid reconstitution in artemis-deficient mice following lentiviral Artemis gene transfer into hematopoietic stem cells. Mol Ther 2008;16(8):1490–9.
43. Bunting KD, Sangster MY, Ihle JN, et al. Restoration of lymphocyte function in Janus kinase 3-deficient mice by retroviral-mediated gene transfer [comments]. Nat Med 1998;4(1):58–64.
44. Adjali O, Vicente RR, Ferrand C, et al. Intrathymic administration of hematopoietic progenitor cells enhances T cell reconstitution in ZAP-70 severe combined immunodeficiency. Proc Natl Acad Sci U S A 2005;102(38):13586–91.
45. Lagresle-Peyrou C, Yates F, Malassis-Seris M, et al. Long-term immune reconstitution in RAG-1-deficient mice treated by retroviral gene therapy: a balance between efficiency and toxicity. Blood 2006;107(1):63–72.
46. Bosticardo M, Marangoni F, Aiuti A, et al. Recent advances in understanding the pathophysiology of Wiskott-Aldrich syndrome. Blood 2009;113(25):6288–95.
47. Klein C, Nguyen D, Liu CH, et al. Gene therapy for Wiskott-Aldrich syndrome: rescue of T-cell signaling and amelioration of colitis upon transplantation of retrovirally transduced hematopoietic stem cells in mice. Blood 2003;101(6):2159–66.
48. Marangoni F, Bosticardo M, Charrier S, et al. Evidence for long-term efficacy and safety of gene therapy for Wiskott-Aldrich syndrome in preclinical models. Mol Ther 2009;17(6):1073–82.
49. Charrier S, Dupre L, Scaramuzza S, et al. Lentiviral vectors targeting WASp expression to hematopoietic cells, efficiently transduce and correct cells from WAS patients. Gene Ther 2007;14(5):415–28.
50. Dupre L, Trifari S, Follenzi A, et al. Lentiviral vector-mediated gene transfer in T cells from Wiskott-Aldrich syndrome patients leads to functional correction. Mol Ther 2004;10(5):903–15.
51. Dupre L, Marangoni F, Scaramuzza S, et al. Efficacy of gene therapy for Wiskott-Aldrich syndrome using a WAS promoter/cDNA-containing lentiviral vector and nonlethal irradiation. Hum Gene Ther 2006;17(3):303–13.
52. Boztuk K, Schmidt M, Schwaezer A, et al. HSC gene therapy in two WAS patients [abstract]. Hum Gene Ther 2009;20:1371.
53. Ozsahin H, Cavazzana-Calvo M, Notarangelo LD, et al. Long-term outcome following hematopoietic stem-cell transplantation in Wiskott-Aldrich syndrome: collaborative study of the European Society for Immunodeficiencies and European Group for Blood and Marrow Transplantation. Blood 2008;111(1):439–45.
54. Fischer A, Latour S, de Saint Basile G. Genetic defects affecting lymphocyte cytotoxicity. Curr Opin Immunol 2007;19(3):348–53.
55. Recchia A, Bonini C, Magnani Z, et al. Retroviral vector integration deregulates gene expression but has no consequence on the biology and function of transplanted T cells. Proc Natl Acad Sci U S A 2006;103(5):1457–62.
56. Ochs HD, Ziegler SF, Torgerson TR. FOXP3 acts as a rheostat of the immune response. Immunol Rev 2005;203:156–64.
57. Kerns HM, Ryu BY, Stirling BV, et al. B-cell-specific lentiviral gene therapy leads to sustained B cell functional recovery in a murine model of X-linked agammaglobulinemia. Blood 2010. [Epub ahead of print].

58. Seger RA. Modern management of chronic granulomatous disease. Br J Haematol 2008;140(3):255–66.
59. Malech HL, Maples PB, Whiting-Theobald N, et al. Prolonged production of NADPH oxidase-corrected granulocytes after gene therapy of chronic granulomatous disease. Proc Natl Acad Sci U S A 1997;94(22):12133–8.
60. Ott MG, Schmidt M, Schwarzwaelder K, et al. Correction of X-linked chronic granulomatous disease by gene therapy, augmented by insertional activation of MDS1-EVI1, PRDM16 or SETBP1. Nat Med 2006;12(4):401–9.
61. Stein S, Ott MG, Schultze-Strasser S, et al. Genomic instability and myelodysplasia with monosomy 7 consequent to EVI1 activation after gene therapy for chronic granulomatous disease. Nat Med 2010;16:198–204.
62. Kang EM, Choi U, Theobald N, et al. Retrovirus gene therapy for X-linked chronic granulomatous disease can achieve stable long-term correction of oxidase activity in peripheral blood neutrophils. Blood 2010;115(4):783–91.
63. Cartier N, Hacein-Bey-Abina S, Bartholomae CC, et al. Hematopoietic stem cell gene therapy with a lentiviral vector in X-linked adrenoleukodystrophy. Science 2009;326(5954):818–23.
64. Bauer TR Jr, Allen JM, Hai M, et al. Successful treatment of canine leukocyte adhesion deficiency by foamy virus vectors. Nat Med 2008;14(1):93–7.
65. Rottman M, Soudais C, Vogt G, et al. IFN-gamma mediates the rejection of haematopoietic stem cells in IFN-gammaR1-deficient hosts. PLoS Med 2008;5(1):e26.
66. van Deutekom JC, Janson AA, Ginjaar IB, et al. Local dystrophin restoration with antisense oligonucleotide PRO051. N Engl J Med 2007;357(26):2677–86.
67. Porteus MH, Carroll D. Gene targeting using zinc finger nucleases. Nat Biotechnol 2005;23(8):967–73.
68. Redondo P, Prieto J, Munoz IG, et al. Molecular basis of xeroderma pigmentosum group C DNA recognition by engineered meganucleases. Nature 2008;456(7218):107–11.
69. Urnov FD, Miller JC, Lee YL, et al. Highly efficient endogenous human gene correction using designed zinc-finger nucleases. Nature 2005;435(7042):646–51.

Hematopoietic Stem Cell Transplantation: An Overview of Infection Risks and Epidemiology

John R. Wingard, MD*, Jack Hsu, MD, John W. Hiemenz, MD

KEYWORDS

• Hematopoietic stem cell transplantation
• Opportunistic infections • GVHD

Hematopoietic stem cell transplantation (HSCT) (also known as "bone marrow transplantation") is associated with a variety of infectious complications that pose serious threats to transplant recipients. The risk of infectious complications, type of pathogens, and timing of infectious threats varies substantially according to type of HSCT and the manner in which it is performed. In recent years there have been a number of changes in transplant practices that have altered the epidemiology of infectious complications.

HSCT is used to treat two categories of medical conditions. The first category consists of nonmalignant diseases that result in failure of bone marrow function or bone marrow–derived cells including aplastic anemia; myelodysplastic syndromes; immunodeficiency syndromes, such as severe combined immunodeficiency or chronic granulomatous disease; genetic diseases, such as the mucopolysaccharidoses or glycogen storage diseases; or the hemoglobinopathies of thalassemia and sickle cell anemia. The second category is far more prevalent and consists of neoplastic diseases, particularly hematopoietic malignancies, such as acute or chronic leukemia, lymphomas, multiple myeloma, and myeloproliferative diseases. In the first category of diseases, the transplant serves to replace a defective tissue, much in the same way kidney transplantation is performed for kidney failure. In the second category of diseases, the transplant serves two functions. The first function is to facilitate the safe use of cytotoxic therapies (intensive chemotherapy with or without total body irradiation) by reversing the myelosuppressive or myeloablative

A version of this article was previously published in the *Infectious Disease Clinics of North America*, 24:2.
Bone Marrow Transplant Program, Division of Hematology/Oncology, University of Florida College of Medicine, PO Box 100278, 1600 SW Archer Road, Gainesville, FL 32610-0278, USA
* Corresponding author.
E-mail address: wingajr@ufl.edu

effects of the cytotoxic therapy; the second function is to provide immune cells to directly attack neoplastic cells that express tumor-specific or tumor-associated antigens.

There are two major types of HSCT: autologous and allogeneic. Autologous refers to the patient serving as his or her own donor. Allogeneic refers to someone else serving as the donor. The hematopoietic stem cells are collected from the autologous patient before the transplant procedure and cryopreserved. The allogeneic hematopoietic stem cells are collected from the donor (a family member, a volunteer donor, or banked cord blood cells) either before or synchronously with the transplant procedure and are infused into the recipient after receiving a pretransplant conditioning regimen. For allogeneic transplantation, stringent HLA matching between donor and recipient is required to minimize the risk for graft rejection; reduce the risk for graft-versus-host disease (GVHD), which can be viewed as the donor immunity attempting to "reject" the recipient; and to facilitate the development of robust donor protective immunity. When cord blood is used as the source of hematopoietic stem cells, less stringent HLA matching is required because of the naive state of the newborn's immunity, in which case greater donor and recipient HLA disparity is tolerated. Rarely, individuals may have an identical twin, allowing for "syngeneic" HSCT. Although this may be the most optimal source of stem cells for many patients with nonmalignant marrow disorders, the lack of an allogeneic graft versus tumor effect makes this less desirable for patients with malignant disorders, particularly the leukemias and some lymphoproliferative disorders. Autologous transplantation is most commonly used in the treatment of malignant diseases to facilitate intensive antineoplastic cytotoxic therapy.

The hematopoietic stem cell graft may be obtained either from harvesting of bone marrow or by apheresis of the peripheral blood. Bone marrow is the traditional source of stem cells used in HSCT, and is collected by needle aspirations of 1 to 1.5 L of bone marrow obtained from the posterior iliac crests. Ordinarily, hematopoietic stem cells rarely traffic in the circulation, but after chemotherapy, or after administration of granulocyte colony–stimulating factor or plerixafor, large numbers of stem cells are "mobilized" from the bone marrow into the circulation and can be collected from peripheral or central veins by apheresis. Peripheral blood grafts contain more lymphocytes and a greater risk for GVHD when this donor source is used. Bone marrow and peripheral blood grafts consist of a mixture of immature hematopoietic cells, mature hematopoietic cells, and immune cells. Hematopoietic potency of the graft is generally measured by enumeration of the cells expressing the CD34 antigen, an antigen expressed on the cell surface of primitive hematopoietic progenitors. The larger the CD34 count, the faster the neutrophil recovery. Immune potency is measured by enumeration of the lymphocytes (the CD3 count). The larger numbers of CD3$^+$ cells, natural killer cells, and dendritic cells, the more rapid is posttransplant immune reconstitution and greater adoptive immunotherapeutic potency. In some cases the graft may be manipulated ex vivo before administration to the recipient. The most common manipulation of allogeneic grafts is T-cell depletion, which is done to reduce the risk of GVHD. An unintended consequence of T-cell depletion is a greater risk of graft rejection, a higher risk for relapse of the cancer being treated, and slower T-cell reconstitution after transplant.

A conditioning regimen is given before intravenous infusion of the hematopoietic stem cell graft. For patients with cancer, the conditioning regimen consists of intensive chemotherapy with or without total body irradiation, with agents chosen to destroy as much residual cancer as possible. For patients undergoing allogeneic HSCT, suppression of the recipient immunity is also a goal of the conditioning regimen. Agents are chosen to optimize therapeutic goals and minimize toxicities. For autologous transplants, the regimens consist of drugs found to be active against the type of cancer being treated, whose toxicities spare as much as possible nonhematopoietic tissues, and where an antitumor dose-response association is demonstrable. There is a wide array of effective regimens used that vary from cancer to cancer and center to center. For allogeneic HSCT, similar antitumor considerations are also important, but even more important is the immunosuppressive properties of the agents selected. The most widely used agents in allogeneic HSCT are cyclophosphamide, total body irradiation, and antithymocyte globulin. In recent years purine analogs with potent immunosuppressive properties, such as fludarabine, pentostatin, and cladrabine, are increasingly used because they have been found to have less severe nonhemato-poietic tissue toxicity. Many elderly individuals and patients with comorbid conditions unrelated to cancer are unable to tolerate intensive conditioning regimens because of high transplant-related morbidity and mortality. With the increasing recognition that much of the anticancer potency of allogeneic HSCT resides in the adoptive immuno-therapeutic effects of the graft and the advent of less toxic immunosuppressive agents, a growing body of experience with reduced-intensity (nonablative) condi-tioning regimens has developed. Increasingly, reduced-intensity regimens are being used in allogeneic HSCT. To facilitate the development of robust anticancer effects, many such nonablative regimens are coupled with acceleration of the tapering of the posttransplant immunosuppressive regimen. Nonablative regimens are associ-ated with shorter times of neutropenia and less injury to the mucosa because the regi-mens have less cytotoxicity to nonlymphohematopoietic tissues. This has allowed many such transplants to be performed in an outpatient setting with a less intense need for multiple transfusions of blood products, antibiotic support, parenteral analge-sics, and fluid and electrolyte supplementation.

After transplantation, a variety of supportive care measures are provided. A tunneled central venous catheter is usually placed for administration of the chemo-therapy, stem cell infusion, intravenous medications, electrolyte supplements, nutri-tional support, and blood products. An immunosuppressive regimen consisting most commonly of a calcineurin inhibitor (cyclosporine or tacrolimus) plus a short course of intravenous methotrexate is given after transplantation both to prevent graft rejection and to prevent GVHD. Other immunosuppressive regimens are sometimes used. After transplantation the immunosuppressive regimen is usually tapered over 4 to 6 months and eventually discontinued, unless GVHD develops and a more pro-longed course of immunosuppressive therapy is required. Because no immunosup-pressive therapy is given after autologous transplant, immune reconstitution occurs much faster, with humoral and T-cell responses recovering in 3 to 9 months. In contrast, immune reconstitution after allogeneic HSCT is much slower and may take a year or longer. Immune reconstitution may be even slower if GVHD occurs. Even in the absence of GVHD, immune reconstitution is slower if a cord blood, T-cell depleted graft, or graft from a mismatched donor is used as the source of hematopoi-etic stem cells.

THE DYNAMIC NATURE OF DAMAGE TO HOST DEFENSES AND RESTORATION OF HOST DEFENSES AND IMMUNITY AFTER HSCT

The risk for infection and the spectrum of infectious syndromes differs by type of trans-plant, type of conditioning regimen, type of stem cell graft, and type of posttransplant therapies and whether or not certain posttransplant complications occur, such as GVHD. **Table 1** illustrates some of these considerations. The risk of infection can be

Table 1
Effect of transplant characteristics on infectious risk

Transplant Parameter	Effect on Host Barriers and Immunity	Infectious Consequences
Type of transplant	Allogeneic: slower B- and T-cell immune reconstitution	Greater risk for infections of all types, but especially invasive fungal and herpesvirus infections; longer interval of risk
Type of allogeneic donor	Unrelated or mismatched donor: slower B- and T-cell immune reconstitution	Greater risk for infections of all types, but especially invasive fungal and herpesvirus infections; longer interval of risk
Type of stem cell graft	Peripheral blood: faster neutrophil engraftment, more chronic GVHD. Cord blood: slower neutrophil engraftment, less GVHD, slower B- and T-cell immune reconstitution	Different risks for infections associated with neutropenia and GVHD
Stem cell graft manipulation	T-cell depletion: greater risk for graft rejection, slower B- and T-cell immune reconstitution	Greater risk for neutropenic infections, lower risk for infections associated with chronic GVHD, greater and longer risk for herpesvirus and invasive fungal infections
Conditioning regimen	Intensive regimens: more mucosal injury, shorter time to neutropenia and longer neutropenia	Greater risk for neutropenic infections, especially typhlitis
Immunosuppressive regimen (allogeneic)	ATG: more profound deficiency of T-cell immunity. Methotrexate: more mucosal injury, longer time to neutrophil recovery	Greater risk for invasive fungal and herpesvirus infections
Central venous catheter	Breach in skin barrier	Greater risk for bacterial and (less frequently) fungal infections

Abbreviations: ATG, antithymocyte globulin; GVHD, graft-versus-host disease.

divided into three time intervals. The time periods and infectious risks are illustrated in **Table 2**.

Early, before engraftment, the major compromises in host defenses are neutropenia and mucosal injury. The duration of neutropenia is 10 to 14 days after autologous HSCT, 15 to 30 days after allogeneic HSCT using an ablative conditioning regimen, and only 5 to 7 days using a nonablative conditioning regimen. The infectious threats are principally the same bacterial and (less commonly) fungal pathogens (eg, *Candida* species and molds) as seen in neutropenic cancer patients who are not transplant

Table 2
Types of infections encountered at various times after HSCT

Type of Infectious Pathogen	Early Preengraftment (First 2–4 wk)	Early Postengraftment (Second and Third Month)	Late Postengraftment (After Second or Third Month)	Time Independent
Bacteria	Gram-negative bacteria (related to mucosal injury and neutropenia) Gram-positive bacteria (related to venous catheters) *Clostridium difficile* (related to neutropenia, antibiotics, antiacid medications)	Gram-positive bacteria (related to venous catheters) Gram-negative bacteria (related to enteric involvement of GVHD, venous catheters)	Encapsulated bacteria (related to poor opsonization with chronic GVHD) *Nocardia* (related to chronic GVHD)	
Fungi	*Candida* (related to mucosal injury and neutropenia)	*Aspergillus*, other molds and *Pneumocystis jirovecii* (related to GVHD)	*Aspergillus*, other molds and *P jirovecii* (related to GVHD)	
Herpesviruses	HSV	CMV (related to GVHD and impaired cellular immunity) EBV (in patients who have T-cell depleted grafts, receive ATG, or whose donor is mismatched)	CMV and VZV (related to GVHD and impaired cellular immunity and viral latency before transplant) EBV (in patients who have T-cell depleted grafts, receive ATG, or whose donor is mismatched)	
Other viruses		BK virus (related to GVHD and cyclophosphamide in conditioning regimen)		Respiratory viruses (temporally tracks with community outbreaks) Adenoviruses

Abbreviations: ATG, antithymocyte globulin; CMV, cytomegalovirus; EBV, Epstein-Barr virus; GVHD, graft-versus-host disease; HSV, herpes simplex virus; VZV, varicella-zoster virus.

recipients. The evaluation and management strategies of these infectious complications are similar to the ones that have been developed for chemotherapy-induced neutropenic fever. Herpes simplex virus (HSV) reactivates in most HSV-seropositive patients during this time period between 1 and 2 weeks after transplantation. Engraftment demarcates the transition to the second time interval.

The early postengraftment period is categorized by progressive recovery in cell-mediated immunity. This occurs much more rapidly after autologous than allogeneic transplant. The infectious threat then recedes dramatically. After autologous HSCT, many early posttransplant infections are associated with the presence of the central venous catheter. Although the venous catheter is generally removed as early as possible, this may be technically challenging in this group of patients and the catheter may need to remain in place if the patient continues to require transfusion support, supplemental medications, nutrition, intravenous fluid, or electrolyte supplements. Gram-positive bacteria are frequent causes of central venous catheter–associated infections, with gram-negative and mixed bacterial infections less common but occasionally seen. After allogeneic HSCT, there is a similar risk for catheter-associated infections, but GVHD also poses an additional risk for bacterial infections. Bacteremias from enteric organisms are especially problematic in patients with GVHD of the intestinal tract. Infections caused by *Candida* species occasionally occur in patients with GVHD, and are often associated with indwelling venous catheters especially in the presence of intravenous administration of nutritional supplementation. *Aspergillus* species and other mold infections and *Pneumocystis jirovecii* pneumonia (PCP) occur in patients with GVHD and in those on high doses of steroids for GVHD treatment. Cytomegalovirus (CMV) viremia occurs chiefly in patients who were seropositive before transplantation and who develop GVHD. Untreated, CMV viremia often is followed by pneumonia or enterocolitis after allogeneic HSCT, which can be associated with substantial morbidity and mortality.

Beyond 3 months, the risk for opportunistic infection in autologous HSCT patients is small. After allogeneic HSCT, there is gradual reconstitution of humoral and cellular immunity, which approaches normality by 1 year if GVHD does not occur. Immunization of the recipient with the childhood vaccines is recommended at that time.[1,2] The development of chronic GVHD leads to delays in immune reconstitution and necessitates prolonged courses of immunosuppressive therapy that compounds the immunodeficiency caused by the GVHD. Late infections in patients are caused by similar pathogens as those in the early posttransplant period (*Candida* species, *Aspergillus* species and other molds, PCP, and CMV) but also include encapsulated bacteria because of poor opsonization and varicella zoster virus (VZV) infections.

COMMON INFECTIOUS SYNDROMES AFTER HSCT AND THEIR ETIOLOGIES
Neutropenic Fever

Fever occurring in the neutropenic transplant recipient is frequent during the pre-engraftment period. Neutropenic fever is less frequent in patients receiving reduced-intensity conditioning regimens. Fever typically occurs 3 to 5 days after the onset of neutropenia and may be the sole manifestation of infection. Bacterial infections are by far the most common infectious causes of the first fever during neutropenia, but in most cases no microbiologic etiology is documented with the prompt initiation of broad-spectrum empiric antibiotic therapy. Likely sites of infection are lungs; skin (especially catheter insertion sites and the perianal area); and genitourinary tract. In addition, the oral cavity and intestinal tract are also possible sites of infection. Gram-positive bacteria are the most frequently isolated bacterial pathogens, with

Staphylococcus epidermidis making up approximately half, viridians streptococci making up approximately one third, and *Staphylococcus aureus* and several other species making up the remainder of episodes. Gram-negative bacteria make up about 30% to 45% of bacterial infections and include *Enterobacter* spp, *Escherichia coli*, *Klebsiella* spp, *Pseudomonas aeruginosa*, and *Stenotrophomonas maltophilia*. Cultures of blood and from suspected sites of infection should be obtained and empiric antibiotics instituted promptly.

Persistent fever is more problematic. Possible explanations included a delayed response to the initial antibiotic regimen, presence of a gram-positive organism not adequately treated with the initial antibiotic regimen, or antibiotic-resistant gram-negative bacteria. In addition, other types of pathogens are also possible explanations, especially invasive fungal infections by *Candida* spp, *Aspergillus* spp, or other molds. A detailed discussion of the evaluation and approaches to management of neutropenic fever is beyond the scope of this article but is discussed in detail in several authoritative guidelines.[3,4]

Nonneutropenic Fever

Most fevers in the neutropenic transplant recipient resolve at the time of neutrophil recovery. Fever may sometimes occur, however, at the time of engraftment. Although an infectious etiology is possible and should be vigorously pursued, fever often is caused by what has been referred to as the "engraftment syndrome," a noninfectious syndrome of uncertain etiology that consists of fever alone or with rash, pneumonitis, hyperbilirubinemia, or diarrhea. Cultures should be obtained and CT scans of the chest and abdomen should be performed as part of the investigation to assess for a possible infectious focus. If the investigation does not reveal an infectious source, a short course of high-dose corticosteroids may be considered and is often very effective.

Later after engraftment, fever sometimes occurs in the absence of other symptoms. CMV infection, occult sinusitis, central venous catheter–associated infection, or occult fungal infection are frequent causes. Evaluation should include elicitation of infectious symptoms and physical signs; blood cultures for bacteria, fungi, and mycobacteria; urine analysis; and blood samples for CMV polymerase chain reaction (PCR) or antigen. Imaging studies with CT scans of the chest, sinuses, and abdomen should also be considered. Medications can cause fever, so discontinuation of discretionary medications is advisable. If fever persists and no etiology can be discerned, one should consider removal of the venous catheter.

Pneumonia and Pulmonary Infiltrates

Pneumonia is a common complication after HSCT.[5] There are both infectious and noninfectious causes of pneumonia and pulmonary infiltrates in the HSCT recipient, and the likely etiologies vary over time (**Table 3**).

The types of pneumonias can be categorized according to their radiologic appearance into diffuse and localized infiltrates. High-resolution CT scans are the most sensitive radiologic procedure[6,7] because standard radiographs are less sensitive. Diffuse infiltrates can be alveolar, interstitial, mixed alveolar interstitial, or diffuse micronodular. Localized infiltrates may present as lobar consolidation; macronodules (>1 cm); cavities; or wedge-shaped infiltrates.

Before engraftment, most episodes of pneumonia and pulmonary infiltrates are not related to infection. Volume overload may occur during this time period. Congestive heart failure from cardiotoxic drugs or the acute respiratory distress syndrome caused by pulmonary toxicity from the pretransplant conditioning regimen, other antecedent

Table 3
Infectious and noninfectious causes of pneumonia after HSCT

Type of Pulmonary Infiltrate		Preengraftment	Early Postengraftment	Late
Diffuse	Noninfectious	Adult respiratory distress syndrome	Idiopathic interstitial pneumonitis	Bronchiolitis obliterans or bronchiolitis obliterans with organizing pneumonia
		Congestive heart failure		
		Fluid overload		
		Hemorrhagic alveolitis	Hemorrhagic alveolitis	
		Respiratory virus		
	Infectious		CMV	CMV
			Respiratory virus	Respiratory virus
			PCP	PCP
			Adenovirus	Adenovirus
Localized	Noninfectious	Aspiration		
		Pulmonary thromboembolism		
		Micronodules caused by chemotherapy		
	Infectious	Bacterial pneumonia	Bacterial pneumonia	Bacterial pneumonia
		Aspergillus or other mold pneumonia	*Aspergillus* or other mold pneumonia	*Aspergillus* or other mold pneumonia
			Nocardia	*Nocardia*

Abbreviations: CMV, cytomegalovirus; PCP, *pneumocystis jirovecii* pneumonia.

therapy, or prior medical conditions are frequent. Hemorrhagic alveolitis may also occur because of toxicity from the conditioning regimen or inflammatory cytokines released as a consequence of the transplant procedure. These noninfectious pulmonary syndromes typically produce diffuse infiltrates. Aspiration pneumonia or bacterial or mold pneumonia also occur but are less frequent and typically produce localized infiltrates. Mold pneumonias are characterized by macronodules, some with halo signs, which later become cavitary. *Aspergillus* spp are by far the most common mold pathogens, with Zygomycetes accounting for 10% to 20% of mold pneumonias, and *Scedosporium* spp, *Fusarium* spp, and other genera accounting for a small percent of mold pneumonias.

Early after engraftment, diffuse pneumonias are evenly divided between infectious and noninfectious causes. Idiopathic pneumonia accounts for half of diffuse pneumonias.[8] The risk for idiopathic pneumonia is associated with higher-intensity conditioning regimens. CMV accounts for approximately 40% of diffuse pneumonias and is most commonly seen in patients with acute GVHD.[9] PCP (if the patient is not taking PCP prophylaxis), legionella, adenovirus, or various respiratory viruses are other possible causes of diffuse pneumonia. Increasingly, respiratory virus infections are being recognized as important causes of diffuse pneumonias.[10–17] Bacterial or mold pneumonias are the most common causes of localized pulmonary infiltrates. The most important risk factor for pulmonary aspergillosis and other mold pneumonias is GVHD.[18,19] Pulmonary aspergillosis most frequently presents as macronodules on CT imaging of the chest. In a large series, 94% of patients had at least one nodule and 79% had multiple nodules.[20] Halo signs, which occur early in infection, were present in 61% of patients with pulmonary aspergillosis. In another single-center series, pulmonary infection with Zygomycetes was observed to have more nodules on CT imaging than commonly occurs in pulmonary aspergillosis.[21]

During the late postengraftment period, there is a more heterogeneous spectrum of infectious causes of pneumonia.[22] Patients with chronic GVHD are particularly susceptible to sinopulmonary infections caused by encapsulated bacteria and increasingly susceptible to mold pneumonias.[23,24] *Nocardia* is an occasional pathogen that can cause pneumonia with similar clinical and radiographic features as infection with *Aspergillus* spp.[25] Bronchiolitis obliterans with organizing pneumonia (cryptogenic organizing pneumonia) is a manifestation of chronic GVHD. PCP may also occur (if the patient is not taking PCP prophylaxis). In the past, CMV pneumonia rarely occurred late, but increasingly, late CMV pneumonia is becoming more common.[26] GVHD and early CMV viremia are risk factors for late CMV pneumonia.

In some cases pneumonias may be caused by multiple pathogens. For example, CMV may be accompanied by superinfection with bacterial pathogens or *Aspergillus* spp. Infection with *Aspergillus* species may similarly be accompanied by bacterial, CMV, or Zygomycetes coinfections. Accordingly, assessment should be thorough and one should not ignore cultures or other tests indicating more than one pathogen.

Although radiology is essential in the assessment of pneumonia, some clinical features suggest certain etiologies. Hemoptysis is suggestive of hemorrhagic alveolitis or thromboembolism. Hemoptysis with pleuritic pain or pleural friction rub is suggestive of infection with *Aspergillus* spp or another mold. Cough is usually nonproductive of sputum with CMV, respiratory virus, PCP, and most noninfectious pneumonias. Although useful, these findings are not sufficiently specific to be diagnostic.

Assessment of diffuse infiltrates should include nasal and throat swabs for viral diagnostic assays with culture or direct fluorescence assay, enzyme-linked immunosorbent assay, or PCR assays for the respiratory viruses. After engraftment, blood should be collected for CMV PCR or antigen assay. Bronchoscopy with bronchoalveolar lavage

(BAL) can be quite useful in further assessment.[27,28] The sensitivity and specificity of testing of BAL fluid for infectious etiologies causing diffuse infiltrates (eg, PCP, CMV, or respiratory viruses) are quite good.

Assessment of localized infiltrates should include blood cultures for bacteria and fungi. Sputum, if available, should be cultured. When infection with *Aspergillus* species is suspected, serum for galactomannan[29–31] can be helpful. One should consider bronchoscopic evaluation with cultures and stains in this setting, although the yield in the investigation of nodular infiltrates is lower. Bronchoscopy with BAL can still be useful because it may detect or exclude certain coinfecting pathogens and allow a more focused antimicrobial therapy. For peripheral nodules or infiltrates, CT-guided needle, video-assisted thoracoscopy guided, or even open lung biopsies may be useful if the patient is not significantly thrombocytopenic.

While evaluation of pneumonia proceeds, one should presumptively initiate therapy for the most likely etiologies because delay in initiating therapy may compromise the prospects for a successful outcome. Presumptive therapy should not be used in lieu of a proper assessment, because the spectrum of possible pathogens is large and toxicities of multiple therapies can lead to harm. Once the etiology is established it is important to discontinue the unneeded therapies. If the etiology has not been definitively established, evaluation should be continued.

Diarrhea

Diarrhea may have multiple etiologies (**Table 4**). Shortly after the conditioning regimen, cytotoxic mucosal injury may result in noninfectious diarrhea. During the pre-engraftment period, typhlitis and *Clostridium difficile* enterocolitis are potentially serious complications. Both infections are typically accompanied by fever, abdominal discomfort, and distention. Guarding and ileus may also be present. CT scan shows bowel wall thickening and may also demonstrate bowel distention. With typhlitis, the ascending colon is often involved but other portions of the large and small intestine may also be involved.[32–34] The microbiologic etiology of typhlitis is rarely determined, but is presumed to be caused mostly by gram-negative and anaerobic bacteria. Invasion of the compromised bowel wall by *Candida* species has been noted.[35,36] Toxic megacolon, perforation, and septic shock may result from severe typhlitis and can result in death.

Enteritis caused by *C difficile* is one of the most common nosocomial infections. Strains that produce highly potent toxins have been noted to cause outbreaks and such infections may result in perforation, shock, and death.[37–41] The use of fluoroquinolones and the use of gastric acid suppressants are risk factors for overgrowth in the bowel and infection with *C difficile*.

Table 4
Infectious and noninfectious causes of diarrhea after HSCT

Preengraftment	Early Postengraftment	Late
Mucosal injury from conditioning regimen	GVHD	GVHD
Neutropenic enterocolitis (typhlitis)	C difficile enterocolitis	C difficile enterocolitis
Clostridium difficile enterocolitis	CMV	CMV
Enteric viruses	Adenovirus	Adenovirus
	Enteric viruses	Enteric viruses

Abbreviations: CMV, cytomegalovirus; GVHD, graft-versus-host disease.

Enteric viruses, including enteroviruses, caliciviruses, and astroviruses, are potential causes of diarrhea[42–45] in the patient undergoing HSCT. Generally, HSCT patients become vulnerable to such pathogens as viral outbreaks occur in the community. Adenoviruses and CMV also can cause diarrhea.[46–48] Infrequently, enteropathic bacteria, such as *Shigella* spp and *Salmonella* spp, protozoa, and helminthic infections can cause enterocolitis.

After engraftment, GVHD is a major noninfectious cause of diarrhea in addition to the previously noted infectious causes. GVHD of the gastrointestinal tract is most commonly associated with the presence of cutaneous GVHD, but occasionally it may occur in the absence of other manifestations of GVHD. GVHD of the gut typically occurs in the early postengraftment period as part of acute GVHD (rather than chronic GVHD). With changing transplant practices, however, which have included the increasing use of peripheral blood as a source of stem cells, donor lymphocyte infusions, and reduced intensity transplant regimens, the spectrum of clinical manifestations of acute and chronic GVHD are blending over time.

Evaluation should include stool samples for assays for *C difficile* antigen or toxin, viral cultures or enzyme-linked immunosorbent assays, CMV antigen or PCR testing, and examination of stool for presence of ova and parasites. For more severe episodes of diarrhea, abdominal CT provides assessment of bowel wall thickening or the development of intra-abdominal abscesses. In patients with typhlitis or severe *C difficile* enterocolitis, serial kidneys-ureter-bladder radiographs can be useful to monitor for evidence of toxic megacolon. For cases where the etiology remains uncertain, colonoscopy should be considered for visual inspection to determine if there are pseudomembranes and to obtain biopsy for histologic examination to assess for GVHD and presence of CMV or other infections by immunostaining, culture, or PCR.

CMV

Decades ago, CMV pneumonia was the predominant infectious life-threatening complication after HSCT. Although pneumonia is the most common CMV syndrome, esophagitis, gastritis, or enterocolitis are other infections that may be caused by CMV. Unlike the patient with severe immunodeficiency caused by infection with HIV, CMV chorioretinitis rarely occurs in patients undergoing HSCT. Although CMV infection occurs after both autologous and allogeneic HSCT, CMV disease is uncommon after autologous HSCT. In allogeneic HSCT patients, seropositivity and GVHD are the major risk factors for CMV reactivation and disease.[49,50] CMV viremia generally precedes pneumonia by 1 to 2 weeks. Because of the adoption of close monitoring for reactivation of CMV and antiviral management strategies routinely used after allogeneic HSCT, CMV disease has receded as a serious threat early after HSCT. In the past, CMV disease most commonly occurred during the early postengraftment period. Recently, however, late-onset CMV disease has been increasing in occurrence.[26] Risk factors for late CMV disease include early viremia posttransplantation and the development of GVHD.

Clinical presentation of CMV pneumonia is low-grade fever, nonproductive cough, and dyspnea. Progressive hypoxia ensues over several days. Examination of the chest may be unrevealing or demonstrate scattered rales. Chest radiographic examination demonstrates alveolar, interstitial, or mixed alveolar-interstitial diffuse infiltrates. Bronchoscopy with BAL specimens for immunostaining or PCR assays is diagnostic with sensitivity and specificity of 90% or higher. Bronchoscopy may also reveal coinfection by bacteria, PCP, or *Aspergillus* spp. For gastrointestinal CMV syndromes, endoscopic examination of the gastrointestinal tract with biopsy should be performed.

Hepatitis

Hepatocellular injury is common after HSCT. Two patterns are seen: cholestasis (elevations of bilirubin and alkaline phosphatase) and hepatitis (elevations of hepatic transaminases). Abnormalities of liver function tests after HSCT are most commonly of noninfectious causes that can give rise to either pattern. These abnormalities can be in the form of cholestasis from hepatic veno-occlusive disease (VOD) (sinusoidal obstruction syndrome) caused by the conditioning regimen, either cholestasis or hepatitis caused by various medications, or cholestasis caused by acute or chronic GVHD. VOD almost always occurs before day 30, GVHD almost always occurs after engraftment. Iron overload from red cell transfusions before the transplant often leads to a hepatocellular injury pattern that can occur at any time after HSCT. Exacerbation of viral hepatitis present before the transplant can produce a hepatitis pattern that may wax and wane periodically after HSCT. This can lead to serious and progressive hepatic injury with tapering of immunosuppressive therapy as immune reconstitution strengthens. In the late postengraftment period, fulminant hepatitis may occur from severe infection with VZV, which may occur even in the absence of vesicular skin lesions. In some cases of hepatic syndromes, the cause may be multifactorial because of multiple etiologies, both infectious and noninfectious. Biliary obstruction caused by a stone may give rise to a cholestatic pattern. Cholecystitis has also been reported to occasionally occur, with an association with busulfan in the conditioning regimen.

Evaluation of liver function abnormalities occurring in the HSCT recipient depends on the type of pattern and time posttransplant. A patient with a cholestatic picture should undergo ultrasonongraphy of the abdomen first to exclude biliary obstruction. A review of medications should be performed and discontinuation of any implicated medications should be considered. Before engraftment cholestasis is frequently caused by VOD. Biopsy is often not possible at this time because of significant thrombocytopenia. After engraftment, GVHD is a strong consideration and biopsy should be performed if possible to confirm the diagnosis. HSCT recipients with the hepatitis pattern should be evaluated with viral hepatitis PCR assays and serum iron studies. Although the latter may be difficult to interpret in the presence of ongoing inflammation, HSCT recipients with a history of multiple red cell transfusions and a serum ferritin in excess of 1000 ng/mL should be considered at risk for iron overload syndrome. Any medications that might be suspected should be discontinued if possible and if the etiology remains uncertain, liver biopsy should be considered.

Rash

Rashes frequently occur after HSCT from a variety of causes. The rash of acute GVHD typically presents as an erythematous maculopapular rash, especially of the palms, soles, and earlobes, but the entire body may be affected along with the mucosal surfaces. In the setting of chronic GVHD, lichenoid or sclerodermatoid changes of skin and mucosal surfaces predominate. Skin involvement by infections usually produces localized lesions. Common manifestations of disseminated infections may include subcutaneous nodules of the skin. These lesions may be macronodular erythematous lesions, sometimes with a necrotic center. Vesicular lesions are characteristic of VZV either in a dermatomal or widely disseminated distribution. Paronychia may be caused by bacteria or yeasts; however, they can commonly be caused by *Fusarium* spp or other molds in the severely immunocompromised HSCT recipient and can lead to life-threatening systemic fungal infection.

Punch biopsy of skin lesions can be diagnostic. If a fungal infection is suspected, special stains for fungal organisms, such as the Gomori methenamine silver stain, are necessary because routine histologic stains, such as hematoxylin and eosin, may not be sufficient to visualize the presence of fungi in the tissues. Where disseminated infection is suspected bacterial and fungal blood cultures should also be part of the evaluation. Vesicles found on the skin should be unroofed with a tuberculin-sized syringe and needle to collect fluid for viral cultures, immunostains, or PCR for VZV and HSV.

PREVENTION AND TREATMENT APPROACHES

Management strategies are beyond the scope of this article. Consensus guidelines for infection prevention for HSCT patients were first published in 2000[51] and recently have been updated.[1] Evaluation and management guidelines for neutropenic fever have been published.[3,4] Prevention and treatment guidelines for *Candida* and *Aspergillus* have been published.[52,53] Discussions of CMV treatment have been published.[49,54]

SUMMARY

HSCT has become a common treatment of bone marrow failure and certain malignancies. Types of transplant, including types of stem cells and conditioning regimens vary, impacting the magnitude and duration of primary risk periods. Risks for infections caused by numerous bacterial, viral, and fungal pathogens can extend over a long period of time, dictating preventative strategies and differential diagnoses.

REFERENCES

1. Tomblyn M, Chiller T, Einsele H, et al. Guidelines for preventing infectious complications among hematopoietic cell transplant recipients: a global perspective. Bone Marrow Transplant 2009;15(10):1143–238.
2. Ljungman P, Engelhard D, Da La Camara R, et al. Vaccination of stem cell transplant recipients: recommendations of the Infectious Diseases Working Party of the EBMT. Bone Marrow Transplant 2005;35:737–46.
3. Hughes WT, Armstrong D, Bodey GP, et al. 2002 guidelines for the use of antimicrobial agents in neutropenic patients with cancer. Clin Infect Dis 2002;34(6):730–51.
4. Friefeld AG, Baden LR, Brown AE, et al. The NCCN fever and neutropenia clinical practice guidelines in oncology. Version 1. 2005.
5. Gosselin MV, Adams RH. Pulmonary complications in bone marrow transplantation. J Thorac Imaging 2002;17(2):132–44.
6. Heussel CP, Kauczor HU, Heussel G, et al. Early detection of pneumonia in febrile neutropenic patients: use of thin-section CT. AJR Am J Roentgenol 1997;169(5):1347–53.
7. Conces DJ Jr. Noninfectious lung disease in immunocompromised patients. J Thorac Imaging 1999;14(1):9–24.
8. Wingard JR, Mellits ED, Sostrin MB, et al. Interstitial pneumonitis after allogeneic bone marrow transplantation: nine-year experience at a single institution. Medicine (Baltimore) 1988;67(3):175–86.
9. Wingard JR, Piantadosi S, Burns WH, et al. Cytomegalovirus infections in bone marrow transplant recipients given intensive cytoreductive therapy. Rev Infect Dis 1990;12(Suppl 7):S793–804.
10. Harrington RD, Hooton TM, Hackman RC, et al. An outbreak of respiratory syncytial virus in a bone marrow transplant center. J Infect Dis 1992;165(6):987–93.

11. Ljungman P. Respiratory virus infections in bone marrow transplant recipients: the European perspective. Am J Med 1997;102(3A):44–7.

12. Whimbey E, Champlin RE, Couch RB, et al. Community respiratory virus infections among hospitalized adult bone marrow transplant recipients. Clin Infect Dis 1996;22(5):778–82.

13. Whimbey E, Englund JA, Couch RB. Community respiratory virus infections in immunocompromised patients with cancer. Am J Med 1997;102(3A):10–8.

14. Bowden RA. Respiratory virus infections after marrow transplant: the Fred Hutchinson Cancer Research Center experience. Am J Med 1997;102(3A): 27–30.

15. Nichols WG, Gooley T, Boeckh M. Community-acquired respiratory syncytial virus and parainfluenza virus infections after hematopoietic stem cell transplantation: the Fred Hutchinson Cancer Research Center experience. Biol Blood Marrow Transplant 2001;7(Suppl):11S–5S.

16. Whimbey E, Vartivarian SE, Champlin RE, et al. Parainfluenza virus infection in adult bone marrow transplant recipients. Eur J Clin Microbiol Infect Dis 1993; 12(9):699–701.

17. Ljungman P. Respiratory virus infections in stem cell transplant patients: the European experience. Biol Blood Marrow Transplant 2001;7(Suppl):5S–7S.

18. De La Rosa GR, Champlin RE, Kontoyiannis DP. Risk factors for the development of invasive fungal infections in allogeneic blood and marrow transplant recipients. Transpl Infect Dis 2002;4(1):3–9.

19. Fukuda T, Boeckh M, Carter RA, et al. Risks and outcomes of invasive fungal infections in recipients of allogeneic hematopoietic stem cell transplants after nonmyeloablative conditioning. Blood 2003;102(3):827–33.

20. Greene RE, Schlamm HT, Oestmann JW, et al. Imaging findings in acute invasive pulmonary aspergillosis: clinical significance of the halo sign. Clin Infect Dis 2007;44(3):373–9.

21. Chamilos G, Marom EM, Lewis RE, et al. Predictors of pulmonary zygomycosis versus invasive pulmonary aspergillosis in patients with cancer. Clin Infect Dis 2005;41(1):60–6.

22. Wingard JR, Santos GW, Saral R. Late-onset interstitial pneumonia following allergenic bone marrow transplantation. Transplantation 1985;39(1):21–3.

23. Marr KA, Carter RA, Boeckh M, et al. Invasive aspergillosis in allogeneic stem cell transplant recipients: changes in epidemiology and risk factors. Blood 2002; 100(13):4358–66.

24. Yamasaki S, Heike Y, Mori S, et al. Infectious complications in chronic graft-versus-host disease: a retrospective study of 145 recipients of allogeneic hematopoietic stem cell transplantation with reduced- and conventional-intensity conditioning regimens. Transpl Infect Dis 2008;10:252–9.

25. Daly AS, McGeer A, Lipton JH. Systemic nocardiosis following allogeneic bone marrow transplantation. Transpl Infect Dis 2003;5:16–20.

26. Boeckh M, Leisenring W, Riddell SR, et al. Late cytomegalovirus disease and mortality in recipients of allogeneic hematopoietic stem cell transplants: importance of viral load and T-cell immunity. Blood 2003;101(2):407–14.

27. Dunagan DP, Baker AM, Hurd DD, et al. Bronchoscopic evaluation of pulmonary infiltrates following bone marrow transplantation. Chest 1997;111(1):135–41.

28. Feller-Kopman D, Ernst A. The role of bronchoalveolar lavage in the immunocompromised host. Semin Respir Infect 2003;18(2):87–94.

29. Maertens J, Theunissen K, Verhoef G, et al. Galactomannan and computed tomography-based preemptive antifungal therapy in neutropenic patients at

high risk for invasive fungal infection: a prospective feasibility study. Clin Infect Dis 2005;41(9):1242–50.

30. Maertens J, Van Eldere J, Verhaegen J, et al. Use of circulating galactomannan screening for early diagnosis of invasive aspergillosis in allogeneic stem cell transplant recipients. J Infect Dis 2002;186(9):1297–306.

31. Pfeiffer CD, Fine JP, Safdar N. Diagnosis of invasive aspergillosis using a galactomannan assay: a meta-analysis. Clin Infect Dis 2006;42:1417–27.

32. Gorschluter M, Mey U, Strehl J, et al. Neutropenic enterocolitis in adults: systematic analysis of evidence quality. Eur J Haematol 2005;75(1):1–13.

33. Cardona AF, Ramos PL, Casasbuenas A. From case reports to systematic reviews in neutropenic enterocolitis. Eur J Haematol 2005;75(5):445–6.

34. Aksoy DY, Tanriover MD, Uzun O, et al. Diarrhea in neutropenic patients: a prospective cohort study with emphasis on neutropenic enterocolitis. Ann Oncol 2007;18(1):183–9.

35. Cardona Zorrilla AF, Reveiz HL, Casasbuenas A, et al. Systematic review of case reports concerning adults suffering from neutropenic enterocolitis. Clin Transl Oncol 2006;8(1):31–8.

36. Gorschluter M, Mey U, Strehl J, et al. Invasive fungal infections in neutropenic enterocolitis: a systematic analysis of pathogens, incidence, treatment and mortality in adult patients. BMC Infect Dis 2006;6:35.

37. Weiss K. Poor infection control, not fluoroquinolones, likely to be primary cause of *Clostridium difficile*-associated diarrhea outbreaks in Quebec. Clin Infect Dis 2006;42(5):725–7.

38. McDonald LC, Killgore GE, Thompson A, et al. An epidemic, toxin gene-variant strain of *Clostridium difficile*. N Engl J Med 2005;353(23):2433–41.

39. Pepin J, Saheb N, Coulombe MA, et al. Emergence of fluoroquinolones as the predominant risk factor for *Clostridium difficile*-associated diarrhea: a cohort study during an epidemic in Quebec. Clin Infect Dis 2005;41(9):1254–60.

40. Kuijper EJ, van den Berg RJ, Debast S, et al. *Clostridium difficile* ribotype 027, toxinotype III, the Netherlands. Emerg Infect Dis 2006;12(5):827–30.

41. Loo VG, Poirier L, Miller MA, et al. A predominantly clonal multi-institutional outbreak of *Clostridium difficile*-associated diarrhea with high morbidity and mortality. N Engl J Med 2005;353(23):2442–9.

42. Yolken RH, Bishop CA, Townsend TR, et al. Infectious gastroenteritis in bone-marrow-transplant recipients. N Engl J Med 1982;306(17):1010–2.

43. Townsend TR, Bolyard EA, Yolken RH, et al. Outbreak of coxsackie A1 gastroenteritis: a complication of bone-marrow transplantation. Lancet 1982;1(8276):820–3.

44. Cox GJ, Matsui SM, Lo RS, et al. Etiology and outcome of diarrhea after marrow transplantation: a prospective study. Gastroenterology 1994;107(5):1398–407.

45. van Kraaij MG, Dekker AW, Verdonck LF, et al. Infectious gastro-enteritis: an uncommon cause of diarrhoea in adult allogeneic and autologous stem cell transplant recipients. Bone Marrow Transplant 2000;26(3):299–303.

46. La Rosa AM, Champlin RE, Mirza N, et al. Adenovirus infections in adult recipients of blood and marrow transplants. Clin Infect Dis 2001;32(6):871–6.

47. Shields AF, Hackman RC, Fife KH, et al. Adenovirus infections in patients undergoing bone-marrow transplantation. N Engl J Med 1985;312(9):529–33.

48. Hale GA, Heslop HE, Krance RA, et al. Adenovirus infection after pediatric bone marrow transplantation. Bone Marrow Transplant 1999;23(3):277–82.

49. Boeckh M, Nichols WG, Papanicolaou G, et al. Cytomegalovirus in hematopoietic stem cell transplant recipients: current status, known challenges, and future strategies. Biol Blood Marrow Transplant 2003;9(9):543–58.

50. Boeckh M, Nichols WG. The impact of cytomegalovirus serostatus of donor and recipient before hematopoietic stem cell transplantation in the era of antiviral prophylaxis and preemptive therapy. Blood 2004;103(6):2003–8.
51. Dykewicz CA, Jaffe HW, Spira TJ, et al. Guidelines for preventing opportunistic infections among hematopoietic stem cell transplant recipients. MMWR Recomm Rep 2000;49(RR-10):1–125.
52. Walsh TJ, Anaissie EJ, Denning DW, et al. Treatment of aspergillosis: clinical practice guidelines of the Infectious Diseases Society of America. Clin Infect Dis 2008;46(3):327–60.
53. Pappas PG, Rex JH, Sobel JD, et al. Infectious Diseases Society of America. Guidelines for treatment of candidiasis. Clin Infect Dis 2004;38(2):161–89.
54. Boeckh M, Ljungman P. How we treat cytomegalovirus in hematopoietic cell transplant recipients. Blood 2009;113(23):5711–9.

Infectious Complications Associated with Immunomodulating Biologic Agents

Sophia Koo, MD[a,b,c],*, Francisco M. Marty, MD[a,b,c], Lindsey R. Baden, MD[a,b,c]

KEYWORDS

• Monoclonal antibodies • Biologic therapies
• Infectious complications

The repertoire of monoclonal antibodies and other biologic therapies targeted at precise components of the immune response continues to expand rapidly. In theory, these therapies should carry fewer infectious risks than traditional immunosuppressive therapies, but with increasing clinical use, it seems that many of these agents have a wide array of unintended, sometimes fatal, infectious consequences. Given the low frequency of these infectious events, an increase in specific infectious risks is often not appreciable in initial randomized controlled trials, and the discernment of these patterns often relies on ongoing surveillance during the postmarketing period, with the accumulation of a larger volume of patient exposures and reporting to national registries or voluntary reporting systems. Because patients who require immunomodulating biologic therapy are usually at higher risk of developing infections at baseline given their underlying disease and prior and concurrent treatment with other immunosuppressive agents, it is often difficult to discern a pattern of infection attributable to the addition of biologic therapies to this background, even when a pattern is present. In addition, biologic therapies may have different target affinities, be used at various

Funding support: none.
A version of this article was previously published in the *Infectious Disease Clinics of North America*, 24:2.
[a] Division of Infectious Diseases, Brigham and Women's Hospital, 75 Francis Street, PBB-A4, Boston, MA 02115, USA
[b] Division of Infectious Diseases, Dana-Farber Cancer Institute, Boston, MA, USA
[c] Harvard Medical School, Boston, MA, USA
* Corresponding author. Division of Infectious Diseases, Brigham and Women's Hospital, 75 Francis Street, PBB-A4, Boston, MA 02115.
E-mail address: skoo@partners.org

Hematol Oncol Clin N Am 25 (2011) 117–138
doi:10.1016/j.hoc.2010.11.009
0889-8588/11/$ – see front matter © 2011 Elsevier Inc. All rights reserved.

dosages, and given with different frequencies, all of which may affect their immuno-suppressive consequences. Furthermore, the use of prophylactic antimicrobial agents (eg, acyclovir and trimethoprim/sulfamethoxazole) or preemptive monitoring (eg, cytomegalovirus [CMV] viral load surveillance) may alter disease diagnosis and presentation. This review describes the range of infectious complications associated to date with each of the immunomodulating biologic therapies approved by the US Food and Drug Administration (FDA). Monoclonal antibodies used to treat infections and to diagnose disease on radiology studies are beyond the scope of this discussion.

B-LYMPHOCYTE DEPLETION: RITUXIMAB

Rituximab is a chimeric murine-human monoclonal IgG1 that targets CD20 on normal and malignant B lymphocytes, with rapid and durable depletion of these cells for 6 to 9 months. Serum immunoglobulin levels remain largely stable, although prolonged hypogammaglobulinemia has been described in some patients with non-Hodgkin lymphoma (nHL) receiving rituximab concurrently with autologous hematopoietic stem cell transplantation (HSCT).[1] Rituximab does not significantly affect CD3, CD4, CD8 or natural killer (NK) T-cell populations, and in theory has minimal effects on cell-mediated immunity.[2]

Rituximab was initially approved by the FDA in 1997 for the treatment of relapsed or refractory low-grade or follicular nHL, and has subsequently been approved for the treatment of several other CD20+ B-cell lymphomas, either alone or in combination with other chemotherapy, and treatment of moderate to severe rheumatoid arthritis (RA) in combination with methotrexate in patients with an inadequate response to tumor necrosis factor α (TNF-α) antagonists. According to the manufacturer, there have been more than a million patient exposures since its approval, giving rituximab the most extensive clinical use of any biologic therapy to date.

No appreciable increase in infectious complications was observed with rituximab therapy over placebo in several randomized controlled trials for the treatment of nHL or B-cell chronic lymphocytic leukemia (CLL),[3,4] although 2 recent meta-analyses of randomized trials of rituximab maintenance therapy in lymphoma patients have reported a higher relative risk (2.90) of grade 3 to 4 infections with rituximab therapy.[5,6]

In some studies of human immunodeficiency virus (HIV)-associated nHL, addition of rituximab to standard chemotherapy was associated with a higher incidence of serious infections, particularly in patients with profound CD4 lymphopenia. A pooled assessment of 3 phase II randomized trials in which patients with HIV-associated nHL and a median CD4 count of 161 cells/μL receiving rituximab with standard chemotherapy reported a 14% incidence of serious opportunistic infections (OIs) within 3 months of chemotherapy completion despite trimethoprim-sulfamethoxazole and fluconazole prophylaxis, with the development of infections typically associated with impaired cellular immunity, including CMV retinitis, tuberculosis (TB), *Pneumocystis jirovecii* pneumonia (PCP), and salmonellosis.[7] Another phase III trial of patients with HIV-associated nHL treated with rituximab or placebo plus cyclophosphamide, hydroxydauno-mycin, oncovin (vincristine), and prednisone (CHOP) reported a significant difference in infectious mortality, 14% with rituximab (R-CHOP) compared with 2% with placebo.[8] Of patients treated with R-CHOP, the incidence of infectious mortality was far higher in patients with baseline CD4 counts less than 50 cells/μL (36%) than patients with CD4 counts 50 cells/μL or greater (6%). Several OIs developed within 6 months of ritux-imab therapy in patients treated with R-CHOP, including PCP, CMV, invasive candidi-asis, and *Mycobacterium avium intercellulare* (MAI), whereas no OIs were observed in the CHOP arm. Using more stringent enrollment criteria (exclusion of patients with

CD4 <100 cells/μL, prior OIs, or poor performance status), a phase II study of R-CHOP in HIV-associated patients with nHL reported a lower incidence of infection.[9] The depletion of B lymphocytes in patients with severe deficits in cellular immunity seems to increase the risk of developing OIs.

Hepatitis B virus (HBV) reactivation has been consistently associated with rituximab treatment in postmarketing reports. Humoral immunity to HBV surface antigen is known to play an important role in the containment of HBV infection, and several reports describe a reverse seroconversion phenomenon, with loss of protective HBV surface antibody and sometimes fulminant reactivation of HBV infection in rituximab recipients, particularly in patients with chronic HBV and detectable surface antigen before treatment.[10,11] A recent study of patients with resolved HBV infection (positive HBV core antibody and negative surface antigen) in an HBV-endemic area receiving R-CHOP or CHOP for nHL described a 23.8% reactivation rate at 6 months in patients receiving R-CHOP, including 1 case of progression to hepatic failure, and 0% reactivation in patients receiving CHOP alone.[12] The investigators associated rituximab exposure, male gender, and a lack of HBV surface antibody with HBV reactivation in this setting. Although most HBV reactivation seems to occur within 6 months of starting rituximab-containing therapy, reactivations as late as a year following therapy have been reported.[13] Assessment of HBV status before starting rituximab-containing chemotherapy is essential in patients from endemic areas or with risk factors for prior HBV infection. Lamivudine prophylaxis during rituximab-containing chemotherapy has been reported to prevent HBV reactivation,[11,14] and some groups recommend prophylactic HBV antiviral therapy in HBV surface antigen-positive patients for at least 6 months after completing chemotherapy.[15] Optimal management of patients with resolved HBV infection receiving rituximab chemotherapy is less well defined, but patients should at a minimum have HBV surface antigen, HBV viral load, and liver function test monitoring every few months to assess for HBV reactivation.

From the initial FDA approval of rituximab in 1997 to 2008, 76 cases of progressive multifocal leukoencephalopathy (PML) associated with rituximab use have been reported to the manufacturer's global safety database.[16] PML is traditionally associated with profound deficits in cellular immunity, and the role of rituximab-induced impairments in humoral immunity in the development of PML is far less clear. Most cases have been reported in patients with lymphoproliferative disorders, although cases have also been reported in patients receiving rituximab therapy for systemic lupus erythematosus, RA, and immune thrombocytopenic purpura.[17] Most of these patients were previously or concurrently exposed to other immunosuppressive therapies. Patients received a median of 6 rituximab doses and were exposed to rituximab for a median of 16 months before their PML diagnosis. The case fatality rate was high (90%), and the clinical course of these patients was rapidly progressive, with a 2-month median time to death after PML diagnosis. In 9 of 14 cases with available data, CD4 counts were less than 500 cells/μL. Although the absolute overall incidence of PML cases in patients exposed to rituximab is low, rituximab has carried a black box warning for PML since 2007, and active postmarketing surveillance is ongoing.

A case-control study of patients with persistent, relapsing *Babesia microti* infection and severe morbidity and death despite repeated courses of antiparasitic therapy identified rituximab treatment as an important factor in the inability to clear this infection. Patients required prolonged courses of antiparasitic therapy for cure, for at least 2 weeks after clearance of parasites on blood smear.[18]

A case series reported a higher rate of PCP infection in patients receiving rituximab in combination with CHOP-based chemotherapy for lymphoma (6%–13%) compared with patients receiving comparable CHOP-based regimens alone (4%). PCP has been linked to rituximab therapy in other case series and reports, although patients concurrently received steroids and other immunosuppressive therapy.[19–21] Although PCP infection has been classically associated with CD4 lymphocyte deficits, B-cell deficient mice are exquisitely sensitive to PCP infection and are unable to generate a protective CD4 memory and effector T-cell response to PCP.[22,23]

There have been several reports of TB and nontuberculous mycobacterial (NTM) infections in association with rituximab. A recent survey-based study of mycobacterial infections reported by members of the Emerging Infections Network identified 3 cases of TB and 5 cases of NTM associated with rituximab use.[24] Severe MAI infection and disseminated M kansasii and M wolinskyi infections have been reported in patients receiving rituximab, although patients in these cases also received other concurrent immunosuppression.[25,26] B lymphocytes seem to be important in the containment of TB in murine infection models, and B-lymphocyte knockout mice are unable to contain TB infections, with an increased pulmonary mycobacterial burden compared with mice with normal B-cell function.[27] B lymphocytes are present in the periphery of tuberculous granulomas in active folliclelike centers associated with antigen-presenting cells and CD4 and CD8 T lymphocytes in human TB infection, and are believed to help orchestrate containment of infection.[28]

Several other severe infections have been linked to rituximab use at a sporadic case report level, including persistent enteroviral meningoencephalitis,[29–31] CMV disease,[32–34] disseminated varicella-zoster virus (VZV),[35,36] pure red cell aplasia from parvovirus B19 infection,[37–39] West Nile virus meningoencephalitis,[40–42] and nocardiosis,[43,44] although all patients received rituximab in combination with other immunosuppressive therapies, and the causal role of rituximab itself is unclear.

ANTI-TNF-α THERAPIES: INFLIXIMAB, ADALIMUMAB, ETANERCEPT, CERTOLIZUMAB PEGOL, GOLIMUMAB

Infliximab, adalimumab, and golimumab are monoclonal antibodies directed against TNF-α, certolizumab pegol is a pegylated fragment antigen-binding (Fab) fragment of a humanized anti-TNF-α monoclonal antibody, and etanercept is a soluble receptor for TNF-α. All of these therapies abrogate TNF-α activity to varying degrees, and are effective treatment modalities for various inflammatory conditions. The monoclonal antibodies bind soluble and cell-surface TNF-α, with fixation of complement and lysis of T lymphocytes and neutrophils expressing surface TNF-α, whereas etanercept is able to bind only to soluble TNF-α and does not seem to have the same lytic effect on cells expressing membrane-bound TNF-α.[45] TNF-α is essential for macrophage activation, phagosome activation, differentiation of monocytes into macrophages, recruitment of neutrophils and macrophages, granuloma formation, and maintenance of granuloma integrity, and therapy with TNF-α blockers is associated with a particularly increased risk of granulomatous and intracellular infections.[46–48]

Infliximab was approved in 1998 for the treatment of RA, psoriatic arthritis and plaque psoriasis, ankylosing spondylitis, ulcerative colitis, and Crohn disease. Adalimumab was approved in 1999, and has the same treatment indications as infliximab, except for ulcerative colitis. Etanercept was approved in 2001 for the treatment of RA, psoriasis and psoriatic arthritis, and ankylosing spondylitis. In 2009, the FDA approved golimumab for RA, psoriatic arthritis, and ankylosing spondylitis, and certolizumab for RA and Crohn disease refractory to conventional therapy.

The overall incidence of serious infections associated with anti-TNF-α therapy has been estimated from comprehensive national registry data of RA patients from the

United Kingdom[49] and Germany[50] at 5.2 to 6.2 per 100 patient-years in patients with infliximab, 6.3 per 100 patient-years with adalimumab, and 5.3 to 6.4 per 100 person-years with etanercept. The German biologics register study adjusted for differences in patient characteristics using propensity scores, and reported an adjusted relative risk for total serious adverse infectious events of 2.2 with etanercept and 3.0 with infliximab use. An observational cohort study of the Swedish biologics register of RA patients assessed the risk of hospitalization with infection with anti-TNF-α therapy, and reported an increased relative risk of 1.43 during the first year, 1.15 during the second year, and no difference in the risk of hospitalization in subsequent years compared with RA patients not receiving anti-TNF-α therapy.[51] A meta-analysis of anti-TNF-α therapy trials in RA reported an odds ratio (OR) of 2.0 for serious infections and 3.3 for malignancy in patients receiving anti-TNF-α therapy, compared with placebo, with only 12 granulomatous infections (10 cases of TB, 1 of histoplasmosis, and 1 of coccidioidomycosis) in 126 serious infections.[52]

An association between anti-TNF-α therapy and TB was noted a few years after the initial approval of infliximab.[53] A query of the FDA MedWatch spontaneous reporting system in 2001 showed 70 TB cases developing a median of 12 weeks after initial infliximab exposure, with a high proportion of extrapulmonary dissemination (57%), and a frequent lack of granuloma formation in patients with biopsy samples. In the United States, the rate of granulomatous and intracellular infection in patients receiving anti-TNF-α therapy has been estimated from the FDA adverse event reporting system, which relies on spontaneous reporting of cases, unlike national registries. These infections were more common in patients receiving infliximab (129 events per 100,000 patients) than etanercept (60 events per 100,000 patients).[54,55] The rate of TB was 54 per 100,000 patients in infliximab patients, with a rate ratio of 1.9 compared with etanercept patients, and the median time to TB was substantially shorter in infliximab patients (17 weeks) than etanercept patients (48 weeks). A case-control study of RA patients in an American pharmaceutical claims database also identified a higher rate ratio in patients treated with biologic therapy (1.5) compared with patients receiving nonbiologic RA therapy, and also reported an earlier median time to TB in patients receiving infliximab (17 weeks) than in patients receiving etanercept (79 weeks).[56] A Monte Carlo simulation of time to reactivation of latent TB calculated a median monthly rate of TB reactivation of 20.8% in patients receiving infliximab, 12.1-fold higher than patients receiving etanercept.[57] There was a clustering of infliximab-associated TB reactivation cases in the first year; the risk of progression of new TB infection to active disease was comparable in infliximab and etanercept patients, suggesting that much of the excess risk of TB with infliximab therapy over etanercept is a consequence of more efficient latent TB reactivation shortly after starting anti-TNF-α therapy, whereas both infliximab and etanercept fairly equally increase the risk of active incident disease. In TB patients receiving anti-TNF-α therapy, an immune reconstitution inflammatory syndrome-like reaction has been described after withdrawal of these agents, sometimes requiring the reinitiation of these agents to control an overly exuberant and deleterious host immune response.[58,59]

NTM infections have also been associated with anti-TNF-α therapy. The rate of NTM in the United States has been estimated at 9 cases per 100,000 patients with infliximab and 6 cases per 100,000 patients with etanercept.[54] A recent survey asking members of the Emerging Infections Network to identify all cases of TB and NTM in patients receiving anti-TNF-α therapy in their clinical practice during the prior 6 months found that reports of NTM (65%) exceeded reports of TB.[24] Most cases were MAI infections, but cases of *M chelonae*, *M abscessus*, *M marinum*, *M fortuitum*, *M haemophilum*, *M kansasii*, and *M scrofulaceum* were also reported. Cases of lepromatous leprosy have been reported in patients from Louisiana, Texas, and the Brazilian Amazon receiving anti-TNF-α therapy for various indications, with high numbers of bacilli on biopsy.[60–62] The progression of disease has been observed to be faster than usual in these patients. A type 1 reversal reaction was described in the 2 North American patients a month after discontinuing anti-TNF-α therapy and starting antibiotic therapy, with exacerbation of skin lesions, malaise, and greater organization of the inflammatory infiltrate on skin biopsy.[61] Severe infections with other rare mycobacterial pathogens, such as M peregrinum,[63] M aurum,[64] M bovis,[65] and M szulgai[66] have been described on a case report level in patients receiving anti-TNF-α therapy.

Histoplasmosis has been associated with anti-TNF-α therapy, with a significantly higher rate in infliximab (19 cases per 100,000 patients) than etanercept recipients (3 cases per 100,000 patients) in the United States.[54] Most cases have been reported within 6 months of initiation of anti-TNF-α therapy,[67] and many of the reported cases have been associated with disseminated disease.[68,69]

Coccidioidomycosis has been reported in association with anti-TNF-α therapy, also with significantly higher rates with infliximab (11 cases per 100,000 patients) than etanercept (1 case per 100,000 patients) exposure in the United States.[54,70] An assessment of patients with inflammatory arthritis living in Coccidioides immitis–endemic areas reported a relative risk of approximately 5 for coccidioidomycosis with infliximab compared with other antirheumatic drugs.[71]

The rate of cryptococcosis in the United States is estimated at 9 cases per 100,000 patients exposed to anti-TNF-α therapy, and there is no notable difference in patients treated with infliximab or etanercept.[54]

TNF-α is essential for normal activation of macrophage phagosomes and clearance of intracellular pathogens, and several intracellular infections have been associated with anti-TNF-α therapy, including Listeria bacteremia and meningitis,[54,72,73] which has been reported at higher rates in infliximab (9 cases per 100,000 patients) than etanercept (1 case per 100,000 patients) recipients, Legionella pneumonia,[54,74,75] and salmonellosis.[54,76,77] Several intracellular protozoal pathogens have been reported in association with anti-TNF-α therapy, including relapsing cutaneous and visceral leishmaniasis in endemic areas,[78–80] overwhelming Plasmodium falciparum parasitemia,[81] and a report of an eventually fatal progressive myositis caused by Brachiola algerae.[82]

TNF-α enhances conidial phagocytosis by alveolar macrophages, augments the effectiveness of polymorphonuclear cells against Aspergillus hyphae, and contributes to the recruitment and activation of neutrophils and mononuclear cells in the lung; anti-TNF-α therapy has been associated with an increased risk of invasive fungal infections, with overall invasive aspergillosis (IA) and invasive candidasis rates of approximately 7 to 8 cases per 100,000 exposed patients.[54,83] A review of invasive fungal infections associated with TNF-α inhibition identified 281 cases, most associated with infliximab therapy, and many associated with concurrent corticosteroid therapy.[70] IA was associated with TNF-α therapy in 64 reports, invasive candidiasis in 64 cases, and zygomycosis in 4 cases. Other fungi that generally cause localized disease, such as Trichophyton rubrum and Sporothrix schenckii infection, have been associated with disseminated disease in recipients of anti-TNF-α therapy.[84,85]

Other infections associated with anti-TNF-α therapy include PCP,[86–88] nocardiosis (~4 cases per 100,000 infliximab recipients),[54] toxoplasmosis (~2 cases per 100,000 infliximab recipients),[54,89] bartonellosis,[54] and brucellosis.[54]

The relationship between TNF-α inhibition and reactivation of latent and chronic viral infections is less well defined. A recent assessment of herpes zoster in the large German biologics registry reported 86 episodes, with a crude incidence rate of

11.1 per 1000 patient-years with monoclonal antibodies (adalimumab, infliximab), 8.9 for etanercept, and 5.6 with conventional disease-modifying antirheumatic therapy. Adjusting for other factors, the hazard ratio of herpes zoster with monoclonal antibody therapy compared with conventional therapy was 1.8, and there was no discernible increase in risk with etanercept.[90] An assessment of large patient databases from the United States and the United Kingdom identified an increased risk of zoster with conventional disease-modifying RA therapy and a higher risk (OR 1.5) in patients receiving biologic therapy.[91] Reactivation of other herpesviruses has not clearly been associated with anti-TNF-α therapy, although 3 cases of herpes simplex virus encephalitis were recently reported in patients receiving infliximab or adalimumab.[92] Several cases of severe HBV reactivation in patients with positive surface antigen at the start of anti-TNF-α therapy have been reported,[93–95] although concurrent lamivudine treatment may decrease the risk of reactivation in these patients.[96]

Allogeneic HSCT recipients with severe steroid-refractory acute graft-versus-host disease (GVHD) have a high risk of invasive fungal disease (IFD) and CMV reactivation, likely because of the loss of normal mucosal barrier integrity and heavy concurrent immune suppression; the addition of anti-TNF-α therapy further increases the risk of these infections. A retrospective evaluation of 21 patients receiving infliximab for steroid-refractory GVHD reported the development of bacterial infections in 81%, viral reactivations in 67% (predominantly CMV), and invasive fungal infections in 48% of patients.[97] Patients receiving infliximab for severe steroid-refractory GVHD at the authors' institution had a high incidence rate of IFD (6.8 cases per 1000 GVHD patient-days) compared with 0.53 cases per 1000 GVHD patient-days in patients not exposed to infliximab.[98] The adjusted hazard ratio for IFD in patients exposed to infliximab was 13.6 compared with patients who were not exposed.

Clinical experience with certolizumab pegol and golimumab is limited. Some studies of certolizumab for Crohn disease and RA have reported an increased incidence of serious infections compared with placebo, including several cases of TB.[99–101] Although many randomized trials of golimumab have shown no increase in the overall incidence of serious infections compared with placebo, a trial in RA patients also treated with methotrexate[102] and a trial in patients with severe asthma refractory to high-dose inhaled steroids and β2 agonists[103] reported a higher incidence of serious infections with golimumab therapy, with 1 case of TB and 1 case of *Legionella* pneumonia. As golimumab is similar in structure to infliximab, it is likely that a comparable pattern of OIs will emerge with further clinical use.

A consensus group statement on the use of biologic agents in patients with RA recommends measures to reduce infectious complications in patients receiving anti-TNF-α therapy, including screening for latent TB infection and assessment for latent or chronic HBV and hepatitis C virus infection before starting therapy.[104]

ANTI-INTERLEUKIN 1 THERAPIES: ANAKINRA, RILONACEPT

The cytokine interleukin 1 (IL-1) is secreted by numerous cell types in response to inflammatory antigens, and has a wide range of biologic activity, including mediation of the febrile response to infection and inflammation, B-cell activation, induction of IL-2 with subsequent stimulation of T-cell maturation, and induction of IL-6, TNF-γ, and IL-8.

Anakinra, a recombinant IL-1 receptor antagonist, was approved for the treatment of moderate to severe RA in 2001. It competitively inhibits binding of IL-1 to IL-1 type I receptor, with a decrease in the response to inflammatory stimuli. The German biologics registry reported a rate of 3.2 serious infections per 100 patient-years in patients exposed to anakinra, although the total number of patients receiving anakinra was small.[50] A meta-analysis of all randomized placebo-controlled trials evaluating anakinra in RA reported a 1.4% incidence of serious infections with anakinra, compared with 0.5% with placebo, and the OR of serious infection was 3.40 in patients treated with high-dose anakinra versus placebo, although this difference was not significant when results were adjusted for underlying comorbidities.[105] Pneumonia and other bacterial infections accounted for most events; no OIs were reported. One case of TB was reported in a patient enrolled in an RA study who had underlying pneumoconiosis from mining,[106] and 1 case of visceral leishmaniasis was reported in a child living in an endemic area of France receiving anakinra for systemic onset juvenile idiopathic arthritis 6 months after starting treatment.[107]

Rilonacept is a dimeric fusion protein of the ligand-binding domain of the extracellular portion of the human IL-1 receptor and IL-1 receptor accessory protein linked to the Fc portion of human IgG1. It acts as a soluble decoy receptor and binds IL-1β, preventing its normal binding to IL-1 receptors. Rilonacept was approved in 2008 for the treatment of cryopyrin-associated periodic syndromes (CAPS), characterized by excessive IL-1β production. In a study of 47 patients with CAPS, rilonacept was associated with upper respiratory infections in 26% of patients, compared with 4% in patients receiving placebo.[108] One case of Streptococcus pneumoniae meningitis developed during the open-label extension period, but was believed not to be related to the study drug. The rilonacept package insert reported a case of MAI olecranon bursitis in a patient receiving rilonacept for an unapproved indication and intra-articular glucocorticoid injections.

ALEMTUZUMAB

Alemtuzumab is a humanized monoclonal IgG1 that targets CD52 on normal and neoplastic B and T lymphocytes, monocytes, macrophages, and NK cells, with lysis of these cell populations and substantial sustained deficits in cell-mediated and humoral immunity. CD4 and CD8 T-lymphocyte counts reach their nadir approximately 4 weeks after administration, and median counts remain at less than 25% of baseline values for approximately 9 months.[109]

Alemtuzumab received accelerated approval by the FDA in 2001 for the treatment of B-cell CLL refractory to alkylating agents and fludarabine, and regular approval for single-agent therapy for B-cell CLL in 2007.

A wide spectrum of infections has been associated with alemtuzumab therapy, particularly herpesvirus reactivations, incident viral infections, and invasive fungal infections. Before the routine use of PCP and herpesvirus prophylaxis in these patients, a phase II study of alemtuzumab for the treatment of fludarabine-refractory CLL reported a 41.7% incidence of OIs, including reactivation of latent herpesviruses (CMV, disseminated VZV) and invasive fungal infections (PCP, IA, candidiasis). Severe infections were reported in 8% of patients in the first, 6% in the second, and 7% in the third month of therapy.[110] Another phase II study of alemtuzumab in this patient population used PCP prophylaxis and valacyclovir herpesvirus prophylaxis but still reported a 20% incidence of CMV reactivation, and cases of disseminated VZV, probable IA, sinus zygomycosis, and disseminated NTM infection.[111] A larger multicenter study in this population mandated PCP and herpesvirus prophylaxis in all patients, and reported a lower incidence of overall grade 3 to 4 infection (26.9%) and CMV reactivation (8%). Several OIs developed after alemtuzumab treatment despite prophylaxis, including PCP, IA, rhinocerebral zygomycosis, cryptococcal pneumonia, invasive candidiasis, herpes zoster, and Listeria meningitis.[112]

A retrospective evaluation of 27 patients receiving alemtuzumab for lymphoproliferative disorders, primarily CLL, at the authors' institution showed a high rate of OIs (33%) and non-OIs (82%) despite PCP and herpesvirus prophylaxis.[113] Patients developed a diverse array of OIs (IA, disseminated histoplasmosis, adenovirus pneumonia, PML, cerebral toxoplasmosis, CMV disease, and disseminated acathamebiasis) a median of 169 days after starting alemtuzumab. Many patients (44%) developed asymptomatic CMV viremia on hybrid-capture assay. Infections contributed to mortality in 7 of 10 patients who died.

A lower incidence of infection has been reported in studies of alemtuzumab as first-line therapy for CLL, compared with studies in patients heavily exposed to prior chemotherapy regimens for refractory CLL. In a phase II study of first-line treatment of patients with symptomatic CLL, only 10% of patients developed CMV reactivation and no patients developed CMV disease.[114] In a large study of treatment-naive CLL patients randomized to either alemtuzumab or chlorambucil single-agent therapy, 15.6% of patients in the alemtuzumab arm developed symptomatic CMV infection without CMV disease, although 52.4% of patients receiving alemtuzumab had asymptomatic CMV viremia, compared with only 7.5% in patients receiving chlorambucil.[115] No other OIs were reported in this study.

Several cases of severe mycobacterial infections have been reported in patients with CLL treated with alemtuzumab, including disseminated MAI,[116] disseminated *M bovis* in a patient concurrently receiving intravesical bacille Calmette-Guérin therapy for localized bladder cancer,[117] cutaneous *M haemophilum* infection,[118] and cutaneous *M chelonae* infection.[119]

The use of alemtuzumab for T-cell depletion in nonmyeloablative allogeneic HSCT is associated with a particularly high incidence of CMV reactivation (50%–85%),[113,120–123] severe adenovirus infection and disease (40%), particularly in patients with low absolute lymphocyte counts,[122] respiratory virus infections, including influenza, parainfluenza, and respiratory syncytial virus (30%), with frequent progression to lower respiratory tract infection,[124] and symptomatic *Human herpesvirus 6* encephalitis (11.6%).[125] A recent large retrospective evaluation of posttransplant lymphoproliferative disorder (PTLD) cases in allogeneic HSCT recipients identified alemtuzumab T-cell depletion as a significant risk factor for the development of PTLD, with a relative risk of 3.1, although the risk of PTLD with alemtuzumab was substantially lower than with other T-cell depleting modalities.[126]

A retrospective assessment of a large number of solid-organ transplant patients receiving alemtuzumab for prevention or treatment of allograft rejection described a 10% incidence of OIs, including CMV disease in 3% of patients, and several cases of BK virus infection, PTLD, esophageal candidiasis, cryptococcosis, other IFDs, nocardiosis, mycobacterial infections, and isolated cases of *Parvovirus B19* infection, *Balamuthia mandrillaris*, and toxoplasmosis. The incidence of OI was higher in patients receiving alemtuzumab for treatment of rejection (21%) compared with patients treated with alemtuzumab for induction (4.5%). The OR for the development of an OI after alemtuzumab exposure was particularly high in lung (3.7) and intestinal transplant (8.3) recipients.[127]

All patients receiving alemtuzumab should receive PCP and herpesvirus prophylaxis. Given the high incidence of CMV infection with alemtuzumab treatment, CMV prophylaxis or close monitoring with preemptive therapy may be warranted. One study reported the effectiveness of prompt initiation of preemptive CMV therapy in preventing CMV disease despite a high rate of CMV reactivation.[128] A recent study randomized patients receiving alemtuzumab for various hematologic malignancies to prophylactic valacyclovir 500 mg daily or valganciclovir 450 mg twice daily, and reported no CMV reactivation in the valganciclovir arm, versus 35% in the acyclovir arm.[129]

BLOCKING ACTIVATED T-LYMPHOCYTE PROLIFERATION: DACLIZUMAB, BASLIXIMAB

Daclizumab and basiliximab are monoclonal antibodies that target CD25, the α chain of the IL-2 receptor complex expressed on activated alloantigen-reactive T lymphocytes, with competitive inhibition of IL-2 binding and abatement of IL-2-mediated lymphocyte proliferation, differentiation, and cytokine release. Antigen-specific alloreactive T cells are depleted, with a blunted response to antigenic challenge. The FDA approved daclizumab in 1997 and basiliximab in 1998 for the prophylaxis of acute allograft rejection in renal transplant recipients in combination with other immunosuppressive therapy.

Daclizumab does not seem to be associated with an increased risk of infectious complications in solid-organ transplantation. In randomized controlled trials of daclizumab in renal transplantation, a decreased incidence of acute rejection has been reported with daclizumab compared with placebo, with a lower requirement for antirejection therapy, and possibly a lower incidence of CMV reactivation.[130,131] Daclizumab for prophylaxis of acute rejection in cardiac transplantation has also been reported to reduce the risk of rejection, with a comparable incidence of serious OI at 6 months (6.9%) compared with placebo.[132] One retrospective study of lung transplant patients at a single national center reported daclizumab use in induction as a risk factor for the development of IA, with an OR of 2.05 compared with polyclonal induction regimens, but this has not been corroborated by other reports.[133]

A high rate of infectious mortality has been reported in allogeneic HSCT recipients receiving daclizumab for steroid-refractory acute GVHD, although a causal role for daclizumab is unclear, given the high baseline risk of OI in this population. In 1 series, 10 of 43 patients died of GVHD and infection and 7 patients died of infection. Three patients, all of whom were T-cell-depleted unrelated-donor HSCT recipients, developed EBV-associated PTLD during or after daclizumab exposure.[134] In a retrospective assessment of patients receiving daclizumab for steroid-refractory GVHD, 95% of patients developed OIs by 6 months, and infection contributed to mortality in 79% of patients who died.[135] Bacterial infections were reported in 88% of all patients, viral infections in 53%, with CMV infection in 35% and EBV-associated PTLD in 7%, and IFD in 51%, with IA in 12% of patients, 1 *Scedosporium apiospermum* infection, and 1 *Cunninghamella* infection. Other OIs reported in this study included 3 MAI infections, and 1 case each of TB, toxoplasmosis, nocardiosis, and *Legionella* infection.

Similar to daclizumab, basiliximab does not seem to be generally associated with an increased risk of serious infection in renal,[136–138] cardiac,[139,140] or liver transplantation.[141,142] A large randomized study comparing basiliximab with antithymocyte globulin identified a higher incidence of acute rejection episodes in patients randomized to basiliximab and a higher incidence of CMV disease in the basiliximab arm (17.5 vs 7.8%) in this context.[143]

Data on basiliximab use for treatment of steroid-refractory acute GVHD are limited; a single prospective phase II study reported infections in 65% of patients, with CMV reactivation in 22% of patients, 2 cases of IFD, and 1 case of cerebral toxoplasmosis.

SELECTIVE T-CELL COSTIMULATION BLOCKADE: ABATACEPT, BELATACEPT

Abatacept and belatacept are soluble fusion proteins comprised of the extracellular domain of anticytotoxic T-lymphocyte-associated antigen 4 and the Fc portion of IgG1. These proteins block the costimulatory engagement of CD80 or CD86 on antigen-presenting cells with CD28 on T lymphocytes, preventing full T-lymphocyte activation. Abatacept was approved by the FDA in 2005 for the treatment of RA, and belatacept is currently being reviewed for approval. Some randomized controlled trials of abatacept in RA have reported a higher incidence of serious infections than placebo, particularly in patients receiving other concurrent biologic therapy,[144–146] with approximately 5 cases of serious infection per 100 patient-years in patients treated with prolonged courses of therapy,[147,148] although a recent meta-analysis of trials in RA patients did not show a statistically significant increase in infections overall.[105] Most of these serious infections are pneumonias and pyogenic bacterial infections, although a single case of IA and a possible case of TB have been reported. Exposure to abatacept confers a lesser risk of TB reactivation than exposure to murine anti-TNF-α therapy in a mouse TB infection model; mice treated with abatacept for 16 weeks were able to control their *M tuberculosis* infection and all animals survived to the end of the experiment, whereas 100% of mice treated with anti-TNF-α therapy died with disseminated TB infection.[149] Mice treated with abatacept had similar activated T-lymphocyte, macrophage, B-lymphocyte, and neutrophil counts compared with mice treated only with the carrier vehicle and produced a comparable IFN-γ response to infection. The clinical experience with belatacept is limited; in a randomized controlled trial of belatacept versus cyclosporine in combination with basiliximab, mycophenolate mofetil, and corticosteroids for induction therapy in patients receiving renal transplantation, 1 patient developed PTLD while receiving intensive belatacept, and 2 additional patients in the belatacept arm developed PTLD after belatacept was replaced with conventional agents.[150]

THERAPIES INTERFERING WITH T-LYMPHOCYTE MIGRATION: NATALIZUMAB, EFALIZUMAB

Natalizumab is a humanized IgG4 that targets the α_4 subunit of $\alpha_4\beta_1$ and $\alpha_4\beta_7$ integrins on the surface of activated T lymphocytes, inhibiting binding to cellular adhesion molecules in the central nervous system and the gastrointestinal tract and blocking migration of T lymphocytes into these tissues. Treatment is associated with a profound decrease in CD4, CD8, and CD19 lymphocytes in the cerebrospinal fluid.[151] Natalizumab was initially approved for the treatment of relapsing multiple sclerosis (MS) in 2004, then withdrawn from the market a few months later after 3 cases of PML were reported in clinical trials in patients with prolonged exposure to natalizumab and interferon β-1a combination therapy,[152–154] with an overall risk of 1 case per 1000 exposed patients treated for an average of 17.9 months.[155] Natalizumab was reintroduced as MS monotherapy in 2006 with a black box warning about the risk of PML. Additional cases of PML in patients receiving prolonged natalizumab monotherapy (12–31 months) have been reported since that time, with an associated mortality of 23%.[16] In addition to PML, other sporadic OIs were reported in natalizumab recipients during the FDA hearing for market reapproval, including viral meningitis and encephalitis, CMV infection, pulmonary IA, PCP pneumonia, VZV pneumonia, and MAI, although many patients were receiving concurrent immunosuppression.[151] Natalizumab was recently approved for the treatment of refractory Crohn disease.

Efalizumab is a monoclonal IgG1 that binds to CD11a, the α-subunit of leukocyte functional antigen 1 (LFA-1) on activated T lymphocytes, inhibiting lymphocyte binding to endothelial cellular adhesion molecules and blocking migration of these cells through the endothelium during inflammation. It was initially approved for the treatment of plaque psoriasis in 2003, and received a black box warning in 2008, when 3 confirmed PML cases and 1 possible case were reported in patients exposed to efalizumab monotherapy for more than 3 years, with a risk of 1 case per 400 exposed patients. None of these patients had other underlying chronic conditions, and patients were not receiving concurrent immunosuppression with other agents.[16] Other sporadic OIs typically associated with impairment in cell-mediated immunity were reported in association with efalizumab therapy, including visceral leishmaniasis in a patient living in an endemic area,[156] disseminated cryptococcosis,[157] and CMV reactivation.[158] Given its unfavorable risk-benefit profile, efalizumab was voluntarily withdrawn from the market in 2009.

ALEFACEPT

Alefacept is a recombinant fusion protein of human lymphocyte function-associated antigen-3 (LFA-3) and a portion of human IgG1. It binds to CD2 receptors on T lymphocytes to block their activation and to FcγRIII on NK cells, with apoptosis of CD2 memory-effector T-lymphocytes and dose-dependent reductions in CD4 and CD8 T-lymphocyte counts for approximately 28 weeks. Despite the depletion of CD4+CD45RO+ and CD8+CD45RO+ cell populations, naive T-cell populations are relatively preserved, and the T-cell-dependent humoral immune response to extrinsic antigens seems to be preserved in patients receiving alefacept challenged with neoantigen (φX174) vaccination.[159] Responses to a recall antigen (tetanus toxoid) were also preserved despite a quantitative loss of memory-effector cells. Alefacept was approved in 2003 for the treatment of moderate to severe plaque psoriasis. A meta-analysis of randomized controlled trials of alefacept for plaque psoriasis reported no discernible increase in serious infections in alefacept recipients compared with placebo.[160] Despite a depletion of CD4 counts, OIs have only rarely been reported in patients receiving alefacept to date: 1 patient receiving alefacept and infliximab concurrently developed disseminated *Nocardia farcinica* infection,[161] and a patient receiving alefacept for psoriasis with a CD4 count of 298 cells/μL developed MAI olecranon bursitis.[162]

PROLONGED NEUTROPENIA: GEMTUZUMAB OZOGAMICIN

Gemtuzumab ozogamicin (GO) is a humanized monoclonal antibody directed at CD33 conjugated to calicheamicin, an antibiotic with potent antitumor activity that cleaves double-stranded DNA at specific sequences. Most myeloid blast cells in acute myelogenous leukemia (AML) express CD33, as do normal hematopoietic progenitor cells. GO was approved in 2000 for the treatment of CD33+ AML in first relapse in patients 60 years of age or older who are not candidates for other cytotoxic chemotherapy. Because it targets normal hematopoietic progenitor cells along with malignant myeloid cells, GO is associated with prolonged myelosuppression, with neutropenia lasting approximately 40 days in patients with a clinical response to GO, accompanied by risk of bacteremia and pneumonia.[163] Despite prolonged neutropenia, an increased risk of IFD has not been described in GO recipients.

SUMMARY

Our understanding of the infectious risks associated with the use of these targeted therapies is nascent. Each biologic target (eg, CD20, CD33) may predispose a different infectious susceptibility. Altering the disease targeted, using the biologic therapy at a different point in the disease process (eg, initial vs salvage therapy) or for off-label indications, and altering the dose or the frequency of administration may all substantively affect the infectious risk engendered with these immunotherapies. Optimal minimization of infectious complications associated with the use of these agents requires vigilance. Patients receiving certain targeted biologic immunomodulators are at higher risk for the reactivation of latent or chronic infections and the acquisition of incident infection than patients not exposed to these therapies. Patients should be screened for latent and chronic infections associated with these biologic agents before starting therapy, and receive prophylactic or preemptive therapy for these infections if screening is positive. Careful assessment for emergent illness is required, as usual presenting symptoms of infection may be altered or absent.

REFERENCES

1. Shortt J, Spencer A. Adjuvant rituximab causes prolonged hypogammaglobulinaemia following autologous stem cell transplant for non-Hodgkin's lymphoma. Bone Marrow Transplant 2006;38:433.
2. McLaughlin P, Grillo-Lopez AJ, Link BK, et al. Rituximab chimeric anti-CD20 monoclonal antibody therapy for relapsed indolent lymphoma: half of patients respond to a four-dose treatment program. J Clin Oncol 1998;16:2825.
3. Byrd JC, Rai K, Peterson BL, et al. Addition of rituximab to fludarabine may prolong progression-free survival and overall survival in patients with previously untreated chronic lymphocytic leukemia: an updated retrospective comparative analysis of CALGB 9712 and CALGB 9011. Blood 2005;105:49.
4. Rafailidis PI, Kakisi OK, Vardakas K, et al. Infectious complications of monoclonal antibodies used in cancer therapy: a systematic review of the evidence from randomized controlled trials. Cancer 2007;109:2182.
5. Aksoy S, Dizdar O, Hayran M, et al. Infectious complications of rituximab in patients with lymphoma during maintenance therapy: a systematic review and meta-analysis. Leuk Lymphoma 2009;50:357.
6. Vidal L, Gafter-Gvili A, Leibovici L, et al. Rituximab maintenance for the treatment of patients with follicular lymphoma: systematic review and meta-analysis of randomized trials. J Natl Cancer Inst 2009;101:248.
7. Spina M, Jaeger U, Sparano JA, et al. Rituximab plus infusional cyclophosphamide, doxorubicin, and etoposide in HIV-associated non-Hodgkin lymphoma: pooled results from 3 phase 2 trials. Blood 2005;105:1891.
8. Kaplan LD, Lee JY, Ambinder RF, et al. Rituximab does not improve clinical outcome in a randomized phase 3 trial of CHOP with or without rituximab in patients with HIV-associated non-Hodgkin lymphoma: AIDS-Malignancies Consortium Trial 010. Blood 2005;106:1538.
9. Boue F, Gabarre J, Gisselbrecht C, et al. Phase II trial of CHOP plus rituximab in patients with HIV-associated non-Hodgkin's lymphoma. J Clin Oncol 2006;24:4123.
10. Dervite I, Hober D, Morel P. Acute hepatitis B in a patient with antibodies to hepatitis B surface antigen who was receiving rituximab. N Engl J Med 2001;344:68.
11. Tsutsumi Y, Tanaka J, Kawamura T, et al. Possible efficacy of lamivudine treatment to prevent hepatitis B virus reactivation due to rituximab therapy in a patient with non-Hodgkin's lymphoma. Ann Hematol 2004;83:58.
12. Yeo W, Chan TC, Leung NW, et al. Hepatitis B virus reactivation in lymphoma patients with prior resolved hepatitis B undergoing anticancer therapy with or without rituximab. J Clin Oncol 2009;27:605.
13. Garcia-Rodriguez MJ, Canales MA, Hernandez-Maraver D, et al. Late reactivation of resolved hepatitis B virus infection: an increasing complication post rituximab-based regimens treatment? Am J Hematol 2008;83:673.
14. Hamaki T, Kami M, Kusumi E, et al. Prophylaxis of hepatitis B reactivation using lamivudine in a patient receiving rituximab. Am J Hematol 2001;68:292.

15. Yeo W, Johnson PJ. Diagnosis, prevention and management of hepatitis B virus reactivation during anticancer therapy. Hepatology 2006;43:209.

16. Carson KR, Focosi D, Major EO, et al. Monoclonal antibody-associated progressive multifocal leucoencephalopathy in patients treated with rituximab, natalizumab, and efalizumab: a review from the Research on Adverse Drug Events and Reports (RADAR) Project. Lancet Oncol 2009;10:816.

17. Carson KR, Evens AM, Richey EA, et al. Progressive multifocal leukoencephalopathy after rituximab therapy in HIV-negative patients: a report of 57 cases from the Research on Adverse Drug Events and Reports project. Blood 2009;113:4834.

18. Krause PJ, Gewurz BE, Hill D, et al. Persistent and relapsing babesiosis in immunocompromised patients. Clin Infect Dis 2008;46:370.

19. Kumar D, Gourishankar S, Mueller T, et al. *Pneumocystis jirovecii* pneumonia after rituximab therapy for antibody-mediated rejection in a renal transplant recipient. Transpl Infect Dis 2009;11:167.

20. Teichmann LL, Woenckhaus M, Vogel C, et al. Fatal *Pneumocystis pneumonia* following rituximab administration for rheumatoid arthritis. Rheumatology (Oxford) 2008;47:1256.

21. Venhuizen AC, Hustinx WN, van Houte AJ, et al. Three cases of *Pneumocystis jirovecii* pneumonia (PCP) during first-line treatment with rituximab in combination with CHOP-14 for aggressive B-cell non-Hodgkin's lymphoma. Eur J Haematol 2008;80:275.

22. Lund FE, Hollifield M, Schuer K, et al. B cells are required for generation of protective effector and memory CD4 cells in response to pneumocystis lung infection. J Immunol 2006;176:6147.

23. Marcotte H, Levesque D, Delanay K, et al. *Pneumocystis carinii* infection in transgenic B cell-deficient mice. J Infect Dis 1996;173:1034.

24. Winthrop KL, Yamashita S, Beekmann SE, et al. Mycobacterial and other serious infections in patients receiving anti-tumor necrosis factor and other newly approved biologic therapies: case finding through the Emerging Infections Network. Clin Infect Dis 2008;46:1738.

25. Chen YC, Jou R, Huang WL, et al. Bacteremia caused by *Mycobacterium wolinskyi*. Emerg Infect Dis 2008;14:1818.

26. Lutt JR, Pisculli ML, Weinblatt ME, et al. Severe nontuberculous mycobacterial infection in 2 patients receiving rituximab for refractory myositis. J Rheumatol 2008;35:1683.

27. Maglione PJ, Xu J, Chan J. B cells moderate inflammatory progression and enhance bacterial containment upon pulmonary challenge with *Mycobacterium tuberculosis*. J Immunol 2007;178:7222.

28. Ulrichs T, Kosmiadi GA, Trusov V, et al. Human tuberculous granulomas induce peripheral lymphoid follicle-like structures to orchestrate local host defence in the lung. J Pathol 2004;204:217.

29. Archimbaud C, Bailly JL, Chambon M, et al. Molecular evidence of persistent echovirus 13 meningoencephalitis in a patient with relapsed lymphoma after an outbreak of meningitis in 2000. J Clin Microbiol 2003;41:4605.

30. Padate BP, Keidan J. Enteroviral meningoencephalitis in a patient with non-Hodgkin's lymphoma treated previously with rituximab. Clin Lab Haematol 2006;28:69.

31. Quartier P, Tournilhac O, Archimbaud C, et al. Enteroviral meningoencephalitis after anti-CD20 (rituximab) treatment. Clin Infect Dis 2003;36:e47.

32. Goldberg SL, Pecora AL, Alter RS, et al. Unusual viral infections (progressive multifocal leukoencephalopathy and cytomegalovirus disease) after high-dose

chemotherapy with autologous blood stem cell rescue and peritransplantation rituximab. Blood 2002;99:1486.

33. Lee MY, Chiou TJ, Hsiao LT, et al. Rituximab therapy increased post-transplant cytomegalovirus complications in non-Hodgkin's lymphoma patients receiving autologous hematopoietic stem cell transplantation. Ann Hematol 2008;87:285.

34. Suzan F, Ammor M, Ribrag V. Fatal reactivation of cytomegalovirus infection after use of rituximab for a post-transplantation lymphoproliferative disorder. N Engl J Med 2001;345:1000.

35. Bermudez A, Marco F, Conde E, et al. Fatal visceral varicella-zoster infection following rituximab and chemotherapy treatment in a patient with follicular lymphoma. Haematologica 2000;85:894.

36. McIlwaine LM, Fitzsimons EJ, Soutar RL. Inappropriate antidiuretic hormone secretion, abdominal pain and disseminated varicella-zoster virus infection: an unusual and fatal triad in a patient 13 months post rituximab and autologous stem cell transplantation. Clin Lab Haematol 2001;23:253.

37. Crowley B, Woodcock B. Red cell aplasia due to parvovirus b19 in a patient treated with alemtuzumab. Br J Haematol 2002;119:279.

38. Isobe Y, Sugimoto K, Shiraki Y, et al. Successful high-titer immunoglobulin therapy for persistent parvovirus B19 infection in a lymphoma patient treated with rituximab-combined chemotherapy. Am J Hematol 2004;77:370.

39. Sharma VR, Fleming DR, Slone SP. Pure red cell aplasia due to parvovirus B19 in a patient treated with rituximab. Blood 2000;96:1184.

40. Huang C, Slater B, Rudd R, et al. First isolation of West Nile virus from a patient with encephalitis in the United States. Emerg Infect Dis 2002;8:1367.

41. Levi ME, Quan D, Ho JT, et al. Impact of rituximab-associated B-cell defects on West Nile virus meningoencephalitis in solid organ transplant recipients. Clin Transplant 2009. [Epub ahead of print].

42. Mawhorter SD, Sierk A, Staugaitis SM, et al. Fatal West Nile Virus infection after rituximab/fludarabine–induced remission for non-Hodgkin's lymphoma. Clin Lymphoma Myeloma 2005;6:248.

43. Flohr TR, Sifri CD, Brayman KL, et al. Nocardiosis in a renal transplant recipient following rituximab preconditioning. Ups J Med Sci 2009;114:62.

44. Kundranda MN, Spiro TP, Muslimani A, et al. Cerebral nocardiosis in a patient with NHL treated with rituximab. Am J Hematol 2007;82:1033.

45. Scallon B, Cai A, Solowski N, et al. Binding and functional comparisons of two types of tumor necrosis factor antagonists. J Pharmacol Exp Ther 2002;301:418.

46. Algood HM, Lin PL, Flynn JL. Tumor necrosis factor and chemokine interactions in the formation and maintenance of granulomas in tuberculosis. Clin Infect Dis 2005;41(Suppl 3):S189.

47. Harris J, Hope JC, Keane J. Tumor necrosis factor blockers influence macrophage responses to *Mycobacterium tuberculosis*. J Infect Dis 2008;198:1842.

48. Roach DR, Bean AG, Demangel C, et al. TNF regulates chemokine induction essential for cell recruitment, granuloma formation, and clearance of mycobacterial infection. J Immunol 2002;168:4620.

49. Dixon WG, Symmons DP, Lunt M, et al. Serious infection following anti-tumor necrosis factor alpha therapy in patients with rheumatoid arthritis: lessons from interpreting data from observational studies. Arthritis Rheum 2007;56:2896.

50. Listing J, Strangfeld A, Kary S, et al. Infections in patients with rheumatoid arthritis treated with biologic agents. Arthritis Rheum 2005;52:3403.

51. Askling J, Fored CM, Brandt L, et al. Time-dependent increase in risk of hospi-
    talisation with infection among Swedish RA patients treated with TNF antago-
    nists. Ann Rheum Dis 2007;66:1339.
52. Bongartz T, Sutton AJ, Sweeting MJ, et al. Anti-TNF antibody therapy in rheuma-
    toid arthritis and the risk of serious infections and malignancies: systematic
    review and meta-analysis of rare harmful effects in randomized controlled trials.
    JAMA 2006;295:2275.
53. Keane J, Gershon S, Wise RP, et al. Tuberculosis associated with infliximab,
    a tumor necrosis factor alpha-neutralizing agent. N Engl J Med 2001;345:1098.
54. Wallis RS, Broder M, Wong J, et al. Granulomatous infections due to tumor
    necrosis factor blockade: correction. Clin Infect Dis 2004;39:1254.
55. Wallis RS, Broder MS, Wong JY, et al. Granulomatous infectious diseases asso-
    ciated with tumor necrosis factor antagonists. Clin Infect Dis 2004;38:1261.
56. Brassard P, Kezouh A, Suissa S. Antirheumatic drugs and the risk of tubercu-
    losis. Clin Infect Dis 2006;43:717.
57. Wallis RS. Mathematical modeling of the cause of tuberculosis during tumor
    necrosis factor blockade. Arthritis Rheum 2008;58:947.
58. Arend SM, Leyten EM, Franken WP, et al. A patient with de novo tuberculosis
    during anti-tumor necrosis factor-alpha therapy illustrating diagnostic pitfalls
    and paradoxical response to treatment. Clin Infect Dis 2007;45:1470.
59. Wallis RS, van Vuuren C, Potgieter S. Adalimumab treatment of life-threatening
    tuberculosis. Clin Infect Dis 2009;48:1429.
60. Oberstein EM, Kromo O, Tozman EC. Type I reaction of Hansen's disease with
    exposure to adalimumab: a case report. Arthritis Rheum 2008;59:1040.
61. Scollard DM, Joyce MP, Gillis TP. Development of leprosy and type 1 leprosy
    reactions after treatment with infliximab: a report of 2 cases. Clin Infect Dis
    2006;43:e19.
62. Vilela Lopes R, Barros Ohashi C, Helena Cavaleiro L, et al. Development of
    leprosy in a patient with ankylosing spondylitis during the infliximab treatment:
    reactivation of a latent infection? Clin Rheumatol 2009;28:615.
63. Marie I, Heliot P, Roussel F, et al. Fatal *Mycobacterium peregrinum* pneumonia in
    refractory polymyositis treated with infliximab. Rheumatology (Oxford) 2005;44:
    1201.
64. Martin-Aspas A, Guerrero-Sanchez F, Garcia-Martos P, et al. Bilateral pneu-
    monia by *Mycobacterium aurum* in a patient receiving infliximab therapy. J Infect
    2008;57:167.
65. Larsen MV, Sorensen IJ, Thomsen VO, et al. Re-activation of bovine tuberculosis
    in a patient treated with infliximab. Eur Respir J 2008;32:229.
66. van Ingen J, Boeree M, Janssen M, et al. Pulmonary *Mycobacterium szulgai*
    infection and treatment in a patient receiving anti-tumor necrosis factor therapy.
    Nat Clin Pract Rheumatol 2007;3:414.
67. Lee JH, Slifman NR, Gershon SK, et al. Life-threatening histoplasmosis compli-
    cating immunotherapy with tumor necrosis factor alpha antagonists infliximab
    and etanercept. Arthritis Rheum 2002;46:2565.
68. Asrani NS. Disseminated histoplasmosis associated with the treatment of rheu-
    matoid arthritis with anticytokine therapy. Ann Intern Med 2008;149:594.
69. Wood KL, Hage CA, Knox KS, et al. Histoplasmosis after treatment with anti-
    tumor necrosis factor-alpha therapy. Am J Respir Crit Care Med 2003;167:
    1279.
70. Tsiodras S, Samonis G, Boumpas DT, et al. Fungal infections complicating tumor
    necrosis factor alpha blockade therapy. Mayo Clin Proc 2008;83:181.

71. Bergstrom L, Yocum DE, Ampel NM, et al. Increased risk of coccidioidomycosis in patients treated with tumor necrosis factor alpha antagonists. Arthritis Rheum 2004;50:1959.

72. Pena-Sagredo JL, Hernandez MV, Fernandez-Llanio N, et al. *Listeria monocytogenes* infection in patients with rheumatic diseases on TNF-alpha antagonist therapy: the Spanish Study Group experience. Clin Exp Rheumatol 2008;26: 854.

73. Slifman NR, Gershon SK, Lee JH, et al. *Listeria monocytogenes* infection as a complication of treatment with tumor necrosis factor alpha-neutralizing agents. Arthritis Rheum 2003;48:319.

74. Li Gobbi F, Benucci M, Del Rosso A. Pneumonitis caused by *Legionella pneumoniae* in a patient with rheumatoid arthritis treated with anti-TNF-alpha therapy (infliximab). J Clin Rheumatol 2005;11:119.

75. Wondergem MJ, Voskuyl AE, van Agtmael MA. A case of legionellosis during treatment with a TNFalpha antagonist. Scand J Infect Dis 2004;36:310.

76. Fu A, Bertouch JV, McNeil HP. Disseminated *Salmonella typhimurium* infection secondary to infliximab treatment. Arthritis Rheum 2004;50:3049.

77. Netea MG, Radstake T, Joosten LA, et al. Salmonella septicemia in rheumatoid arthritis patients receiving anti-tumor necrosis factor therapy: association with decreased interferon-gamma production and toll-like receptor 4 expression. Arthritis Rheum 2003;48:1853.

78. Bagalas V, Kioumis I, Argyropoulou P, et al. Visceral leishmaniasis infection in a patient with rheumatoid arthritis treated with etanercept. Clin Rheumatol 2007;26:1344.

79. Fabre S, Gibert C, Lechiche C, et al. Visceral leishmaniasis infection in a rheumatoid arthritis patient treated with infliximab. Clin Exp Rheumatol 2005;23:891.

80. Mueller MC, Fleischmann E, Grunke M, et al. Relapsing cutaneous leishmaniasis in a patient with ankylosing spondylitis treated with infliximab. Am J Trop Med Hyg 2009;81:52.

81. Geraghty EM, Ristow B, Gordon SM, et al. Overwhelming parasitemia with *Plasmodium falciparum* infection in a patient receiving infliximab therapy for rheumatoid arthritis. Clin Infect Dis 2007;44:e82.

82. Coyle CM, Weiss LM, Rhodes LV 3rd, et al. Fatal myositis due to the microsporidian *Brachiola algerae*, a mosquito pathogen. N Engl J Med 2004; 351:42.

83. Roilides E, Dimitriadou-Georgiadou A, Sein T, et al. Tumor necrosis factor alpha enhances antifungal activities of polymorphonuclear and mononuclear phagocytes against *Aspergillus fumigatus*. Infect Immun 1998;66:5999.

84. Gottlieb GS, Lesser CF, Holmes KK, et al. Disseminated sporotrichosis associated with treatment with immunosuppressants and tumor necrosis factor-alpha antagonists. Clin Infect Dis 2003;37:838.

85. Lowther AL, Somani AK, Camouse M, et al. Invasive *Trichophyton rubrum* infection occurring with infliximab and long-term prednisone treatment. J Cutan Med Surg 2007;11:84.

86. Harigai M, Koike R, Miyasaka N. *Pneumocystis pneumonia* associated with infliximab in Japan. N Engl J Med 2007;357:1874.

87. Kaur N, Mahl TC. *Pneumocystis jiroveci* (*carinii*) pneumonia after infliximab therapy: a review of 84 cases. Dig Dis Sci 2007;52:1481.

88. Takeuchi T, Tatsuki Y, Nogami Y, et al. Postmarketing surveillance of the safety profile of infliximab in 5000 Japanese patients with rheumatoid arthritis. Ann Rheum Dis 2008;67:189.

89. Garcia-Vidal C, Rodriguez-Fernandez S, Teijon S, et al. Risk factors for opportunistic infections in infliximab-treated patients: the importance of screening in prevention. Eur J Clin Microbiol Infect Dis 2009;28:331.

90. Strangfeld A, Listing J, Herzer P, et al. Risk of herpes zoster in patients with rheumatoid arthritis treated with anti-TNF-alpha agents. JAMA 2009;301:737.

91. Smitten AL, Choi HK, Hochberg MC, et al. The risk of herpes zoster in patients with rheumatoid arthritis in the United States and the United Kingdom. Arthritis Rheum 2007;57:1431.

92. Bradford RD, Pettit AC, Wright PW, et al. Herpes simplex encephalitis during treatment with tumor necrosis factor-alpha inhibitors. Clin Infect Dis 2009;49:924.

93. Esteve M, Saro C, Gonzalez-Huix F, et al. Chronic hepatitis B reactivation following infliximab therapy in Crohn's disease patients: need for primary prophylaxis. Gut 2004;53:1363.

94. Michel M, Duvoux C, Hezode C, et al. Fulminant hepatitis after infliximab in a patient with hepatitis B virus treated for an adult onset still's disease. J Rheumatol 2003;30:1624.

95. Zingarelli S, Frassi M, Bazzani C, et al. Use of tumor necrosis factor-alpha-blocking agents in hepatitis B virus-positive patients: reports of 3 cases and review of the literature. J Rheumatol 2009;36:1188.

96. Roux CH, Brocq O, Breuil V, et al. Safety of anti-TNF-alpha therapy in rheumatoid arthritis and spondylarthropathies with concurrent B or C chronic hepatitis. Rheumatology (Oxford) 2006;45:1294.

97. Couriel D, Saliba R, Hicks K, et al. Tumor necrosis factor-alpha blockade for the treatment of acute GVHD. Blood 2004;104:649.

98. Marty FM, Lee SJ, Fahey MM, et al. Infliximab use in patients with severe graft-versus-host disease and other emerging risk factors of non-*Candida* invasive fungal infections in allogeneic hematopoietic stem cell transplant recipients: a cohort study. Blood 2003;102:2768.

99. Keystone E, Heijde D, Mason D Jr, et al. Certolizumab pegol plus methotrexate is significantly more effective than placebo plus methotrexate in active rheumatoid arthritis: findings of a fifty-two-week, phase III, multicenter, randomized, double-blind, placebo-controlled, parallel-group study. Arthritis Rheum 2008; 58:3319.

100. Schreiber S, Khaliq-Kareemi M, Lawrance IC, et al. Maintenance therapy with certolizumab pegol for Crohn's disease. N Engl J Med 2007;357:239.

101. Smolen J, Landewe RB, Mease P, et al. Efficacy and safety of certolizumab pegol plus methotrexate in active rheumatoid arthritis: the RAPID 2 study. A randomised controlled trial. Ann Rheum Dis 2009;68:797.

102. Keystone EC, Genovese MC, Klareskog L, et al. Golimumab, a human antibody to tumour necrosis factor {alpha} given by monthly subcutaneous injections, in active rheumatoid arthritis despite methotrexate therapy: the GO-FORWARD Study. Ann Rheum Dis 2009;68:789.

103. Wenzel SE, Barnes PJ, Bleecker ER, et al. A randomized, double-blind, placebo-controlled study of tumor necrosis factor-alpha blockade in severe persistent asthma. Am J Respir Crit Care Med 2009;179:549.

104. Furst DE, Keystone EC, Kirkham B, et al. Updated consensus statement on biological agents for the treatment of rheumatic diseases. Ann Rheum Dis 2008; 67(Suppl 3): iii2.

105. Salliot C, Dougados M, Gossec L. Risk of serious infections during rituximab, abatacept and anakinra treatments for rheumatoid arthritis: meta-analyses of randomised placebo-controlled trials. Ann Rheum Dis 2009;68:25.

106. Le Loet X, Nordstrom D, Rodriguez M, et al. Effect of anakinra on functional status in patients with active rheumatoid arthritis receiving concomitant therapy with traditional disease modifying antirheumatic drugs: evidence from the OMEGA Trial. J Rheumatol 2008;35:1538.

107. Lequerre T, Quartier P, Rosellini D, et al. Interleukin-1 receptor antagonist (anakinra) treatment in patients with systemic-onset juvenile idiopathic arthritis or adult onset still disease: preliminary experience in France. Ann Rheum Dis 2008;67:302.

108. Hoffman HM, Throne ML, Amar NJ, et al. Efficacy and safety of rilonacept (interleukin-1 Trap) in patients with cryopyrin-associated periodic syndromes: results from two sequential placebo-controlled studies. Arthritis Rheum 2008;58:2443.

109. Morris EC, Rebello P, Thomson KJ, et al. Pharmacokinetics of alemtuzumab used for in vivo and in vitro T-cell depletion in allogeneic transplantations: relevance for early adoptive immunotherapy and infectious complications. Blood 2003;102:404.

110. Rai KR, Freter CE, Mercier RJ, et al. Alemtuzumab in previously treated chronic lymphocytic leukemia patients who also had received fludarabine. J Clin Oncol 2002;20:3891.

111. Ferrajoli A, O'Brien SM, Cortes JE, et al. Phase II study of alemtuzumab in chronic lymphoproliferative disorders. Cancer 2003;98:773.

112. Keating MJ, Flinn I, Jain V, et al. Therapeutic role of alemtuzumab (Campath-1H) in patients who have failed fludarabine: results of a large international study. Blood 2002;99:3554.

113. Martin SI, Marty FM, Fiumara K, et al. Infectious complications associated with alemtuzumab use for lymphoproliferative disorders. Clin Infect Dis 2006;43:16.

114. Lundin J, Kimby E, Bjorkholm M, et al. Phase II trial of subcutaneous anti-CD52 monoclonal antibody alemtuzumab (Campath-1H) as first-line treatment for patients with B-cell chronic lymphocytic leukemia (B-CLL). Blood 2002;100:768.

115. Hillmen P, Skotnicki AB, Robak T, et al. Alemtuzumab compared with chlorambucil as first-line therapy for chronic lymphocytic leukemia. J Clin Oncol 2007;25:5616.

116. Saadeh CE, Srkalovic G. *Mycobacterium avium* complex infection after alemtuzumab therapy for chronic lymphocytic leukemia. Pharmacotherapy 2008;28:281.

117. Abad S, Gyan E, Moachon L, et al. Tuberculosis due to *Mycobacterium bovis* after alemtuzumab administration. Clin Infect Dis 2003;37:e27.

118. Kamboj M, Louie E, Kiehn T, et al. *Mycobacterium haemophilum* infection after alemtuzumab treatment. Emerg Infect Dis 2008;14:1821.

119. Dungarwalla M, Field-Smith A, Jameson C, et al. Cutaneous *Mycobacterium chelonae* infection in chronic lymphocytic leukaemia. Haematologica 2007;92:e5.

120. Chae YS, Sohn SK, Kim JG, et al. Impact of alemtuzumab as conditioning regimen component on transplantation outcomes in case of CMV-seropositive recipients and donors. Am J Hematol 2008;83:649.

121. Chakrabarti S, Mackinnon S, Chopra R, et al. High incidence of cytomegalovirus infection after nonmyeloablative stem cell transplantation: potential role of Campath-1H in delaying immune reconstitution. Blood 2002;99:4357.

122. Ho AY, Pagliuca A, Kenyon M, et al. Reduced-intensity allogeneic hematopoietic stem cell transplantation for myelodysplastic syndrome and acute myeloid leukemia with multilineage dysplasia using fludarabine, busulphan, and alemtuzumab (FBC) conditioning. Blood 2004;104:1616.

123. Perez-Simon JA, Kottaridis PD, Martino R, et al. Nonmyeloablative transplantation with or without alemtuzumab: comparison between 2 prospective studies in
patients with lymphoproliferative disorders. Blood 2002;100:3121.
124. Chakrabarti S, Avivi I, Mackinnon S, et al. Respiratory virus infections in transplant recipients after reduced-intensity conditioning with Campath-1H: high incidence but low mortality. Br J Haematol 2002;119:1125.
125. Vu T, Carrum G, Hutton G, et al. Human herpesvirus-6 encephalitis following
allogeneic hematopoietic stem cell transplantation. Bone Marrow Transplant
2007;39:705.
126. Landgren O, Gilbert ES, Rizzo JD, et al. Risk factors for lymphoproliferative
disorders after allogeneic hematopoietic cell transplantation. Blood 2009;113:
4992.
127. Peleg AY, Husain S, Kwak EJ, et al. Opportunistic infections in 547 organ transplant recipients receiving alemtuzumab, a humanized monoclonal CD-52 antibody. Clin Infect Dis 2007;44:204.
128. Laurenti L, Piccioni P, Cattani P, et al. Cytomegalovirus reactivation during alemtuzumab therapy for chronic lymphocytic leukemia: incidence and treatment
with oral ganciclovir. Haematologica 2004;89:1248.
129. O'Brien S, Ravandi F, Riehl T, et al. Valganciclovir prevents cytomegalovirus reactivation in patients receiving alemtuzumab-based therapy. Blood 2008;111:1816.
130. Hengster P, Pescovitz MD, Hyatt D, et al. Cytomegalovirus infections after treatment with daclizumab, an anti IL-2 receptor antibody, for prevention of renal allograft rejection. Roche Study Group. Transplantation 1999;68:310.
131. Vincenti F, Kirkman R, Light S, et al. Interleukin-2-receptor blockade with daclizumab to prevent acute rejection in renal transplantation. Daclizumab Triple
Therapy Study Group. N Engl J Med 1998;338:161.
132. Hershberger RE, Starling RC, Eisen HJ, et al. Daclizumab to prevent rejection
after cardiac transplantation. N Engl J Med 2005;352:2705.
133. Iversen M, Burton CM, Vand S, et al. Aspergillus infection in lung transplant
patients: incidence and prognosis. Eur J Clin Microbiol Infect Dis 2007;26:879.
134. Przepiorka D, Kernan NA, Ippoliti C, et al. Daclizumab, a humanized anti-inter-
leukin-2 receptor alpha chain antibody, for treatment of acute graft-versus-host
disease. Blood 2000;95:83.
135. Perales MA, Ishill N, Lomazow WA, et al. Long-term follow-up of patients treated
with daclizumab for steroid-refractory acute graft-vs-host disease. Bone Marrow
Transplant 2007;40:481.
136. Keown P, Balshaw R, Khorasheh S, et al. Meta-analysis of basiliximab for immunoprophylaxis in renal transplantation. BioDrugs 2003;17:271.
137. Lawen JG, Davies EA, Mourad G, et al. Randomized double-blind study of immunoprophylaxis with basiliximab, a chimeric anti-interleukin-2 receptor monoclonal antibody, in combination with mycophenolate mofetil-containing triple
therapy in renal transplantation. Transplantation 2003;75:37.
138. Sheashaa HA, Bakr MA, Ismail AM, et al. Basiliximab induction therapy for live
donor kidney transplantation: a long-term follow-up of prospective randomized
controlled study. Clin Exp Nephrol 2008;12:376.
139. Mattei MF, Redonnet M, Gandjbakhch I, et al. Lower risk of infectious deaths in
cardiac transplant patients receiving basiliximab versus anti-thymocyte globulin
as induction therapy. J Heart Lung Transplant 2007;26:693.
140. Mehra MR, Zucker MJ, Wagoner L, et al. A multicenter, prospective, randomized, double-blind trial of basiliximab in heart transplantation. J Heart Lung
Transplant 2005;24:1297.

141. Lupo L, Panzera P, Tandoi F, et al. Basiliximab versus steroids in double therapy immunosuppression in liver transplantation: a prospective randomized clinical trial. Transplantation 2008;86:925.

142. Neuhaus P, Clavien PA, Kittur D, et al. Improved treatment response with basiliximab immunoprophylaxis after liver transplantation: results from a double-blind randomized placebo-controlled trial. Liver Transpl 2002;8:132.

143. Brennan DC, Daller JA, Lake KD, et al. Rabbit antithymocyte globulin versus basiliximab in renal transplantation. N Engl J Med 2006;355:1967.

144. Kremer JM, Genant HK, Moreland LW, et al. Effects of abatacept in patients with methotrexate-resistant active rheumatoid arthritis: a randomized trial. Ann Intern Med 2006;144:865.

145. Weinblatt M, Combe B, Covucci A, et al. Safety of the selective costimulation modulator abatacept in rheumatoid arthritis patients receiving background biologic and nonbiologic disease-modifying antirheumatic drugs: a one-year randomized, placebo-controlled study. Arthritis Rheum 2006;54:2807.

146. Weinblatt M, Schiff M, Goldman A, et al. Selective costimulation modulation using abatacept in patients with active rheumatoid arthritis while receiving etanercept: a randomised clinical trial. Ann Rheum Dis 2007;66:228.

147. Genovese MC, Becker JC, Schiff M, et al. Abatacept for rheumatoid arthritis refractory to tumor necrosis factor alpha inhibition. N Engl J Med 2005;353:1114.

148. Genovese MC, Schiff M, Luggen M, et al. Efficacy and safety of the selective costimulation modulator abatacept following 2 years of treatment in patients with rheumatoid arthritis and an inadequate response to anti-tumour necrosis factor therapy. Ann Rheum Dis 2008;67:547.

149. Bigbee CL, Gonchoroff DG, Vratsanos G, et al. Abatacept treatment does not exacerbate chronic *Mycobacterium tuberculosis* infection in mice. Arthritis Rheum 2007;56:2557.

150. Vincenti F, Larsen C, Durrbach A, et al. Costimulation blockade with belatacept in renal transplantation. N Engl J Med 2005;353:770.

151. Goodin DS, Cohen BA, O'Connor P, et al. Assessment: the use of natalizumab (Tysabri) for the treatment of multiple sclerosis (an evidence-based review): report of the Therapeutics and Technology Assessment Subcommittee of the American Academy of Neurology. Neurology 2008;71:766.

152. Kleinschmidt-DeMasters BK, Tyler KL. Progressive multifocal leukoencephalopathy complicating treatment with natalizumab and interferon beta-1a for multiple sclerosis. N Engl J Med 2005;353:369.

153. Langer-Gould A, Atlas SW, Green AJ, et al. Progressive multifocal leukoencephalopathy in a patient treated with natalizumab. N Engl J Med 2005;353:375.

154. Van Assche G, Van Ranst M, Sciot R, et al. Progressive multifocal leukoencephalopathy after natalizumab therapy for Crohn's disease. N Engl J Med 2005;353:362.

155. Yousry TA, Major EO, Ryschkewitsch C, et al. Evaluation of patients treated with natalizumab for progressive multifocal leukoencephalopathy. N Engl J Med 2006;354:924.

156. Balato A, Balato N, Patruno C, et al. Visceral leishmaniasis infection in a patient with psoriasis treated with efalizumab. Dermatology 2008;217:360.

157. Tuxen AJ, Yong MK, Street AC, et al. Disseminated cryptococcal infection in a patient with severe psoriasis treated with efalizumab, methotrexate and ciclosporin. Br J Dermatol 2007;157:1067.

158. Miquel FJ, Colomina J, Marii JI, et al. Cytomegalovirus infection in a patient treated with efalizumab for psoriasis. Arch Dermatol 2009;145:961.
159. Gottlieb AB, Casale TB, Frankel E, et al. CD4+ T-cell-directed antibody responses are maintained in patients with psoriasis receiving alefacept: results of a randomized study. J Am Acad Dermatol 2003;49:816.
160. Brimhall AK, King LN, Licciardone JC, et al. Safety and efficacy of alefacept, efalizumab, etanercept and infliximab in treating moderate to severe plaque psoriasis: a meta-analysis of randomized controlled trials. Br J Dermatol 2008; 159:274.
161. Al-Tawfiq JA, Al-Khatti AA. Disseminated systemic *Nocardia farcinica* infection complicating alefacept and infliximab therapy in a patient with severe psoriasis. Int J Infect Dis 2009;14:e153.
162. Prasertsuntarasai T, Bello EF. *Mycobacterium avium* complex olecranon bursitis in a patient treated with alefacept. Mayo Clin Proc 2005;80:1532.
163. Sievers EL, Larson RA, Stadtmauer EA, et al. Efficacy and safety of gemtuzumab ozogamicin in patients with CD33-positive acute myeloid leukemia in first relapse. J Clin Oncol 2001;19:3244.

Infections in Pediatric Transplant Recipients: Not Just Small Adults

Marian G. Michaels, MD, MPH*, Michael Green, MD, MPH

KEYWORDS

- Immunocompromised children • Pediatric transplantation
- Cytomegalovirus • Epstein-Barr virus • Vaccinations

Transplantation increasingly is being used as treatment for children with end-stage organ diseases, hematopoietic rescue from therapy used to treat malignancies, and as a cure of primary immune deficiencies. The numbers of transplant procedures performed on children is substantially less than those performed on adults, with recipients under the age of 18 years accounting for only 7.7% of all solid organ transplants performed in the United States.[1] Because the numbers are limited, data on specific infections more often are based on retrospective reviews from single institutions and less rigorously defined than data for adults. In addition, data on infections from adult studies often are extrapolated to assist with the management of pediatric patients. Although this approach is reasonable in many cases, it may be less reliable for situations where the underlying disease influences the risk for infection and where age of the recipient has substantial impact upon the risk for infectious complications. This article reviews some of the major concepts of infections that complicate pediatric transplantation, highlighting differences of epidemiology, evaluation, treatment and prevention for children compared with adult recipients.

SOLID ORGAN TRANSPLANTATION

Over the last 20 years, increasing numbers of children have undergone transplantation of kidney, liver, heart, lungs, pancreas, and intestines with survival continuing to improve over time. For example, children who undergo heart transplantation and survive the first year have a median survival well over 15 years.[2] Although both patient

A version of this article was previously published in the *Infectious Disease Clinics of North America*, 24:2.
Department of Pediatrics and Surgery, Children's Hospital of Pittsburgh, One Children's Hospital Drive, 4401 Penn Avenue, Pittsburgh, PA 15224, USA
* Corresponding author.
E-mail address: marian.michaels@chp.edu

Hematol Oncol Clin N Am 25 (2011) 139–150
doi:10.1016/j.hoc.2010.11.010
0889-8588/11/$ – see front matter © 2011 Elsevier Inc. All rights reserved.

and graft survival varies by type of organ and by age of the recipient, observed survival for pediatric solid organ transplantation (SOT) recipients is often as good, if not better than that of adults. For example, in the United States, pediatric kidney transplant recipients have a survival over 97% compared with adult 3-year survival of 91%.[3] Infections, however, remain a major cause of morbidity and mortality in these patients. To understand the types of infections that might occur after transplantation, it is useful to consider several sets of key principles related to infectious complications. The first principle is that the type of infection present in an SOT recipient is predicted by the time period after transplantation in which the patient presents. In general, the pattern and timing of infections are similar in both adults and children.[4] Although the actual breakpoints of a time line are indistinct, one can consider the general timing of presentation after SOT to help predict the types of infections that might be occurring in a given child based on stereotypical patterns:

The early period (0 to 4 weeks) is one in which postoperative bacterial surgical infections predominate.

The middle period (generally 1 to 6 months) is the time wherein opportunistic infections and reactivation of latent infections in the recipient or from the donor are prominent.

The late period (usually after 6 months) is a period when community-acquired viruses and infections associated with chronic graft dysfunction predominate.[4–7]

This concept, put forward in the early era of SOT, is generally true today.[7] Not only does it inform the evaluation of fevers in a patient after SOT, but it likewise has led to the tailoring of preventive strategies for specific time periods and patients.[8]

The second major principle informing the understanding of infectious complications of SOT is that there is a defined set of key risk factors that predispose to infection in these children. These risk factors can be categorized as those present before transplantation, those relating to the transplant procedure itself, and postoperative risk factors that are influenced most heavily by the immunosuppression required to prevent rejection. A careful examination of these risk factors identifies the major differences in types and outcome of infection between pediatric and adult recipients.

Pretransplant Risk Factors

The age of the child at the time of undergoing SOT is an important factor that influences the types of infections they may experience after transplantation. Age impacts upon the chance of having had prior exposure to infectious agents. The presence of prior infection can have both negative and positive influences on the transplant recipient. For example, older candidates are more likely to have encountered pathogens that establish lifelong latent infection such as herpes simplex virus (HSV), cytomegalovirus (CMV), tuberculosis, as well as certain endemic fungi. This can be negative, as these microbes can reactivate under the pressure of immune suppression with significant clinical consequences. Accordingly, strategies have been developed to screen for or prevent reactivation of these potential pathogens following transplantation.[4–7] On the positive side, disease associated with reactivation of latent pathogens (or even reinfection with a new strain of a given latent pathogen) tends to be less aggressive than that associated with primary infection occurring after SOT, as the person has some baseline immunity.[4–9] In some cases (eg, Epstein-Barr virus [EBV]), this pre-existing immunity provides a high degree of protection against clinical disease after transplantation.[9,10]

The age of a child at the time of SOT impacts on the likelihood that he or she will have acquired immunity against potential pathogens from natural infection. Certain pathogens appear to specifically cause infections in younger SOT recipients. For instance, children who receive a heart transplant before 2 years of age have been noted to be at increased risk for recurrent *Streptococcus pneumoniae* disease including bacteremia, even when they are older and have normal splenic function.[11] It is hypothesized that this may occur because of lack of normal antibody function.[12] Children receiving a transplant before 1 year of age often will not have had exposures to common respiratory pathogens until after transplantation. Respiratory syncytial virus (RSV), influenza, and parainfluenza have been shown to be more severe in the very young transplant recipient who is less than a year of age compared with older individuals.[13–15]

Age also impacts on the likelihood that children undergoing SOT will have had the opportunity to receive their full compliment of immunizations.[16–19] Accordingly, young children who receive a transplant before receiving their routine primary vaccinations will be at higher risk for vaccine-preventable infections. In addition, the authors have found that even with increasing age children who have underlying diseases that require transplantation often miss the opportunity to receive their age-appropriate vaccinations because of time spent in the hospital or primary attention being diverted from routine childhood care (Michaels MG, unpublished observation, 2009).

A second pretransplant factor influencing the risk of infectious complications following SOT is the underlying cause of organ dysfunction. The causes of organ failure in children are typically different than adults. Accordingly, this leads to differences in the risk of infection between pediatric and adult SOT recipients. For example, hepatitis C virus (HCV) is a leading cause of liver disease requiring transplantation in adults, but is rare in the pediatric population. For this reason, recurrent HCV infection following liver transplantation is not typically an issue in pediatric recipients. On the other hand, children are more likely to have congenital anomalies (eg, Biliary atresia) as a cause of end-stage liver disease. These malformations may predispose to recurrent episodes of infection (eg, cholangitis) that might predispose to infection with multidrug-resistant bacteria following the organ transplant. Congenital heart defects that require neonatal transplantation do so at a time when the child is particularly vulnerable to bacterial infections. For example, neonates requiring heart transplantation are at increased risk for mediastinitis caused by gram-negative bacteria compared with older children and adults.[20,21] Small bowel transplantation in childhood is more often associated with neonatal catastrophic events such as necrotizing enterocolitis from prematurity or complicated gastroschisis. These children have been hospitalized for significant periods of their life and have numerous prior intravascular line associated infections and exposures to antibiotics. Accordingly, they often are colonized with bacteria that have resistance to multiple antibiotics.[22]

Intraoperative Factors

In contrast to adult SOT recipients, pediatric patients more often receive organs from adult donors, with a resultant discrepancy in their size because of the relative paucity of pediatric donors. This size discrepancy can lead to an increased risk for anastomotic complications with the potential consequence of leakage, thrombosis, or necrosis, or the potential to leave the body cavity (abdomen or chest) open for a prolonged period of time. In these cases, the child is at an increased risk of bacteria and yeast infections postoperatively.[5,6,22]

Children are also at increased risk for donor-associated transmission of pathogens, as they more frequently lack immunity to this set of organisms. In particular, children are much more likely to be EBV seronegative before transplant, placing them at an increased likelihood of being in a mismatched state and at a marked increased risk of developing post-transplant lymphoproliferative disorders (PTLDs) compared with adult recipients. This in large part explains the much higher frequency of EBV/PTLDs observed in children compared with adults.[9,10,22–24] This is also true for CMV; accordingly primary CMV infections also are seen much more frequently in pediatric recipients compared with adult recipients.[23,25–29]

Post-transplant Risk Factors

As with adult recipients, immunosuppression is the major post-transplant risk factor for infection in children undergoing SOT. Unlike adults, this immunosuppressive therapy can have a substantial impact on growth and development, including the developing immune system. Children requiring higher levels of immune suppression because of rejection are at increased risk for developing more severe infection. This is true not only for common transplant associated pathogens (eg, CMV, EBV), but also for community-acquired viral pathogens such as RSV, parainfluenza, and influenza. Because children are more likely to be immunologically naïve to community pathogens, disease attributable to these agents tends to be more severe in children than adults.[5,6]

The general requirement for immunosuppression also results in decreased immunogenicity of vaccinations that are provided following SOT.[16–19,30–34] Although there are inadequate studies addressing the use of vaccines in pediatric SOT recipients, it is very likely that those children requiring higher levels of immune suppression are less likely to experience the full benefit of these vaccinations. Accordingly, they will be at increased risk of developing vaccine-associated diseases compared with both adults and children requiring lower levels of immunosuppression after transplant. Further, live virus vaccines remain generally contraindicated after transplant.[16–18,35] Although a growing number of transplant centers will administer varicella vaccine and measles-mumps-rubella vaccine after SOT, the numbers of children studied are small, and potential risks of vaccine-associated disease are not inconsequential.[36–39]

Finally, young children, whether immunosuppressed or not, are more likely than adults to share potentially infectious secretions with one another. Children who undergo SOT therefore are more likely to have infectious exposures from their siblings, playmates, and classmates. Their imperfect hygienic practices create an increased risk for exposure to community-acquired pathogens compared with adults.

Prevention

Recommendations for the prevention of infection following SOT are generally similar for both pediatric and adult organ transplant recipients.[4–7] Along with routine serologic screening for human immunodeficiency virus (HIV), hepatitis B virus (HBV), HCV, and syphilis, pediatric transplant centers should evaluate immunity to EBV, CMV, and HSV. In addition, organ candidates who are old enough to have been immunized or have had wild-type infection should have antibody measured against measles and varicella. Results of serologic assays should be interpreted, taking into account the potential of passive antibody presence from the mother (children under 12 to 15 months of age) or from blood products.

One important opportunity to improve post-transplant outcome can be accomplished during the pretransplant evaluation of potential pediatric candidates of SOT. A history of vaccination should be evaluated as early as possible in these candidates, and accelerated schedules should be encouraged to give them as many protective vaccines as possible before transplantation. Primary vaccine series can be started as early as 6 weeks of age and subsequent primary immunizations given every

4 weeks.[18,35] Varicella vaccination and measles-mumps-rubella vaccination should be given at least a month before transplantation.

Following SOT, children with herpes simplex seropositivity should be given acyclovir prophylaxis until the maximal period of immunosuppression has past (generally several months).[5,6] The decision to use prophylaxis against CMV versus virologic monitoring of patients at risk to inform pre-emptive antiviral therapy is similar to decisions used for adult recipients.[28,29,40] In contrast to adults, however, children are more likely to be at risk of developing primary CMV infection. Accordingly, many pediatric transplant centers will use chemoprophylaxis against CMV, as many experts believe this is the preferred strategy for high-risk mismatched patients (seronegative recipients of seropositive donors).[28,41] Finally, because most children are EBV seronegative, many centers have employed strategies of EBV viral load monitoring to inform preemptive reductions in immune suppression in an effort to prevent complications associated with this pathogen.[42,43]

HEMATOPOIETIC STEM CELL TRANSPLANTATION

Replacement of the bone marrow in children can be as a rescue measure after intense chemotherapy or radiation required to eradicate certain malignancies, or for replacement of a deficient bone marrow as seen with primary immune deficiencies, primary bone marrow failure, inborn errors of metabolism, or an assortment of genetic disorders.[44–46] Overall, there are fewer differences in the infections seen between pediatric and adult hematopoietic stem cell transplantation (HSCT) than that for SOT, since both adults and children are rendered immunologically naïve in preparation for the transplant. The source of cells can be autologous (from the individual's own cells) or allogeneic (from another person), and it can be from bone marrow (related or unrelated), peripheral blood that has been stimulated to be enriched for stem cells, or from cord blood. The risk for infection varies with both the underlying reason for HSCT and with the type of donor used, as well as how the cells have been prepared. For example, people undergoing autologous HSCT will have risks for infection before engraftment but fewer risks afterwards. Patients receiving HSCT with a T-cell depleted stem cell product may have less risk of graft-versus-host disease (GVHD) but some increased risk of infection. Cord blood transplants may take longer to engraft, with concomitant increased risks for infection during the pre-engraftment period. In addition to these risk factors, both GVHD and the medications to prevent or treat GVHD put the child at risk for infections. Finally, infections following HSCT can be classified according to specific time periods after transplantation similar to SOT recipients.[44–46] These time periods include the pretransplantation period, pre-engraftment period (0 to 1 month), postengraftment period (1 to 3 months), and the late post-transplantation period (>3 months). Children and adults have specific defects in host defenses that vary during these periods and predispose to infection. The presence of indwelling catheters or mucositis that may occur secondary to radiation or chemotherapy interrupts the normal anatomic barriers creating defects in this important host defense that may be present anytime following transplantation but tend to predominate in the early periods.

Pretransplantation Period

Children come to HSCT with various underlying diseases, differing exposures to chemotherapy, and variable histories of prior infections and amount of immunosuppression. Infections that are present in these children before transplantation, whether because of neutropenia or bone marrow dysfunction from immune or genetic disorders, or the presence of invasive catheters, should be recognized and addressed prior to transplantation. During the pretransplant period, children undergoing autologous HSCT are at similar risk for infection as those undergoing allogeneic transplantation, as the major risks during this period are neutropenia and breaks in the normal barriers of the skin and oropharyngeal and gastrointestinal (GI) mucous membranes.[47] Infection with circulating community viral infections (RSV, influenza, adenovirus) can have an important negative impact.[48–51] Accordingly, having infection control policies to prevent the spread of viruses to these children is imperative.

Pre-engraftment Period

During this period, neutropenia and breeches in the normal anatomic barriers of the body comprise the greatest risk factors for infection. Bacterial infections predominate, with bacteremia being the most commonly documented. Both gram-positive and gram-negative organisms occur. Gram-negative bacilli increase in frequency when the mucosal lining of the GI tract is interrupted.[44–47] Oral mucositis predisposes to the presence of S viridans, which can be associated with antibiotic resistance.[44–47,52] Likewise, the presence of extended-spectrum β-lactamase production in the gram-negative bacilli is being noted increasingly.[45,46] Fungal infections occurring during this phase most often are caused by Candida species, but Aspergillus subspecies are increased in frequency with prolonged neutropenia. More recently, mucormycosis also has been identified in those who have had prolonged neutropenia before HSCT.[53–56]

Viral infections also occur during the pre-engraftment period. Although reactivation of HSV is observed commonly after HSCT in adults,[57] it is less frequent in children, who are less frequently seropositive before transplantation. As noted in the section concerning prevention, children who have had prior infection with HSV should receive prophylaxis to prevent reactivation. Nosocomial or community exposures to circulating viral pathogens represent an important potential source of infection for these children.[48–51] There is growing evidence that community-acquired viruses cause increased morbidity and mortality for HSCT recipients during this time period. Adenovirus is a particularly important viral pathogen that may present earlier in children, although it typically presents after engraftment.[58–60]

Postengraftment Period

The predominant defect in host defenses in the early phase after engraftment is altered cell-mediated immunity.[46] Infectious risks are potentiated by the presence of GVHD. This risk is especially accentuated 50 to 100 days after HSCT, when host immunity is lost and donor immunity is not yet established.[44–46] Opportunistic pathogens predominate during this time period. Without the use of appropriate prophylaxis Pneumocystis jiroveci pneumonia presents in this phase early after engraftment.[61] Aspergillus is a prominent cause of fungal infection during this period; in addition, other opportunistic mycoses also are being recognized increasingly.[53,55,56] Hepatosplenic candidiasis frequently presents during the postengraftment period, although seeding likely occurred during the neutropenic phase.[62] Reactivation of Toxoplasma gondii, a rare cause of disease among pediatric HSCT recipients, also may present after engraftment.[63]

CMV is one of the most important causes of morbidity and mortality among HSCT recipients, and it typically presents during this early postengraftment phase; it is covered in detail in an article on CMV in this journal. Although primary infection from the donor can cause disease, the most prominent problems from CMV after HSCT are caused by reactivation in an HSCT recipient whose donor was naïve to the virus.[64–66] For this reason, the older HSCT patient is at greater risk by virtue of more likely having acquired CMV before transplantation. Disease risk from CMV after HSCT also is increased in recipients of donors who are unrelated, or T-cell depleted and children whose course is complicated by GVHD.[44–46,65] Similar to adults, children with CMV disease present with fevers, with or without associated symptoms including hepatitis, esophagitis, or gastroenteritis, and life-threatening interstitial pneumonitis. Asymptomatic shedding or viremia also can occur. Prophylaxis and monitoring with institution of pre-emptive treatment have helped to decrease the risk of serious fatal disease.[67,68]

Adenovirus is the second most important viral infection during this period in children undergoing HSCT, causing disease in approximately 30% of stem cell recipients.[44] Similar to CMV, children receiving grafts from HLA-matched donors or cord blood cell transplants have an increased risk for disease, along with those who had total body irradiation.[44,45] Polyomaviruses, such as BK virus, are recognized as a cause of hemorrhagic cystitis and renal dysfunction following HSCT.[44,45] Nosocomial acquisition of circulating community-acquired pathogens likewise can occur during this time period.

Late Post-transplantation Period

Late after HSCT, in the absence of GVHD, infections are less of a problem. When present, however, chronic GVHD significantly affects the humoral and cell-mediated immune function and causes a breakdown of some anatomic barriers such as is seen with chronic GVHD of the GI tract or lungs. Encapsulated bacteria such as S pneumoniae and Haemophilus influenzae have been noted to cause disease during this period.[44–47] Viral infections, in particular reactivation of varicella–zoster virus (VZV), also accounts for infections during this time period.[44–46] Fungal infections are less frequent during the late post-transplantation time period.

Prevention

Similar to preventive strategies for children who are going to undergo SOT, children being evaluated for HSCT should have a thorough history reviewed of their past infections and their risk for infections. Also similar to SOT, many of the decisions on prophylaxis have been derived from studies in adult recipients. Serology should be obtained to determine the prior presence of latent or persistent viruses such as members of the herpesvirus family (HSV, VZV, CMV, EBV), HIV, HBV, HCV, hepatitis A virus (HAV), and syphilis. Many centers also will screen for antibody against T gondii, because it can reactivate in seropositive individuals. Similar to adults, the use of prophylaxis is advised to prevent reactivation of specific viruses such as HSV. For those with past disease, acyclovir (either intravenously or orally depending on the patient's clinical status) should be used during the highest periods of immunosuppression. A study in adults suggests a year of prophylaxis is beneficial without adverse side effects.[69] This therapy is also useful for prophylaxis against reactivation of varicella. Although prophylaxis against CMV is efficacious, ganciclovir (the best studied medication) is toxic to the bone marrow. Accordingly, many centers opt to use a stringent monitoring protocol and institute pre-emptive treatment when the viral load is positive.[46,70] Children who are negative for CMV before HSCT also should receive leukocyte-reduced blood products in an effort to avoid exposure to and infection with this pathogen.[46]

Fungal prophylaxis and bacterial prophylaxis usually are instituted during the period of neutropenia with variation on the specific type of drug based on the infectious disease history of the individual child and the type of HSCT he or she is receiving (eg, autologous vs allogeneic).[44–46,71,72] Intravenous immunoglobulin use is somewhat controversial. However, it is used at many centers through the early engraftment phase or when there is significant chronic GVHD.[44–46] Trimethoprim sulfamethoxazole is the mostly widely employed prophylaxis against *P jiroveci* pneumonia (PCP). Because of myelosuppression associated with its use, it usually is given before HSCT and then held until engraftment, at which time it is reinstituted.[44–46]

Vaccination is particularly important among children undergoing HSCT as they may not have even had their full complement of primary vaccines before beginning chemotherapy. The timing to restart vaccination after HCST is based on the risk of disease, the ability for the immune system to respond to the antigen, and the safety of the vaccine. These issues are impacted upon by the type of transplant and donor's immunity, the presence of ongoing GVHD, and the use of passive immunoglobulin. In general, the recipient will acquire the immunity that is found in the donor. Antibody titers to vaccine antigens, however, tend not be long-lasting, and repeat vaccination is warranted.[44–46] Live virus vaccines are the ones that have the potential to cause serious vaccine-associated disease when given to an immunosuppressed host. Recommendations do exist to repeat or reissue non-live vaccines at 12, 14, and 24 months after HSCT.[35,44–46] Studies in children who have undergone HSCT show that vaccinations against measles, mumps, and rubella as a single vaccine have been given safely to children 2 years after HSCT if they do not have chronic GVHD or receipt of ongoing immunosuppressive medication.[35,44,45] While these recommendations are set forward, some experts believe that rather than having one guideline for all HSCT recipients, recommendations should be individualized based on the ability of a particular recipient to mount a response.

SUMMARY

In summary, children undergoing SOT and HSCT are at risk of developing infectious complications following these procedures. Although these children may experience similar types and timing of infections as adults undergoing transplantation, their younger age, lack of immunologic experience, and potential increased likelihood of exposure to community-acquired pathogens require careful attention to the differences in infectious diseases seen in pediatric transplant recipients compared with adults undergoing these procedures.

REFERENCES

1. Available at: http://www.optn.transplant.hrsa.gov/latestData/rptData.asp. Accessed August 30, 2009.
2. Boucek MM, Aurora P, Edwards LB, et al. Registry of the international society for heart and lung transplantation: tenth official pediatric heart transplantation report—2007. J Heart Lung Transplant 2007;8:796–807.
3. Available at: http://www.ustransplant.org/csr/current/nationalViewer.aspx?o=KI&t=11. Accessed January 9, 2009.
4. Fishman JA. Infection in solid organ transplant recipients. N Engl J Med 2007; 357:2601.
5. Green M, Michaels MG. Infections in solid organ transplant recipients. In: Long SS, Prober CG, Pickering LK, editors. Principles & practice of pediatric infectious diseases. 3rd edition. New York: Churchill Livingstone; 2008. p. 551–7.
6. Keough WL, Michaels MG. Infectious complications in pediatric solid organ transplantation. Pediatr Clin North Am 2003;50(6):1451–69.
7. Fishman JA, Rubin RH. Infection in organ-transplant recipients. N Engl J Med 1998;338(24):1741–51.

8. Green M, Michaels MG. Infectious complications of immunosuppressive medications in organ transplant recipients. Pediatr Infect Dis J 2007;26:443–4.

9. Green M, Michaels MG, Webber SA, et al. The management of Epstein-Barr virus associated post-transplant lymphoproliferative disorders in pediatric solid organ transplant recipients. Pediatr Transplant 1999;3(4):271–81.

10. Boyle GJ, Michaels MG, Webber SA, et al. Post-transplant lymphoproliferative disorders in pediatric thoracic organ recipients. J Pediatr 1997;131:309–13.

11. Stovall SH, Ainley KA, Mason EO Jr, et al. Invasive pneumococcal infections in pediatric cardiac transplant patients. Pediatr Infect Dis J 2001;20(10):946–50.

12. Gennery AR, Cant AJ, Baldwin CI, et al. Characterization of the impaired antipneumococcal polysaccharide antibody production in immunosuppressed pediatric patients following cardiac transplantation. J Clin Immunol 2001;21:43–50.

13. Pohl C, Green M, Wald ER, et al. Respiratory syncytial virus infections in pediatric liver transplant recipients. J Infect Dis 1992;165(1):166–9.

14. Apalsch AM, Green M, Ledesma-Medina J, et al. Parainfluenza and influenza virus infections in pediatric organ transplant recipients. Clin Infect Dis 1995;20(2):394–9.

15. Green M, Michaels MG. Community-acquired respiratory viruses. Amer J Transplantation 2004;4:S105–9.

16. Burroughs M, Moscona A. Immunization of pediatric solid organ transplant candidates and recipients. Clin Infect Dis 2000;30(6):857–69.

17. Campbell AL, Herold BC. Immunization of pediatric solid organ transplantation candidates: immunizations in transplant candidates. Pediatr Transplant 2005;9(5):652–61.

18. Avery RK, Michaels MG. Update on immunizations in solid organ transplant recipients: what clinicians need to know. Amer J Transplantation 2008;1:9–14.

19. Benden C, Danziger-Isakov LA, Astor T, et al. Variability in immunization guidelines in children before and after lung transplantation. Pediatr Transplant 2007;11:882–7.

20. Webber SA, Fricker FJ, Michaels M, et al. Orthotopic heart transplantation in children with congenital heart disease. Ann Thorac Surg 1994;58:1664–9.

21. Doelling NR, Kanter KR, Sullivan KM, et al. Medium-term results of pediatric patients undergoing orthotopic heart transplantation. J Heart Lung Transpl 1997;16(12):1225–30.

22. Green M, Bueno J, Sigurdsson L, et al. Unique aspects of the infectious complications of intestinal transplantation. Curr Opin Organ Transplant 1999;4:361–7.

23. Breinig MK, Zitelli B, Starzl TE, et al. Epstein-Barr virus, cytomegalovirus, and other viral infections in children after liver transplantation. J Infect Dis 1987;156(2):273–9.

24. Paya CV, Fung JJ, Nalesnik MA, et al. Epstein-Barr virus-induced post-transplant lymphoproliferative disorders. ASTS/ASTP EBV-PTLD Task Force and The Mayo Clinic Organized International Consensus Development Meeting. Transplantation 1999;68(10):1517–25.

25. Allen U, Herbert D, Moore D, et al. Canadian PTLD Survey Group—1998. Epstein Barr virus-related post-transplant lymphoproliferative disease in solid organ transplant recipients, 1988–97: a Canadian multi-center experience. Pediatr Transplant 2001;5(3):198–203.

26. Danziger-Isakov LA, Worley S, Michaels MG, et al. The risk, prevention & outcome of cytomegalovirus after pediatric lung transplantation. Transplantation 2009;87(10):1541–8.

27. Bowman JS, Green M, Scantlebury VP. OKT3 and viral disease in pediatric liver transplant recipients. Clin Transplant 1991;5:294–300.
28. Preiksaitis JK, Brennan DC, Fishman J, et al. Canadian society of transplantation consensus workshop on cytomegalovirus management in solid organ transplantation final report. Amer J Transpl 2005;5(2):218–27.
29. Green M, Michaels MG. Pre-emptive therapy of CMV disease in pediatric transplant recipients. Pediatr Infect Dis J 2000;19:875–7.
30. Blumberg EA, Brozena SC, Stutman P, et al. Immunogenicity of pneumococcal vaccine in heart transplant recipients. Clin Infect Dis 2001;32(2):307–10.
31. McCashland TM, Preheim LC, Gentry MJ. Pneumococcal vaccine response in cirrhosis and liver transplantation. J Infect Dis 2000;181(2):757–60.
32. Blumberg EA, Albano C, Pruett T, et al. The immunogenicity of influenza virus vaccine in solid organ transplant recipients. Clin Infect Dis 1996;22(2):295–302.
33. Kumar D, Welsh B, Siegal D, et al. Immunogenicity of pneumococcal vaccine in renal transplant recipients—three-year follow-up of a randomized trial. Am J Transplant 2007;7(3):633–8.
34. Lin PL, Michaels MG, Green M, et al. Safety and immunogenicity of the American Academy of Pediatrics—recommended sequential pneumococcal conjugate and polysaccharide vaccine schedule in pediatric solid organ transplant recipients. Pediatrics 2005;116(1):160–7.
35. American Academy of Pediatrics. Immunizations. In: Pickering LK, editor. Red book: 2009 report of the Committee on Infectious Diseases. 28th editon. Elk Grove Village (IL): American Academy of Pediatrics; 2009. p. 68–104.
36. Weinberg A, Horslen SP, Kaufman SS, et al. Safety and immunogenicity of varicella-zoster virus vaccine in pediatric liver and intestine transplant recipients. Am J Transplant 2006;6(3):565–8.
37. Khan S, Erlichman J, Rand EB. Live virus immunization after orthotopic liver transplantation. Pediatr Transplant 2006;10(1):78–82.
38. Kraft JN, Shaw JC. Varicella infection caused by Oka strain vaccine in a heart transplant recipient. Arch Dermatol 2006;142(7):943–5.
39. Levitsky J, Te HS, Faust TW, et al. Varicella infection following varicella vaccination in a liver transplant recipient. Am J Transplant 2002;2(9):880–2.
40. Humar A, Siegal D, Moussa G, et al. A prospective assessment of valganciclovir for the treatment of cytomegalovirus infection and disease in transplant recipients. J Infect Dis 2005;192(7):1154–7.
41. Danziger-Isakov LA, Faro A, Sweet S, et al. Variability in standard care for cytomegalovirus prevention in pediatric lung transplantation: survey of eight pediatric lung transplant programs. Pediatr Transplant 2003;7:469–73.
42. Green M, Webber SA. EBV viral load monitoring: unanswered questions. Am J Transplant 2002;2:894–5.
43. Lee TC, Savoldo B, Rooney CM, et al. Quantitative EBV viral loads and immunosuppression alterations can decrease PTLD incidence in pediatric liver transplant recipients. Am J Transplant 2005;5(9):2222–8.
44. Lujan-Zibermann L. Infections in hematopoietic stem cell transplant recipients. In: Long SS, Prober CG, Pickering LK, editors. Principles & practice of pediatric infectious diseases. 3rd edition. New York: Churchill Livingstone; 2008. p. 558–62.
45. Patrick CC. Opportunistic infections in hematopoietic stem cell transplantation. In: Feigin R, Cherry JD, Demmler G, et al, editors. Textbook of pediatric infectious diseases. 6th edition. Philadelphia: WB Saunders; 2009. p. 1037–47.

46. Centers for Disease Control and Prevention (CDC). Guidelines for preventing opportunistic infections among hematopoietic stem cell transplant recipients. MMWR Recomm Rep 2000;49:1–125.
47. Mullen CA, Nair J, Sandesh S, et al. Fever and neutropenia in pediatric hematopoietic stem cell transplant patients. Bone Marrow Transplant 2000;25: 59–65.
48. Champlin RE, Whimbey E. Community respiratory virus infections in bone marrow transplant recipients: the M.D. Anderson Cancer Center experience. Biol Blood Marrow Transplant 2001;7(Suppl):8S.
49. Couch RB, Englund JA, Whimbey E. Respiratory viral infections in immunocompetent and immunocompromised persons. Am J Med 1997;102:2.
50. Bowden RA. Respiratory virus infections after marrow transplantation: The Fred Hutchison Cancer Research Center Experience. Am J Med 1997;102:27.
51. Ljungman P. Respiratory virus infections in bone marrow transplant recipients: the European perspective. Am J Med 1997;102:44.
52. Bochud PY, Calandra T, Francioli P. Bacteremia due to viridans streptococci in neutropenic patients: a review. Am J Med 1994;97:256.
53. Meyers JD. Fungal infections in bone marrow transplant patients. Semin Oncol 1990;17:10.
54. Zollner-Schwetz I, Auner HW, Paulitsch A, et al. Oral and intestinal *Candida* colonization in patients undergoing hematopoietic stem-cell transplantation. J Infect Dis 2008;198:150.
55. Boutati EI, Anaissie EJ. Fusarium, a significant emerging pathogen in patients with hematologic malignancy: ten years' experience at a cancer center and implications for management. Blood 1997;90:999.
56. Morrison VA, Haake RJ, Weisdorf DJ. Non-*Candida* fungal infections after bone marrow transplantation: risk factors and outcome. Am J Med 1994; 96:497.
57. Wingard JR. Infections in allogeneic bone marrow transplant recipients. Semin Oncol 1993;20:80.
58. Wasserman R, August CS, Plotkin SA. Viral infections in pediatric bone marrow transplant patients. Pediatr Infect Dis J 1988;7:109.
59. Shields AF, Hackman RC, Fife KH, et al. Adenovirus infections in patients undergoing bone-marrow transplantation. N Engl J Med 1985;312:529.
60. Hale GA, Helsop HE, Krance RA, et al. Adenovirus infection after pediatric bone marrow transplantation. Bone Marrow Transplant 1999;23:277–82.
61. De Castro N, Neuville S, Sarfati C, et al. Occurrence of *Pneumocystis jiroveci* pneumonia after allogeneic stem cell transplantation: a 6-year retrospective study. Bone Marrow Transplant 2005;36:879.
62. Klingspor L, Stintzing G, Fasth A, et al. Deep *Candida* infection in children receiving allogeneic bone marrow transplants: incidence, risk factors and diagnosis. Bone Marrow Transplant 1996;17:1043–9.
63. Slavin MA, Meyers JD, Remington JS, et al. *Toxoplasma gondii* infection in marrow transplant recipients: a 20-year experience. Bone Marrow Transplant 1994;13(5):549–57.
64. Boeckh M, Bowden RA, Goodrich JM, et al. Cytomegalovirus antigen detection in peripheral blood leukocytes after allogeneic marrow transplantation. Blood 1992; 80:1358.
65. Enright H, Haake R, Weisdorf D, et al. Cytomegalovirus pneumonia after bone marrow transplantation. Risk factors and response to therapy. Transplantation 1993;55:1339.

66. Meyers JD, Ljungman P, Fisher LD. Cytomegalovirus excretion as a predictor of cytomegalovirus disease after marrow transplantation: importance of cytomegalovirus viremia. J Infect Dis 1990;162:373.

67. Schmidt GM, Horak DA, Niland JC, et al. Randomized controlled trial of prophylactic ganciclovir for cytomegalovirus pulmonary infection in recipients of allogeneic bone marrow transplants. N Engl J Med 1991;324(15):1005–11.

68. Goodrich JM, Bowden RA, Fisher L, et al. Ganciclovir prophylaxis to prevent cytomegalovirus disease after allogeneic marrow transplant. Ann Intern Med 1993; 118(3):173–8.

69. Erard V, Wald A, Corey L, et al. Use of long-term suppressive acyclovir after hematopoietic stem-cell transplantation: impact on herpes simplex virus (HSV) disease and drug-resistant HSV disease. J Infect Dis 2007;196:266.

70. Boeckh M, Leisenring W, Riddell SR, et al. Late cytomegalovirus disease and mortality in recipients of allogeneic hematopoietic stem cell transplants: importance of viral load and T-cell immunity. Blood 2003;101:407.

71. Marr KA, Siedel K, Slavin MA, et al. Prolonged fluconazole propylaxis is associated with persistent protection against candidiasis-related death in allogeneic marrow transplant recipients: long-term follow-up of a randomized, placebo-controlled trial. Blood 2000;96:2055.

72. Slavin MA, Osborne B, Adams R, et al. Efficacy and safety of fluconazole prophylaxis for fungal infections after marrow transplantation—a prospective, randomized, double-blind study. J Infect Dis 1995;171:1545.

Cytomegalovirus in Hematopoietic Stem Cell Transplant Recipients

Per Ljungman, MD, PhD[a,b,*], Morgan Hakki, MD[c],
Michael Boeckh, MD[d,e]

KEYWORDS

- Adoptive immunotherapy • Antiviral therapy • Cytomegalovirus
- Hematopoietic stem cell transplantation

Human cytomegalovirus (CMV) is a betaherpesvirus in the same family as human herpesvirus-6 and -7. CMV is a large virus including approximately 200 proteins. CMV has been found in a wide range of cells, including endothelial cells, epithelial cells, blood cells including neutrophils, and smooth muscle cells.[1] The presence of CMV in these cells may be caused by active replication within the cell, phagocytosis of CMV proteins, or abortive (incomplete) replication, and likely contributes to dissemination and transmission. As the other herpesviruses, CMV remains in the human body after primary infection for life. Little is known about the site or mechanisms of CMV latency and persistence. Several studies indicate that cells of the granulocyte-monocyte lineage carry CMV[2–4] and these might be one site for latency and persistence. Transplantation of solid organs clearly can transmit CMV, so it is possible that cells other than those mentioned can harbor and transmit the virus. Whether the infected cell type in these organs is blood cells, macrophages, or other cell types, however, has not been clarified.

Per Ljungman had support from the Karolinska Institute research funds, the European Leukemia Net, and the Swedish Children's Cancer Fund. Michael Boeckh had support from the National Institute of Health (NIH CA 18029).

A version of this article was previously published in the *Infectious Disease Clinics of North America*, 24:2.

[a] Department of Hematology, Karolinska University Hospital, S-14186 Stockholm, Sweden
[b] Divison of Hematology, Department of Medicine Huddinge, Karolinska Institutet, S-14186 Stockholm, Sweden
[c] Division of Infectious Diseases, Oregon Health and Science University, Portland, OR, USA
[d] University of Washington, Seattle, WA, USA
[e] Vaccine and Infectious Disease Institute, Fred Hutchinson Cancer Research Center, 1100 Fairview Avenue N, Seattle, WA 98109–4417, USA
* Corresponding author. Division of Hematology, Department of Medicine Huddinge, Karolinska Institutet, S-14186 Stockholm, Sweden.
E-mail address: Per.Ljungman@ki.se

T-cell mediated cellular immunity is the most important factor in controlling CMV replication. CMV induces a strong CD8+ cytotoxic T-lymphocyte (CTL) response, and the proportion of circulating CD8+ T cells in healthy individuals that are specific for CMV antigens ranges from 10% to 40% increasing with age.[5–10] Several CMV proteins are targeted by the CD8+ T-cell response including IE-1, IE-2, and pp65.[7,10–16] Lack of CMV-specific CD8+ CTL responses predisposes to CMV infection, whereas reconstitution of CMV-specific CD8+ CTL responses after hematopoietic cell transplantation correlates with protection from CMV and improved outcome of CMV disease.[17–21] After hematopoietic stem cell transplantation (HSCT), CMV-specific CD4+ responses are associated with protection from CMV disease.[17,22–24] The lack of CMV-specific CD4+ cells is associated with late CMV disease and death in patients who have undergone HSCT.[25] The role of humoral immunity in controlling CMV replication is not clear. Although antibodies to gB and gH can neutralize the virus in cell culture, they do not seem to prevent primary infection in adults, but rather may function to limit disease severity.[26,27]

The innate immune system also seems to be involved in controlling CMV replication. CMV triggers cellular inflammatory cytokine production on binding to the target cell, mediated in part by the interaction of gB and gH with toll-like receptor 2.[28–30] Polymorphisms in toll-like receptor 2 have been associated with CMV infection after liver transplantation.[31] In humans, natural killer cell responses increase during CMV infection after renal transplantation, and a deficiency in natural killer cells is associated with severe CMV infection (among other herpesviruses).[32,33] The genotype of the donor-activating killer immunoglobulin-like receptor, which regulates NK cell function, has recently been demonstrated to influence the development of CMV infection after allogeneic HSCT.[34–36] Finally, polymorphisms in chemokine receptor 5 and interleukin-10 have been associated with CMV disease, whereas polymorphisms in monocyte chemoattractant protein 1 are associated with reactivation after allogeneic HSCT.[37]

DIAGNOSTIC METHODS

The serologic determination of CMV-specific antibodies (IgG and IgM) is important for determining a patient's risk for CMV infection after transplantation but cannot be used for the diagnosis of CMV infection or disease. Growth of CMV in tissue culture takes several weeks, making this technique obsolete for diagnosis of CMV in HSCT recipients. The shell vial (rapid culture/DEAFF) technique, in which monoclonal antibodies are used to detect CMV immediate-early proteins in cultured cells, is not sensitive enough to use for routine blood monitoring,[38] but is highly useful on bronchoalveolar lavage (BAL) fluid in the diagnosis of CMV pneumonia.[39]

The detection of the CMV pp65 in peripheral blood leukocytes (antigenemia) is a rapid and semiquantitative method of diagnosing CMV infection. A positive CMV pp65 assay is predictive for the development of invasive disease in transplant patients.[40,41]

Polymerase chain reaction (PCR) is the most sensitive method for detecting CMV.[42] Quantitative PCR (qPCR) relies on the amplification and quantitative measurement of CMV DNA, while at the same time maintaining high specificity. High levels of DNA in blood (whole blood or plasma) is a good predictor of CMV disease in HSCT recipients.[25,43–46] Although PCR has been used on BAL fluid,[47] viral-load cut-offs have not been defined, and although the sensitivity and negative predictive values are very high, the specificity and positive predictive values are not known.

The detection of CMV mRNA by nucleic acid sequence-based amplification on blood samples is similarly useful as DNA qPCR or pp65 antigenemia for guiding preemptive therapy after HSCT.[48,49] This method is less frequently used, however, compared with the other techniques.

The presence of characteristic CMV "owl's eye" nuclear inclusions in histopathology specimens is useful in the diagnosis of invasive CMV disease. This method has relatively low sensitivity, but can be enhanced by use of immunohistochemical techniques.

CLINICAL MANIFESTATIONS

CMV infection is defined as the detection of CMV, typically by DNA PCR, pp65 antigenemia, or mRNA nucleic acid sequence-based amplification, from plasma or whole blood in a CMV-seronegative patient (primary infection) or a CMV-seropositive patient (reactivation of latent or persistent virus or superinfection with another strain of CMV).[50,51] International definitions of CMV disease, requiring the presence of symptoms and signs compatible with CMV end-organ involvement together with the detection of CMV using a validated method in the appropriate clinical specimen, have been published.[52] Almost any organ can be involved in CMV disease. Fever is a common manifestation, but may be absent in patients receiving high-dose immunosuppression.

CMV pneumonia is the most serious manifestation of CMV in HSCT recipients with a mortality of more than 50%.[53–55] CMV pneumonia often manifests with fever, nonproductive cough, hypoxia, and infiltrates commonly interstitial on radiography. The diagnosis of CMV pneumonia is established by detection of CMV by shell-vial, culture, or histology in BAL or lung biopsy specimens, in the presence of compatible clinical signs and symptoms. Pulmonary shedding of CMV is common, and CMV detection in BAL from asymptomatic patients who underwent routine BAL screening at day 35 after HSCT was predictive of subsequent CMV pneumonia in only approximately two thirds of cases.[56] The presence of CMV in a BAL specimen in the absence of clinical evidence of CMV disease is not proof of CMV pneumonia, but the patient needs to be carefully followed. The relevance of PCR testing on BAL fluid is doubtful because there are little data correlating CMV DNA detection by PCR in BAL fluid with CMV pneumonia. Because of the high negative predictive value afforded by its high sensitivity, however, a negative PCR result can be used to rule out the diagnosis of CMV pneumonia.[47] It is possible that qPCR on BAL might provide additional information, allowing this technique to be used for the diagnosis of CMV pneumonia in the future.

CMV can affect the entire gastrointestinal (GI) tract. Ulcers extending deep into the submucosal layers are seen on endoscopy, but can be macroscopically confused with other disorders including graft-versus-host disease (GVHD) and adenovirus disease. The diagnosis of GI disease relies on detection of CMV in biopsy specimens by culture or histology and can occur in the absence of CMV detection in the blood, even by PCR.[57,58] CMV and GVHD are also frequently seen concomitantly, making the assessment of each disorder's contribution to the symptomatology difficult.

Retinitis is relatively uncommon after transplantation, although its incidence seems to be increasing.[59–62] Decreased visual acuity and blurred vision are early symptoms, and approximately 60% of patients have involvement of both eyes.[60] Untreated, the risk for loss of vision on the affected eye is high. Other manifestations including hepatitis and encephalitis do occur, but are rare.

RISK FACTORS
Allogeneic HSCT Recipients

In allogeneic HSCT recipients, the most important risk factors for CMV disease are the serologic status of the donor and recipient. CMV-seronegative patients receiving stem cells from a CMV-seronegative donor (D-/R-) have a very low risk of primary infection if

CMV-safe blood products are used. Approximately 30% of seronegative recipients transplanted from a seropositive donor (D+/R-) develop primary CMV infection. Although the risk of CMV disease is low because of preemptive treatment of CMV infection, mortality caused by bacterial and fungal infections in these patients is higher than in similarly matched D-/R- transplants (18.3% vs 9.7%, respectively),[63] possibly because of the immunosuppressive effects of CMV or its therapy.

Without prophylaxis, approximately 80% of CMV-seropositive patients experience CMV infection after allogeneic HSCT. Current preventive strategies have decreased the incidence of CMV disease, which had historically occurred in 20% to 35% of these patients.[64] Although a CMV-seropositive recipient is at higher risk for transplant-related mortality than a seronegative recipient,[65,66] the impact of donor serostatus on nonrelapse mortality and survival when the recipient is seropositive remains controversial.[67–78] This combination, however, has been reported as a risk factor for delayed CMV-specific immune reconstitution,[79–82] repeated CMV reactivations,[80,83] late CMV recurrence,[84] and development of CMV disease.[46,80,85]

Other risk factors for CMV infection after allogeneic HSCT include the use of high-dose corticosteroids, T-cell depletion, acute and chronic GVHD, and the use of mismatched or unrelated donors.[43,46,85–89] The use of sirolimus for GVHD prophylaxis seems to have a protective effect against CMV infection, possibly because of the inhibition of cellular signaling pathways that are co-opted by CMV during infection for synthesis of viral proteins.[85,90] The use of nonmyeloablative conditioning regimens generally has been reported to result in a lower rate of CMV infection and disease early after HSCT compared with standard myeloablative regimens.[87,91] By 1 year after HSCT, however, the risks of CMV infection and disease are comparable.[91,92] Umbilical cord blood transplantation (CBT) is an increasingly used technology for HSCT.[93] Because most infants are born without CMV infection, the transplanted allograft is almost always CMV-negative. Among CMV-seropositive recipients who do not receive antiviral prophylaxis, the rate of CMV infection after CBT is 40% to 80%, with one study reporting 100%.[94–98] When patients receive prophylaxis with high-dose valacyclovir after CBT, it does not seem that CBT entails a significantly greater risk of CMV infection and disease than does peripheral blood stem cell or bone marrow transplantation.[89]

Alemtuzumab is an anti-CD52 monoclonal antibody that results in CD4+ and CD8+ lymphopenia that can last for up to 9 months after administration. Patients who received alemtuzumab experienced a higher rate of CMV infection compared with matched controls not receiving alemtuzumab.[99,100]

Late CMV Infection After Allogeneic HSCT

Today, with the use of preemptive ganciclovir therapy, CMV disease has become a more significant problem after day 100 following allogeneic HSCT.[25,84,101] The risk varies a lot between different centers, presumably because of factors related to patient and donor selection and the choices of transplantation modalities used at the different centers (stem cell source, GVHD prophylaxis and treatment, conditioning regimens). Late CMV infection is strongly associated with nonrelapse mortality.[84] Several factors predict the development of late CMV disease[17,23,25,84,86] and extended monitoring and antiviral therapy are warranted in patients with risk factors to reduce the risk.[25,91,102]

Autologous HSCT

After autologous HSCT, approximately 40% of seropositive patients develop CMV infection.[53,103] Although CMV disease is rare after autologous HSCT,[104–107] the outcome of CMV pneumonia is similar to that after allogeneic HSCT.[53,108,109] Risk factors for CMV disease after autologous HSCT include CD34+ selection, high-dose corticosteroids, and the use of total-body irradiation or fludarabine as part of the conditioning regimen.[106]

PREVENTION OF CMV INFECTION AND DISEASE

CMV serology should be assessed as early as possible when a patient is considered a candidate for HSCT and safe blood products should be used in CMV-seronegative candidates to reduce the risk for primary CMV infection. To reduce the risk for transmission of CMV, blood products from CMV-seronegative donors or leukocyte-reduced, filtered blood products should be used.[110–112] Recipients who are CMV seronegative before allogeneic HSCT should ideally receive a graft from a CMV-negative donor. Weighing the factor of donor CMV serostatus compared with other relevant donor factors, such as HLA-match, is difficult. No data exist indicating whether HLA-matching is more important compared with CMV serostatus in affecting a good outcome for the patient. For lesser degrees of mismatch, (allele-mismatches or mismatches on HLA-C, DQ, or DP), the CMV serostatus of the donor should be considered in the selection process.

Intravenous immunoglobulin (IVIG) is not reliably effective as prophylaxis against primary CMV infection. Likewise, the effect of immunoglobulin on reducing CMV infection in seropositive patients is modest.[113–118] The prophylactic use of immunoglobulin is not recommended. Future possibilities for prevention might include a CMV vaccine, and different vaccines are currently in development.[119]

Antiviral Prophylaxis and Preemptive Therapy

Antiviral prophylaxis is defined as the routine administration of an antiviral agent to all patients at risk. Preemptive therapy is initiated when CMV infection is detected, but before the development of CMV-associated symptoms. Both strategies have their benefits and drawbacks (**Table 1**). If an effective antiviral is used for prophylaxis, it could be argued that monitoring would not be required. Additionally, prophylaxis may potentially prevent the indirect effects associated with CMV infection. Prophylaxis by definition results in some patients receiving the drug unnecessarily, however, exposing them to potential drug-related toxicities. The success of the preemptive treatment strategy is largely dependent on the early detection of CMV in blood. By allowing a limited amount of viral replication, preemptive therapy may stimulate immune responses and thereby promote CMV-specific immune reconstitution.[17] Because both strategies are equally effective in preventing CMV disease,[120] most transplant centers have moved toward preemptive strategies as pp65 antigenemia and DNA PCR-based assays have become readily available.[121–123]

More recently, there has been great interest in using methods to determine CMV-specific immune reconstitution after HSCT as an additional means to determine the risk of CMV infection and disease. The usefulness of measuring T-cell responses as a guide for withholding therapy was evaluated in a small pilot study involving HSCT recipients more than 100 days after transplant.[79] Although promising, this strategy requires validation in larger, randomized trials.

Antiviral Agents

High-dose acyclovir reduces the risk for CMV infection and possibly disease.[124,125] Valacyclovir is the prodrug of acyclovir and is better absorbed, resulting in higher serum-concentration. High-dose valacyclovir is more effective than acyclovir in

Table 1
Strategies for preemptive therapy and prophylaxis after HCT

Prevention Strategy	Patient Population	Timing Post-HCT	Initiation	First-line Choice: Induction	First-line Choice: Maintenance	Alternatives	Duration
Preemptive	Allogeneic HSCT recipients	<100 d	At first detection of CMV infection	GCV 5 mg/kg IV bid × 7–14 d and declining viral load	GCV 5 mg/kg IV qd	Foscarnet Valganciclovir Cidofovir	Indicator test negative and minimum 2–3 wk
	Allogeneic HSCT or GVHD requiring steroid therapy or Early CMV infection	>100 d	pp65 Ag ≥5 cells/slide or ≥2 consecutively positive PCR/viremia	GCV 5 mg/kg IV bid × 7–14 d and declining viral load	GCV 5 mg/kg IV qd	Valganciclovir Foscarnet	Until indicator assay negative and minimum 2–3 wk therapy
	Autologous HSCT and CMV seropositive and at high risk[a]	<100 d	pp65 Ag ≥5 cells/slide (or at any level if CD34 ± selected graft)	GCV 5 mg/kg IV bid × 7 d and declining viral load	GCV 5 mg/kg IV qd	Foscarnet Valganciclovir Cidofovir	Until indicator assay negative and minimum 2 wk therapy
Prophylaxis	Allogeneic HSCT recipients	<100 d	At engraftment	GCV 5 mg/kg IV bid × 5–7 d	GCV 5 mg/kg IV qd	Foscarnet Acyclovir[b] Valacyclovir[b]	Day 100 after HCT

Abbreviations: CMV, cytomegalovirus; GCV, ganciclovir; GVHD, graft-versus-host disease; HSCT, hematopoietic stem cell transplantation; PCR, polymerase chain reaction.
[a] Includes use of TBI in conditioning, recent fludarabine, or 2-chlorodeoxyadenosine, high-dose corticosteroids.
[b] Must be combined with active surveillance for CMV infection.

reducing CMV infection and the need for preemptive therapy with ganciclovir after HSCT, although there is no impact on survival.[126] Routine monitoring for CMV infection is required if valacyclovir or acyclovir prophylaxis is used.

Ganciclovir is currently the first-line agent for CMV prophylaxis and preemptive treatment. Intravenous ganciclovir has been demonstrated to reduce the risk of CMV infection and disease compared with placebo, but does not improve overall survival.[120,127–129] Neutropenia occurs in up to 30% of HSCT recipients during ganciclovir therapy[130] increasing the risk of invasive bacterial and fungal infections.[120,127,130] Therapeutic drug monitoring can be helpful to guide therapy and reduce the risk for toxicity, especially in the situation of pre-existing renal impairment.

Valganciclovir is an orally available prodrug of ganciclovir and administration achieves serum concentrations at least equivalent to intravenous ganciclovir.[131–133] The results of several uncontrolled studies suggest that valganciclovir is comparable with intravenous ganciclovir in terms of efficacy and safety when used as preemptive therapy after allogeneic HSCT.[131,134–136] Preliminary data from a randomized trial have been presented indicating little or no difference in efficacy or toxicity compared with intravenous ganciclovir.[137] Until more data are available, however, caution should be exercised when choosing valganciclovir as preemptive therapy.

Foscarnet is as effective as ganciclovir for preemptive therapy after allogeneic transplantation.[138] The commonly encountered toxicities of foscarnet make this drug a second-line agent, most appropriate when ganciclovir is contraindicated or not tolerated.

Cidofovir is a "broad-spectrum" antiviral with a long half-life allowing a once-per-week dosing schedule. The major toxicity with cidofovir, acute renal tubular necrosis, limits its use after HSCT.[139]

Monitoring for CMV Infection and Initiation of Preemptive Therapy

qPCR assays for CMV DNA are increasingly used because of their performance characteristics allowing the development of institution-specific viral load thresholds for initiation of preemptive treatment, thereby avoiding unnecessary treatment of patients who are at low risk of progression to disease. It has been reported that the initial viral load and the viral load kinetics are important as risk factors for CMV disease.[140] Currently, several different variations are used, making it difficult to establish validated universal viral load thresholds because of differences in assay performance and testing material (whole blood vs plasma).[141]

If the preemptive therapy strategy is used, all patients who have undergone allogeneic HSCT should be monitored up to day 100 posttransplant on a weekly basis for CMV infection. Although CMV infection is rare in D-/R- patients, routine monitoring was effective in identifying CMV infection and preventing disease in a large cohort.[112] The ideal duration and frequency of CMV monitoring later after HSCT have not been determined.[91,102]

Various durations of preemptive antiviral treatment have been explored. Most centers now continue antiviral treatment until the designated viral marker is negative and the patient has received at least 2 weeks of antiviral therapy. If an assay less sensitive than DNA PCR, such as the pp65 antigenemia assay, is used, then preemptive therapy should be continued until two negative results are obtained.[138] If a patient is still positive by PCR or pp65 antigenemia assay after 2 weeks of therapy, treatment should be extended until clearance is achieved. It has been shown that a low rate of viral load decrease is a risk factor for later-occurring CMV disease.[46]

Special Populations

Patients with CMV disease occurring before planned allogeneic HSCT have a very high risk of mortality.[142] After transplantation, a patient with documented pretransplant CMV disease should either be monitored for CMV very closely (ie, twice weekly), or be given prophylaxis with ganciclovir or foscarnet.

The optimal approach to CMV after CBT is not clear. One study described successful preemptive treatment with ganciclovir,[98] whereas another combined high-dose valacyclovir prophylaxis with continued monitoring and preemptive therapy.[89]

ANTIVIRAL RESISTANCE

Risk factors for drug resistance include prolonged (months) antiviral therapy, intermittent low-level viral replication in the presence of drug caused by profound immunosuppression or suboptimal drug levels, and lack of prior immunity to CMV.[143] Drug resistance should be suspected in patients who have increasing quantitative viral loads for more than 2 weeks despite antiviral therapy. After start of antiviral therapy in treatment-naive patients, an increase in the viral load occurs in approximately one third of patients and is likely caused by the underlying immunosuppression (clinical resistance), not true drug resistance caused by mutations in the target genes for the antiviral agent used.[41] If the viral load increases in patients who have received previous antiviral therapy, drug resistance should, however, be suspected.

Ganciclovir resistance most often is caused by mutations in the UL97 gene, but mutations in the UL54-encoded DNA polymerase can also occur. Several UL97 mutations that confer resistance have been described.[144] Because different UL97 mutations confer varying degrees of ganciclovir resistance, however, some cases of genotypically defined ganciclovir-resistant CMV may still respond to therapy.[145]

If ganciclovir resistance is documented or suspected, foscarnet is generally the second-line agent of choice. Unlike ganciclovir, foscarnet activity is not dependent on phosphorylation by the UL97 gene product.[146] Resistance to foscarnet can occur and is caused by mutations in UL54. Because cidofovir is not phosphorylated by the CMV UL97 gene product, it is also active against ganciclovir-resistant UL97 mutants. Certain UL54 mutations, however, can confer cross-resistance between ganciclovir and cidofovir.[146,147] Additional genotype testing of UL54 is indicated to evaluate for potential cross-resistance conferring mutations.

Drugs under evaluation, such as maribavir, may provide therapeutic options in the future. Maribavir inhibits the CMV UL97 kinase and is active against wild-type and ganciclovir-resistant CMV strains[148] and has shown promising results in a small series of patients failing therapy with other antiviral agents either because of toxicity or resistance. Other drugs with possible anti-CMV activity include the arthritis drug leflunomide and the antimalaria compound artesunate.[149–151]

MANAGEMENT OF CMV DISEASE

Several studies established the current standard of care for CMV pneumonia, which is treatment with ganciclovir (or foscarnet as an alternative agent) in combination with IVIG.[152–155] These studies showed improved survival rates compared with historical controls. There does not seem to be a specific advantage of CMV-specific immunoglobulin (CMV-Ig) compared with pooled immunoglobulin.[153] In specific clinical situations, however, such as volume overload, CMV-Ig may be preferred. Several studies have raised doubt regarding the beneficial effect of concomitant IVIG,[156,157] but it is still considered as standard-of-care at most centers.

For GI disease, the standard therapy is most often intravenous ganciclovir for 3 to 4 weeks followed by several weeks of maintenance. Shorter courses of induction therapy (2 weeks) are not as effective.[158] There is no role for concomitant IVIG in the treatment of GI disease.[159] Recurrence may occur in approximately 30% of patients in the setting of continued immunosuppression and such patients may benefit from secondary prophylaxis until immunosuppression has been reduced. Foscarnet can be used as an alternative if neutropenia is present. Valganciclovir as maintenance treatment for GI disease has not been well studied.

CMV retinitis is typically treated with systemic ganciclovir, foscarnet, or cidofovir, with or without intraocular ganciclovir injections or implants.[60,160–162] Fomivirsen is an antisense RNA molecule that targets mRNA encoded by CMV and is approved as second-line therapy for CMV retinitis in patients with AIDS.[163]

Other manifestations of CMV disease, such as hepatitis and encephalitis, are uncommon and are typically managed with intravenous ganciclovir. The duration of therapy for these manifestations has not been well-established and should be tailored to the individual patient.

ADOPTIVE IMMUNOTHERAPY

CMV-specific T cells can be generated by several different mechanisms to restore cellular immunity passively after transplantation.[5] Several groups have reported a beneficial impact of adoptive immunotherapy on CMV viral loads in patients who had undergone HSCT.[164] Despite these seemingly promising results, scientific questions remain unanswered (eg, the optimal cell type and dose for infusion) and technical hurdles persist (availability of clinical grade reagents) that preclude adoptive immunotherapy from becoming a routine clinical procedure at the current time.

REFERENCES

1. Sinzger C, Digel M, Jahn G. Cytomegalovirus cell tropism. Curr Top Microbiol Immunol 2008;325:63–83.
2. Bolovan-Fritts CA, Mocarski ES, Wiedeman JA. Peripheral blood CD14(+) cells from healthy subjects carry a circular conformation of latent cytomegalovirus genome. Blood 1999;93(1):394–8.
3. Kondo K, Kaneshima H, Mocarski ES. Human cytomegalovirus latent infection of granulocyte-macrophage progenitors. Proc Natl Acad Sci U S A 1994;91(25): 11879–83.
4. Taylor-Wiedeman J, Sissons JG, Borysiewicz LK, et al. Monocytes are a major site of persistence of human cytomegalovirus in peripheral blood mononuclear cells. J Gen Virol 1991;72(Pt 9):2059–64.
5. Crough T, Khanna R. Immunobiology of human cytomegalovirus: from bench to bedside. Clin Microbiol Rev 2009;22(1):76–98 [table of contents].
6. Gillespie GM, Wills MR, Appay V, et al. Functional heterogeneity and high frequencies of cytomegalovirus-specific CD8(+) T lymphocytes in healthy seropositive donors. J Virol 2000;74(17):8140–50.
7. Khan N, Cobbold M, Keenan R, et al. Comparative analysis of CD8+ T cell responses against human cytomegalovirus proteins pp65 and immediate early 1 shows similarities in precursor frequency, oligoclonality, and phenotype. J Infect Dis 2002;185(8):1025–34.
8. Khan N, Hislop A, Gudgeon N, et al. Herpesvirus-specific CD8 T cell immunity in old age: cytomegalovirus impairs the response to a coresident EBV infection. J Immunol 2004;173(12):7481–9.

9. Ouyang Q, Wagner WM, Wikby A, et al. Large numbers of dysfunctional CD8+ T lymphocytes bearing receptors for a single dominant CMV epitope in the very old. J Clin Immunol 2003;23(4):247–57.

10. Sylwester AW, Mitchell BL, Edgar JB, et al. Broadly targeted human cytomegalovirus-specific CD4+ and CD8+ T cells dominate the memory compartments of exposed subjects. J Exp Med 2005;202(5):673–85.

11. Elkington R, Walker S, Crough T, et al. Ex vivo profiling of CD8+-T-cell responses to human cytomegalovirus reveals broad and multispecific reactivities in healthy virus carriers. J Virol 2003;77(9):5226–40.

12. Kern F, Bunde T, Faulhaber N, et al. Cytomegalovirus (CMV) phosphoprotein 65 makes a large contribution to shaping the T cell repertoire in CMV-exposed individuals. J Infect Dis 2002;185(12):1709–16.

13. Kern F, Surel IP, Faulhaber N, et al. Target structures of the CD8(+)-T-cell response to human cytomegalovirus: the 72-kilodalton major immediate-early protein revisited. J Virol 1999;73(10):8179–84.

14. Khan N, Best D, Bruton R, et al. T cell recognition patterns of immunodominant cytomegalovirus antigens in primary and persistent infection. J Immunol 2007; 178(7):4455–65.

15. Khan N, Bruton R, Taylor GS, et al. Identification of cytomegalovirus-specific cytotoxic T lymphocytes in vitro is greatly enhanced by the use of recombinant virus lacking the US2 to US11 region or modified vaccinia virus Ankara expressing individual viral genes. J Virol 2005;79(5):2869–79.

16. Kondo E, Akatsuka Y, Kuzushima K, et al. Identification of novel CTL epitopes of CMV-pp65 presented by a variety of HLA alleles. Blood 2004;103(2): 630–8.

17. Li CR, Greenberg PD, Gilbert MJ, et al. Recovery of HLA-restricted cytomegalovirus (CMV)-specific T-cell responses after allogeneic bone marrow transplant: correlation with CMV disease and effect of ganciclovir prophylaxis. Blood 1994; 83(7):1971–9.

18. Polic B, Hengel H, Krmpotic A, et al. Hierarchical and redundant lymphocyte subset control precludes cytomegalovirus replication during latent infection. J Exp Med 1998;188(6):1047–54.

19. Quinnan GV Jr, Kirmani N, Rook AH, et al. Cytotoxic t cells in cytomegalovirus infection: HLA-restricted T-lymphocyte and non-T-lymphocyte cytotoxic responses correlate with recovery from cytomegalovirus infection in bone-marrow-transplant recipients. N Engl J Med 1982;307(1):7–13.

20. Reusser P, Cathomas G, Attenhofer R, et al. Cytomegalovirus (CMV)-specific T cell immunity after renal transplantation mediates protection from CMV disease by limiting the systemic virus load. J Infect Dis 1999;180(2):247–53.

21. Reusser P, Riddell SR, Meyers JD, et al. Cytotoxic T-lymphocyte response to cytomegalovirus after human allogeneic bone marrow transplantation: pattern of recovery and correlation with cytomegalovirus infection and disease. Blood 1991;78(5):1373–80.

22. Hebart H, Daginik S, Stevanovic S, et al. Sensitive detection of human cytomegalovirus peptide-specific cytotoxic T-lymphocyte responses by interferon-gamma-enzyme-linked immunospot assay and flow cytometry in healthy individuals and in patients after allogeneic stem cell transplantation. Blood 2002;99(10):3830–7.

23. Krause H, Hebart H, Jahn G, et al. Screening for CMV-specific T cell proliferation to identify patients at risk of developing late onset CMV disease. Bone Marrow Transplant 1997;19(11):1111–6.

24. Ljungman P, Aschan J, Azinge JN, et al. Cytomegalovirus viraemia and specific T-helper cell responses as predictors of disease after allogeneic marrow transplantation. Br J Haematol 1993;83(1):118–24.

25. Boeckh M, Leisenring W, Riddell SR, et al. Late cytomegalovirus disease and mortality in recipients of allogeneic hematopoietic stem cell transplants: importance of viral load and T-cell immunity. Blood 2003;101(2):407–14.

26. Boppana SB, Britt WJ. Antiviral antibody responses and intrauterine transmission after primary maternal cytomegalovirus infection. J Infect Dis 1995; 171(5):1115–21.

27. Jonjic S, Pavic I, Lucin P, et al. Efficacious control of cytomegalovirus infection after long-term depletion of CD8+ T lymphocytes. J Virol 1990;64(11): 5457–64.

28. Boehme KW, Guerrero M, Compton T. Human cytomegalovirus envelope glycoproteins B and H are necessary for TLR2 activation in permissive cells. J Immunol 2006;177(10):7094–102.

29. Compton T, Kurt-Jones EA, Boehme KW, et al. Human cytomegalovirus activates inflammatory cytokine responses via CD14 and Toll-like receptor 2. J Virol 2003;77(8):4588–96.

30. Juckem LK, Boehme KW, Feire AL, et al. Differential initiation of innate immune responses induced by human cytomegalovirus entry into fibroblast cells. J Immunol 2008;180(7):4965–77.

31. Kijpittayarit S, Eid AJ, Brown RA, et al. Relationship between Toll-like receptor 2 polymorphism and cytomegalovirus disease after liver transplantation. Clin Infect Dis 2007;44(10):1315–20.

32. Biron CA, Byron KS, Sullivan JL. Severe herpesvirus infections in an adolescent without natural killer cells. N Engl J Med 1989;320(26):1731–5.

33. Venema H, van den Berg AP, van Zanten C, et al. Natural killer cell responses in renal transplant patients with cytomegalovirus infection. J Med Virol 1994;42(2): 188–92.

34. Chen C, Busson M, Rocha V, et al. Activating KIR genes are associated with CMV reactivation and survival after non-T-cell depleted HLA-identical sibling bone marrow transplantation for malignant disorders. Bone Marrow Transplant 2006;38(6):437–44.

35. Cook M, Briggs D, Craddock C, et al. Donor KIR genotype has a major influence on the rate of cytomegalovirus reactivation following T-cell replete stem cell transplantation. Blood 2006;107(3):1230–2.

36. Zaia JA, Sun JY, Gallez-Hawkins GM, et al. The effect of single and combined activating killer immunoglobulin-like receptor genotypes on cytomegalovirus infection and immunity after hematopoietic cell transplantation. Biol Blood Marrow Transplant 2009;15(3):315–25.

37. Loeffler J, Steffens M, Arlt EM, et al. Polymorphisms in the genes encoding chemokine receptor 5, interleukin-10, and monocyte chemoattractant protein 1 contribute to cytomegalovirus reactivation and disease after allogeneic stem cell transplantation. J Clin Microbiol 2006;44(5):1847–50.

38. Einsele H, Ehninger G, Hebart H, et al. Polymerase chain reaction monitoring reduces the incidence of cytomegalovirus disease and the duration and side effects of antiviral therapy after bone marrow transplantation. Blood 1995; 86(7):2815–20.

39. Crawford SW, Bowden RA, Hackman RC, et al. Rapid detection of cytomegalovirus pulmonary infection by bronchoalveolar lavage and centrifugation culture. Ann Intern Med 1988;108(2):180–5.

40. Boeckh M, Bowden RA, Goodrich JM, et al. Cytomegalovirus antigen detection in peripheral blood leukocytes after allogeneic marrow transplantation. Blood 1992;80(5):1358–64.

41. Nichols WG, Corey L, Gooley T, et al. Rising pp65 antigenemia during preemptive anticytomegalovirus therapy after allogeneic hematopoietic stem cell transplantation: risk factors, correlation with DNA load, and outcomes. Blood 2001; 97(4):867–74.

42. Boeckh M, Huang M, Ferrenberg J, et al. Optimization of quantitative detection of cytomegalovirus DNA in plasma by real-time PCR. J Clin Microbiol 2004; 42(3):1142–8.

43. Einsele H, Hebart H, Kauffmann-Schneider C, et al. Risk factors for treatment failures in patients receiving PCR-based preemptive therapy for CMV infection. Bone Marrow Transplant 2000;25(7):757–63.

44. Emery VC, Griffiths PD. Prediction of cytomegalovirus load and resistance patterns after antiviral chemotherapy. Proc Natl Acad Sci U S A 2000;97(14): 8039–44.

45. Gor D, Sabin C, Prentice HG, et al. Longitudinal fluctuations in cytomegalovirus load in bone marrow transplant patients: relationship between peak virus load, donor/recipient serostatus, acute GVHD and CMV disease. Bone Marrow Transplant 1998;21(6):597–605.

46. Ljungman P, Perez-Bercoff L, Jonsson J, et al. Risk factors for the development of cytomegalovirus disease after allogeneic stem cell transplantation. Haematologica 2006;91(1):78–83.

47. Cathomas G, Morris P, Pekle K, et al. Rapid diagnosis of cytomegalovirus pneumonia in marrow transplant recipients by bronchoalveolar lavage using the polymerase chain reaction, virus culture, and the direct immunostaining of alveolar cells. Blood 1993;81(7):1909–14.

48. Gerna G, Lilleri D, Baldanti F, et al. Human cytomegalovirus immediate-early mRNAemia versus pp65 antigenemia for guiding pre-emptive therapy in children and young adults undergoing hematopoietic stem cell transplantation: a prospective, randomized, open-label trial. Blood 2003;101(12):5053–60.

49. Hebart H, Ljungman P, Klingebiel T, et al. Prospective comparison of PCR-based versus late mRNA-based preemptive antiviral therapy for HCMV infection in patients after allogeneic stem cell transplantation. Blood 2003;102(11):195a.

50. Collier AC, Chandler SH, Handsfield HH, et al. Identification of multiple strains of cytomegalovirus in homosexual men. J Infect Dis 1989;159(1):123–6.

51. Manuel O, Pang XL, Humar A, et al. An assessment of donor-to-recipient transmission patterns of human cytomegalovirus by analysis of viral genomic variants. J Infect Dis 2009;199(11):1621–8.

52. Ljungman P, Griffiths P, Paya C. Definitions of cytomegalovirus infection and disease in transplant recipients. Clin Infect Dis 2002;34(8):1094–7.

53. Boeckh M, Stevens-Ayers T, Bowden RA. Cytomegalovirus pp65 antigenemia after autologous marrow and peripheral blood stem cell transplantation. J Infect Dis 1996;174(5):907–12.

54. Konoplev S, Champlin RE, Giralt S, et al. Cytomegalovirus pneumonia in adult autologous blood and marrow transplant recipients. Bone Marrow Transplant 2001;27(8):877–81.

55. Ljungman P. Cytomegalovirus pneumonia: presentation, diagnosis, and treatment. Semin Respir Infect 1995;10(4):209–15.

56. Schmidt GM, Horak DA, Niland JC, et al. A randomized, controlled trial of prophylactic ganciclovir for cytomegalovirus pulmonary infection in recipients

of allogeneic bone marrow transplants. The City of Hope-Stanford-Syntex CMV Study Group. N Engl J Med 1991;324(15):1005–11.

57. Jang EY, Park SY, Lee EJ, et al. Diagnostic performance of the cytomegalovirus (CMV) antigenemia assay in patients with CMV gastrointestinal disease. Clin Infect Dis 2009;48(12):e121–4.

58. Mori T, Okamoto S, Matsuoka S, et al. Risk-adapted pre-emptive therapy for cytomegalovirus disease in patients undergoing allogeneic bone marrow transplantation. Bone Marrow Transplant 2000;25(7):765–9.

59. Coskuncan NM, Jabs DA, Dunn JP, et al. The eye in bone marrow transplantation. VI. Retinal complications. Arch Ophthalmol 1994;112(3):372–9.

60. Crippa F, Corey L, Chuang EL, et al. Virological, clinical, and ophthalmologic features of cytomegalovirus retinitis after hematopoietic stem cell transplantation. Clin Infect Dis 2001;32(2):214–9.

61. Eid AJ, Bakri SJ, Kijpittayarit S, et al. Clinical features and outcomes of cytomegalovirus retinitis after transplantation. Transpl Infect Dis 2008;10(1):13–8.

62. Larsson K, Lonnqvist B, Ringden O, et al. CMV retinitis after allogeneic bone marrow transplantation: a report of five cases. Transpl Infect Dis 2002;4(2):75–9.

63. Nichols WG, Corey L, Gooley T, et al. High risk of death due to bacterial and fungal infection among cytomegalovirus (CMV)-seronegative recipients of stem cell transplants from seropositive donors: evidence for indirect effects of primary CMV infection. J Infect Dis 2002;185(3):273–82.

64. Boeckh M. Current antiviral strategies for controlling cytomegalovirus in hematopoietic stem cell transplant recipients: prevention and therapy. Transpl Infect Dis 1999;1(3):165–78.

65. Broers AE, van Der Holt R, van Esser JW, et al. Increased transplant-related morbidity and mortality in CMV- seropositive patients despite highly effective prevention of CMV disease after allogeneic T-cell-depleted stem cell transplantation. Blood 2000;95(7):2240–5.

66. Craddock C, Szydlo RM, Dazzi F, et al. Cytomegalovirus seropositivity adversely influences outcome after T- depleted unrelated donor transplant in patients with chronic myeloid leukaemia: the case for tailored graft-versus-host disease prophylaxis. Br J Haematol 2001;112(1):228–36.

67. Behrendt CE, Rosenthal J, Bolotin E, et al. Donor and recipient CMV serostatus and outcome of pediatric allogeneic HSCT for acute leukemia in the era of CMV-preemptive therapy. Biol Blood Marrow Transplant 2009;15(1):54–60.

68. Boeckh M, Nichols WG. The impact of cytomegalovirus serostatus of donor and recipient before hematopoietic stem cell transplantation in the era of antiviral prophylaxis and preemptive therapy. Blood 2004;103(6):2003–8.

69. Bordon V, Bravo S, Van Renterghem L, et al. Surveillance of cytomegalovirus (CMV) DNAemia in pediatric allogeneic stem cell transplantation: incidence and outcome of CMV infection and disease. Transpl Infect Dis 2008;10(1):19–23.

70. Cwynarski K, Roberts IA, Iacobelli S, et al. Stem cell transplantation for chronic myeloid leukemia in children. Blood 2003;102(4):1224–31.

71. Erard V, Guthrie KA, Riddell S, et al. Impact of HLA A2 and cytomegalovirus serostatus on outcomes in patients with leukemia following matched-sibling myeloablative allogeneic hematopoietic cell transplantation. Haematologica 2006;91(10):1377–83.

72. Grob JP, Grundy JE, Prentice HG, et al. Immune donors can protect marrow-transplant recipients from severe cytomegalovirus infections. Lancet 1987;1(8536):774–6.

73. Jacobsen N, Badsberg JH, Lonnqvist B, et al. Graft-versus-leukaemia activity associated with CMV-seropositive donor, post-transplant CMV infection, young donor age and chronic graft-versus-host disease in bone marrow allograft recipients. The Nordic Bone Marrow Transplantation Group. Bone Marrow Transplant 1990;5(6):413–8.

74. Kollman C, Howe CW, Anasetti C, et al. Donor characteristics as risk factors in recipients after transplantation of bone marrow from unrelated donors: the effect of donor age. Blood 2001;98(7):2043–51.

75. Ljungman P, Einsele H, Frassoni F, et al. Donor CMV serological status influences the outcome of CMVseropositive recipients after unrelated donor stem cell transplantation. An EBMT Megafile analysis. Blood 2003;102: 4255–60.

76. Nachbaur D, Clausen J, Kircher B. Donor cytomegalovirus seropositivity and the risk of leukemic relapse after reduced-intensity transplants. Eur J Haematol 2006;76(5):414–9.

77. Ringden O, Schaffer M, Le Blanc K, et al. Which donor should be chosen for hematopoietic stem cell transplantation among unrelated HLA-A, -B, and -DRB1 genomically identical volunteers? Biol Blood Marrow Transplant 2004;10(2):128–34.

78. Gustafsson Jernberg A, Remberger M, Ringden O, et al. Risk factors in pediatric stem cell transplantation for leukemia. Pediatr Transplant 2004;8(5): 464–74.

79. Avetisyan G, Aschan J, Hagglund H, et al. Evaluation of intervention strategy based on CMV-specific immune responses after allogeneic SCT. Bone Marrow Transplant 2007;40(9):865–9.

80. Ganepola S, Gentilini C, Hilbers U, et al. Patients at high risk for CMV infection and disease show delayed CD8+ T-cell immune recovery after allogeneic stem cell transplantation. Bone Marrow Transplant 2007;39(5):293–9.

81. Lilleri D, Fornara C, Chiesa A, et al. Human cytomegalovirus-specific CD4+ and CD8+ T-cell reconstitution in adult allogeneic hematopoietic stem cell transplant recipients and immune control of viral infection. Haematologica 2008;93(2): 248–56.

82. Moins-Teisserenc H, Busson M, Scieux C, et al. Patterns of cytomegalovirus reactivation are associated with distinct evolutive profiles of immune reconstitution after allogeneic hematopoeitic stem cell transplantation. J Infect Dis 2008; 198(6):818–26.

83. Lin TS, Zahrieh D, Weller E, et al. Risk factors for cytomegalovirus reactivation after CD6+ T-cell-depleted allogeneic bone marrow transplantation. Transplantation 2002;74(1):49–54.

84. Ozdemir E, Saliba R, Champlin R, et al. Risk factors associated with late cytomegalovirus reactivation after allogeneic stem cell transplantation for hematological malignancies. Bone Marrow Transplant 2007;40(2):125–36.

85. Marty FM, Bryar J, Browne SK, et al. Sirolimus-based graft-versus-host disease prophylaxis protects against cytomegalovirus reactivation after allogeneic hematopoietic stem cell transplantation: a cohort analysis. Blood 2007;110(2):490–500.

86. Ljungman P, Aschan J, Lewensohn-Fuchs I, et al. Results of different strategies for reducing cytomegalovirus-associated mortality in allogeneic stem cell transplant recipients. Transplantation 1998;66(10):1330–4.

87. Martino R, Rovira M, Carreras E, et al. Severe infections after allogeneic peripheral blood stem cell transplantation: a matched-pair comparison of unmanipulated and CD34+ cell-selected transplantation. Haematologica 2001;86(10): 1075–86.

88. Miller W, Flynn P, McCullough J, et al. Cytomegalovirus infection after bone marrow transplantation: an association with acute graft-v-host disease. Blood 1986;67(4):1162–7.

89. Walker CM, van Burik JA, De For TE, et al. Cytomegalovirus infection after allogeneic transplantation: comparison of cord blood with peripheral blood and marrow graft sources. Biol Blood Marrow Transplant 2007;13(9):1106–15.

90. Kudchodkar SB, Yu Y, Maguire TG, et al. Human cytomegalovirus infection alters the substrate specificities and rapamycin sensitivities of raptor- and rictor-containing complexes. Proc Natl Acad Sci U S A 2006;103(38):14182–7.

91. Junghanss C, Boeckh M, Carter RA, et al. Incidence and outcome of cytomegalovirus infections following nonmyeloablative compared with myeloablative allogeneic stem cell transplantation: a matched control study. Blood 2002; 99(6):1978–85.

92. Nakamae H, Kirby KA, Sandmaier BM, et al. Effect of conditioning regimen intensity on CMV infection in allogeneic hematopoietic cell transplantation. Biol Blood Marrow Transplant 2009;15(6):694–703.

93. Schoemans H, Theunissen K, Maertens J, et al. Adult umbilical cord blood transplantation: a comprehensive review. Bone Marrow Transplant 2006;38(2): 83–93.

94. Albano MS, Taylor P, Pass RF, et al. Umbilical cord blood transplantation and cytomegalovirus: posttransplantation infection and donor screening. Blood 2006;108(13):4275–82.

95. Matsumura T, Narimatsu H, Kami M, et al. Cytomegalovirus infections following umbilical cord blood transplantation using reduced intensity conditioning regimens for adult patients. Biol Blood Marrow Transplant 2007;13(5):577–83.

96. Saavedra S, Sanz GF, Jarque I, et al. Early infections in adult patients undergoing unrelated donor cord blood transplantation. Bone Marrow Transplant 2002;30(12):937–43.

97. Takami A, Mochizuki K, Asakura H, et al. High incidence of cytomegalovirus reactivation in adult recipients of an unrelated cord blood transplant. Haematologica 2005;90(9):1290–2.

98. Tomonari A, Takahashi S, Ooi J, et al. Preemptive therapy with ganciclovir 5 mg/kg once daily for cytomegalovirus infection after unrelated cord blood transplantation. Bone Marrow Transplant 2008;41(4):371–6.

99. Delgado J, Pillai S, Benjamin R, et al. The effect of in vivo T cell depletion with alemtuzumab on reduced-intensity allogeneic hematopoietic cell transplantation for chronic lymphocytic leukemia. Biol Blood Marrow Transplant 2008;14(11): 1288–97.

100. Martin SI, Marty FM, Fiumara K, et al. Infectious complications associated with alemtuzumab use for lymphoproliferative disorders. Clin Infect Dis 2006;43(1): 16–24.

101. Nguyen Q, Champlin R, Giralt S, et al. Late cytomegalovirus pneumonia in adult allogeneic blood and marrow transplant recipients. Clin Infect Dis 1999;28(3): 618–23.

102. Peggs KS, Preiser W, Kottaridis PD, et al. Extended routine polymerase chain reaction surveillance and pre-emptive antiviral therapy for cytomegalovirus after allogeneic transplantation. Br J Haematol 2000;111(3):782–90.

103. Hebart H, Schroder A, Loffler J, et al. Cytomegalovirus monitoring by polymerase chain reaction of whole blood samples from patients undergoing autologous bone marrow or peripheral blood progenitor cell transplantation. J Infect Dis 1997;175(6):1490–3.

104. Bilgrami S, Aslanzadeh J, Feingold JM, et al. Cytomegalovirus viremia, viruria and disease after autologous peripheral blood stem cell transplantation: no need for surveillance. Bone Marrow Transplant 1999;24(1):69–73.

105. Boeckh M, Gooley TA, Reusser P, et al. Failure of high-dose acyclovir to prevent cytomegalovirus disease after autologous marrow transplantation. J Infect Dis 1995;172(4):939–43.

106. Holmberg LA, Boeckh M, Hooper H, et al. Increased incidence of cytomegalovirus disease after autologous CD34-selected peripheral blood stem cell transplantation. Blood 1999;94(12):4029–35.

107. Singhal S, Powles R, Treleaven J, et al. Cytomegaloviremia after autografting for leukemia: clinical significance and lack of effect on engraftment. Leukemia 1997;11(6):835–8.

108. Enright H, Haake R, Weisdorf D, et al. Cytomegalovirus pneumonia after bone marrow transplantation: risk factors and response to therapy. Transplantation 1993;55(6):1339–46.

109. Reusser P, Fisher LD, Buckner CD, et al. Cytomegalovirus infection after autologous bone marrow transplantation: occurrence of cytomegalovirus disease and effect on engraftment. Blood 1990;75(9):1888–94.

110. Bowden R, Cays M, Schoch G, et al. Comparison of filtered blood (FB) to seronegative blood products (SB) for prevention of cytomegalovirus (CMV) infection after marrow transplant. Blood 1995;86:3598–603.

111. Ljungman P, Larsson K, Kumlien G, et al. Leukocyte depleted, unscreened blood products give a low risk for CMV infection and disease in CMV seronegative allogeneic stem cell transplant recipients with seronegative stem cell donors. Scand J Infect Dis 2002;34(5):347–50.

112. Nichols WG, Price TH, Gooley T, et al. Transfusion-transmitted cytomegalovirus infection after receipt of leukoreduced blood products. Blood 2003;101(10):4195–200.

113. Bass E, Powe N, Goodman S, et al. Efficacy of immune globulin in preventing complications of bone marrow transplantation: a meta-analysis. Bone Marrow Transplant 1993;12:179–83.

114. Messori A, Rampazzo R, Scroccaro G, et al. Efficacy of hyperimmune anti-cytomegalovirus immunoglobulins for the prevention of cytomegalovirus infection in recipients of allogeneic bone marrow transplantation: a meta analysis. Bone Marrow Transplant 1994;13:163–8.

115. Raanani P, Gafter-Gvili A, Paul M, et al. Immunoglobulin prophylaxis in patients undergoing haematopoietic stem cell transplantation: systematic review and meta-analysis [abstract O267]. Bone Marrow Transplant 2008; 41(S1):S46.

116. Sullivan KM, Kopecky KJ, Jocom J, et al. Immunomodulatory and antimicrobial efficacy of intravenous immunoglobulin in bone marrow transplantation. N Engl J Med 1990;323(11):705–12.

117. Winston DJ, Ho WG, Lin CH, et al. Intravenous immune globulin for prevention of cytomegalovirus infection and interstitial pneumonia after bone marrow transplantation. Ann Intern Med 1987;106(1):12–8.

118. Zikos P, Van Lint MT, Lamparelli T, et al. A randomized trial of high dose polyvalent intravenous immunoglobulin (HDIgG) vs. cytomegalovirus (CMV) hyperimmune IgG in allogeneic hemopoietic stem cell transplants (HSCT). Haematologica 1998;83(2):132–7.

119. Wloch MK, Smith LR, Boutsaboualoy S, et al. Safety and immunogenicity of a bivalent cytomegalovirus DNA vaccine in healthy adult subjects. J Infect Dis 2008;197(12):1634–42.

120. Boeckh M, Gooley TA, Myerson D, et al. Cytomegalovirus pp65 antigenemia-guided early treatment with ganciclovir versus ganciclovir at engraftment after allogeneic marrow transplantation: a randomized double-blind study. Blood 1996;88(10):4063–71.

121. Avery RK, Adal KA, Longworth DL, et al. A survey of allogeneic bone marrow transplant programs in the United States regarding cytomegalovirus prophylaxis and pre-emptive therapy. Bone Marrow Transplant 2000;26(7):763–7.

122. Ljungman P. CMV infections after hematopoietic stem cell transplantation. Bone Marrow Transplant 2008;42(Suppl 1):S70–2.

123. Ljungman P, Reusser P, de la Camara R, et al. Management of CMV infections: recommendations from the infectious diseases working party of the EBMT. Bone Marrow Transplant 2004;33(11):1075–81.

124. Meyers JD, Reed EC, Shepp DH, et al. Acyclovir for prevention of cytomegalovirus infection and disease after allogeneic marrow transplantation. N Engl J Med 1988;318(2):70–5.

125. Prentice HG, Gluckman E, Powles RL, et al. Impact of long-term acyclovir on cytomegalovirus infection and survival after allogeneic bone marrow transplantation. European Acyclovir for CMV Prophylaxis Study Group. Lancet 1994; 343(8900):749–53.

126. Ljungman P, de la Camara R, Milpied N, et al. Randomized study of valacyclovir as prophylaxis against cytomegalovirus reactivation in recipients of allogeneic bone marrow transplants. Blood 2002;99(8):3050–6.

127. Goodrich JM, Bowden RA, Fisher L, et al. Ganciclovir prophylaxis to prevent cytomegalovirus disease after allogeneic marrow transplant. Ann Intern Med 1993;118(3):173–8.

128. Winston DJ, Ho WG, Bartoni K, et al. Ganciclovir prophylaxis of cytomegalovirus infection and disease in allogeneic bone marrow transplant recipients: results of a placebo- controlled, double-blind trial. Ann Intern Med 1993;118(3):179–84.

129. Winston DJ, Yeager AM, Chandrasekar PH, et al. Randomized comparison of oral valacyclovir and intravenous ganciclovir for prevention of cytomegalovirus disease after allogeneic bone marrow transplantation. Clin Infect Dis 2003; 36(6):749–58.

130. Salzberger B, Bowden RA, Hackman RC, et al. Neutropenia in allogeneic marrow transplant recipients receiving ganciclovir for prevention of cytomegalovirus disease: risk factors and outcome. Blood 1997;90(6):2502–8.

131. Busca A, de Fabritiis P, Ghisetti V, et al. Oral valganciclovir as preemptive therapy for cytomegalovirus infection post allogeneic stem cell transplantation. Transpl Infect Dis 2007;9(2):102–7.

132. Einsele H, Reusser P, Bornhauser M, et al. Oral valganciclovir leads to higher exposure to ganciclovir than intravenous ganciclovir in patients following allogeneic stem cell transplantation. Blood 2006;107(7):3002–8.

133. Winston DJ, Baden LR, Gabriel DA, et al. Pharmacokinetics of ganciclovir after oral valganciclovir versus intravenous ganciclovir in allogeneic stem cell transplant patients with graft-versus-host disease of the gastrointestinal tract. Biol Blood Marrow Transplant 2006;12(6):635–40.

134. Allice T, Busca A, Locatelli F, et al. Valganciclovir as pre-emptive therapy for cytomegalovirus infection post-allogenic stem cell transplantation: implications for the emergence of drug-resistant cytomegalovirus. J Antimicrob Chemother 2009;63(3):600–8.

135. Ayala E, Greene J, Sandin R, et al. Valganciclovir is safe and effective as preemptive therapy for CMV infection in allogeneic hematopoietic stem cell transplantation. Bone Marrow Transplant 2006;37(9):851–6.
136. Takenaka K, Eto T, Nagafuji K, et al. Oral valganciclovir as preemptive therapy is effective for cytomegalovirus infection in allogeneic hematopoietic stem cell transplant recipients. Int J Hematol 2009;89(2):231–7.
137. Volin L, Barkholt L, Nihtinen A, et al. An open-label randomised study of oral valganciclovir versus intravenous ganciclovir for pre-emptive therapy of cytomegalovirus infection after allogeneic stem cell transplantation. Bone Marrow Transplant 2008;42(Suppl 1):S47.
138. Reusser P, Einsele H, Lee J, et al. Randomized multicenter trial of foscarnet versus ganciclovir for preemptive therapy of cytomegalovirus infection after allogeneic stem cell transplantation. Blood 2002;99(4):1159–64.
139. Ljungman P, Deliliers GL, Platzbecker U, et al. Cidofovir for cytomegalovirus infection and disease in allogeneic stem cell transplant recipients. The Infectious Diseases Working Party of the European Group for Blood and Marrow Transplantation. Blood 2001;97(2):388–92.
140. Emery VC, Sabin CA, Cope AV, et al. Application of viral-load kinetics to identify patients who develop cytomegalovirus disease after transplantation. Lancet 2000;355(9220):2032–6.
141. Pang XL, Fox JD, Fenton JM, et al. Interlaboratory comparison of cytomegalovirus viral load assays. Am J Transplant 2009;9(2):258–68.
142. Fries BC, Riddell SR, Kim HW, et al. Cytomegalovirus disease before hematopoietic cell transplantation as a risk for complications after transplantation. Biol Blood Marrow Transplant 2005;11(2):136–48.
143. Chou SW. Cytomegalovirus drug resistance and clinical implications. Transpl Infect Dis 2001;3(Suppl 2):20–4.
144. Chou S. Cytomegalovirus UL97 mutations in the era of ganciclovir and maribavir. Rev Med Virol 2008;18(4):233–46.
145. Iwasenko JM, Scott GM, Rawlinson WD, et al. Successful valganciclovir treatment of post-transplant cytomegalovirus infection in the presence of UL97 mutation N597D. J Med Virol 2009;81(3):507–10.
146. Prichard MN, Britt WJ, Daily SL, et al. Human cytomegalovirus UL97 kinase is required for the normal intranuclear distribution of pp65 and virion morphogenesis. J Virol 2005;79(24):15494–502.
147. Chou S, Lurain NS, Thompson KD, et al. Viral DNA polymerase mutations associated with drug resistance in human cytomegalovirus. J Infect Dis 2003;188(1):32–9.
148. Drew WL, Miner RC, Marousek GI, et al. Maribavir sensitivity of cytomegalovirus isolates resistant to ganciclovir, cidofovir or foscarnet. J Clin Virol 2006;37(2):124–7.
149. Avery RK, Bolwell BJ, Yen-Lieberman B, et al. Use of leflunomide in an allogeneic bone marrow transplant recipient with refractory cytomegalovirus infection. Bone Marrow Transplant 2004;34(12):1071–5.
150. Battiwalla M, Paplham P, Almyroudis NG, et al. Leflunomide failure to control recurrent cytomegalovirus infection in the setting of renal failure after allogeneic stem cell transplantation. Transpl Infect Dis 2007;9(1):28–32.
151. Efferth T, Romero M, Wolf D, et al. The antiviral activities of artemisinin and artesunate. Clin Infect Dis 2008;47:804–11.
152. Emanuel D, Cunningham I, Jules-Elysee K, et al. Cytomegalovirus pneumonia after bone marrow transplantation successfully treated with the combination of

ganciclovir and high-dose intravenous immune globulin. Ann Intern Med 1988; 109(10):777–82.

153. Ljungman P, Engelhard D, Link H, et al. Treatment of interstitial pneumonitis due to cytomegalovirus with ganciclovir and intravenous immune globulin: experience of European Bone Marrow Transplant Group. Clin Infect Dis 1992;14(4): 831–5.

154. Reed EC, Bowden RA, Dandliker PS, et al. Treatment of cytomegalovirus pneumonia with ganciclovir and intravenous cytomegalovirus immunoglobulin in patients with bone marrow transplants. Ann Intern Med 1988;109(10):783–8.

155. Schmidt GM, Kovacs A, Zaia JA, et al. Ganciclovir/immunoglobulin combination therapy for the treatment of human cytomegalovirus-associated interstitial pneumonia in bone marrow allograft recipients. Transplantation 1988;46(6):905–7.

156. Erard V, Gutherie KA, Smith J, et al. Cytomegalovirus pneumonia (CMV-IP) after hematopoeitic cell transplantation (HCT): outcomes and factors associated with mortality [abstract V-1379]. 47th interscience conference on antimicrobial agents and chemotherapy; September 17–20; Chicago (IL) 2007.

157. Machado CM, Dulley FL, Boas LS, et al. CMV pneumonia in allogeneic BMT recipients undergoing early treatment of pre-emptive ganciclovir therapy. Bone Marrow Transplant 2000;26(4):413–7.

158. Reed EC, Wolford JL, Kopecky KJ, et al. Ganciclovir for the treatment of cytomegalovirus gastroenteritis in bone marrow transplant patients: a randomized, placebo-controlled trial. Ann Intern Med 1990;112(7):505–10.

159. Ljungman P, Cordonnier C, Einsele H, et al. Use of intravenous immune globulin in addition to antiviral therapy in the treatment of CMV gastrointestinal disease in allogeneic bone marrow transplant patients: a report from the European Group for Blood and Marrow Transplantation (EBMT). Infectious Diseases Working Party of the EBMT. Bone Marrow Transplant 1998;21(5):473–6.

160. Chang M, Dunn JP. Ganciclovir implant in the treatment of cytomegalovirus retinitis. Expert Rev Med Devices 2005;2(4):421–7.

161. Okamoto T, Okada M, Mori A, et al. Successful treatment of severe cytomegalovirus retinitis with foscarnet and intraocular infection of ganciclovir in a myelosuppressed unrelated bone marrow transplant patient. Bone Marrow Transplant 1997;20(9):801–3.

162. Ganly PS, Arthur C, Goldman JM, et al. Foscarnet as treatment for cytomegalovirus retinitis following bone marrow transplantation. Postgrad Med J 1988; 64(751):389–91.

163. Biron KK. Antiviral drugs for cytomegalovirus diseases. Antiviral Res 2006; 71(2–3):154–63.

164. Einsele H, Kapp M, Grigoleit GU. CMV-specific T cell therapy. Blood Cells Mol Dis 2008;40(1):71–5.

Herpes Viruses in Transplant Recipients: HSV, VZV, Human Herpes Viruses, and EBV

Kevin Shiley, MD*, Emily Blumberg, MD

KEYWORDS

- Herpes virus • PTLD • Kaposi sarcoma • Zoster • HHV-6
- HHV-7

The herpes viruses comprise a large group of enveloped DNA-containing viruses that characteristically cause latent infection in their respective hosts. There are 8 known herpes family viruses associated with human infection: herpes simplex virus (HSV) types 1 and 2, varicella zoster virus (VZV), Epstein-Barr virus (EBV), *Cytomegalovirus* (CMV), *Human herpesvirus 6* (HHV-6), *Human herpesvirus 7* (HHV-7), and *Human herpesvirus 8* (HHV-8). Of these, CMV has received the most attention as a cause of morbidity and mortality among transplant recipients and is discussed separately in articles by Ljungman, Strasfeld, Hirsch, and Einsele in this issue. The remaining herpes viruses are also responsible for significant disease in the transplant patient population. The role of each of these viruses as a cause of disease in the transplant population is discussed in this article.

HSV-1 AND HSV-2

The α-herpes viruses, HSV-1 and HSV-2, are responsible for oral and genital mucocutaneous ulcers in the general population. HSV-2 is generally considered to be sexually transmitted and primarily infects the urogenital mucosa, whereas HSV-1 predominantly affects the oral mucosa and is often transmitted through nonsexual contact. Both

Dr Shiley has no financial disclosures.

Dr Blumberg receives financial support from Roche Pharmaceuticals for research support and consulting services. She also receives research support from Viropharma as a site investigator in a multicenter trial.

A version of this article was previously published in the *Infectious Disease Clinics of North America*, 24:2.

Division of Infectious Diseases, Hospital of the University of Pennsylvania, 3rd Floor Silverstein Pavilion, Suite E, 3400 Spruce Street, Philadelphia, PA 19104, USA

* Corresponding author.

E-mail address: shileyk@uphs.upenn.edu

viruses are neurotropic and primarily infect neurons in their latent forms. Reactivation of HSV is common among transplant recipients, and is the second most common cause of viral infection after transplantation.[1-3]

Most HSV-1 and HSV-2 infections occur in the setting of reactivation rather than primary infection, although primary HSV infections are well documented, particularly among younger patients.[4] Primary infection from transplanted tissue is uncommon but has been observed in renal transplant recipients.[5,6] The high percentage of cases attributed to reactivation is undoubtedly a result of a high baseline population seroprevalence of HSV-1 and HSV-2. Seroprevalence increases with age and varies by geographic, racial, socioeconomic, and ethnic characteristics among the general population. Antibodies to HSV-1 were found in 50% to 96% of people in previous seroprevalence studies.[7-9] Analysis of Americans from the National Health and Nutrition Examination Survey showed the seroprevalence of HSV-1 to be 65% and HSV-2 to be 26% by age 49 years.[10] Higher rates of seropositivity were found in women and minorities in the same survey. The greatest risk factor for reactivation of HSV following transplantation is lack of antiviral prophylaxis.[4,11-15]

Before the introduction of acyclovir, reactivation of HSV infection was estimated to occur in up to 80% of patients receiving hematopoetic stem cell transplant.[13-15] Lower, but still substantial, reactivation rates were described in solid-organ transplant recipients in the years before effective antiviral prophylaxis.[5,16-19] The clinical manifestations of HSV infection range from limited mucocutaneous outbreaks to disseminated infections involving visceral organs and the central nervous system (CNS).

The most common manifestations of HSV are mucocutaneous outbreaks, usually involving the oral and genitourinary mucosa.[20] These infections, which can lead to extensive mucosal involvement, typically occur in the first 30 days following transplantation if prophylaxis is not administered.[1,14,15,18,21] Less common manifestations of HSV involving the lungs and viscera are also described. Pneumonia as a result of HSV-1 and HSV-2 is typically preceded by gingivostomatitis, however pulmonary involvement from disseminated infection and airway manipulation may also occur.[22-28] The diagnosis of HSV pneumonia is complicated because viral shedding within the airways is common in immunosuppressed and critically ill adults and does not necessarily reflect true pneumonia.[29-33] The use of acyclovir in critically ill patients with HSV isolated from respiratory secretions has not been shown to influence mortality, ventilator dependence, or length of hospitalization.[33,34] Therefore, caution should be taken in interpreting results from viral cultures, direct fluorescent antibody staining, and nucleic acid assays without associated cytopathic evidence of infection on tissue biopsy.

Hepatitis is an uncommon manifestation of HSV that is described in several case reports and case series.[17,35-40] When HSV presents with hepatitis there is often evidence of disseminated disease with involvement of the skin and mucous membranes.[36,39] Patients may seem well initially, with elevated liver function tests as the only sign of infection.[37] More often, patients present with nonspecific flulike symptoms of fever, malaise, and myalgias. Increasing levels of aspartate aminotransferase and alanine aminotransferase, sometimes 10 to 20 times the upper limit of normal, are often observed. Cross-sectional imaging may appear normal, but in some cases liver infiltration with microabscesses has been observed.[35] Most cases occur within 30 days of transplant, however some cases have occurred years after transplant.[40] Nearly all HSV hepatitis cases in the literature occurred in patients while off antiviral prophylaxis. Diagnosis is made by liver biopsy with culture and antibody staining for HSV-1 and HSV-2. Pathology typically reveals necrotic hepatitis with loss of lobular architecture.[38] Other visceral manifestations of HSV infection in immunosuppressed hosts include esophagitis, gastritis, and colitis.[41-48]

Encephalitis as a result of HSV infection is rare in the transplant population.[49] On presentation, confusion, fever, and behavioral changes are the predominant findings. Up to one-third of patients present with seizure and one-fifth with focal neurologic findings.[50] Cerebrospinal fluid (CSF) typically has a lymphocytic pleocytosis and increased protein level.[50] The diagnosis of HSV encephalitis is now usually made by polymerase chain reaction (PCR) from CSF rather than brain biopsy.[51] In the general population, on which most research on HSV encephalitis has been conducted, significant neurologic compromise is common following HSV encephalitis.[50] The early initiation of high-dose acyclovir was shown to significantly decrease the morbidity and mortality from HSV encephalitis.[52] In a large cohort of immunocompetent and immunosuppressed patients, long-term neurologic deficits were common despite antiviral treatment.[50] There are insufficient data in the era of antiviral prophylaxis to know if outcomes are worse in transplant recipients.

The introduction of oral and intravenous acyclovir in the 1980s markedly decreased the incidence of serious HSV infections following transplantation. Several small randomized trials demonstrated intravenous and oral acyclovir to be safe and effective as a prophylactic regimen against HSV infections.[1,14,15,18,21] Acyclovir appeared to abbreviate viral shedding and expedite healing from mucocutaneous outbreaks in hematopoetic stem cell transplant recipients.[53] Since the introduction of acyclovir, related compounds such as valacyclovir and famciclovir have also been used successfully for treatment of HSV and varicella zoster infections following transplantation. Ganciclovir also has activity against HSV, and its use in the posttransplant population has been shown to significantly decrease rates of reactivation.[11,12] Resistance to acyclovir and its derivatives does occur and typically reflects prolonged exposure to inadequate dosing of acyclovir at the time of viral reactivation. The highest rates of acyclovir resistance are found in allogeneic stem cell transplant recipients with estimates ranging from 1% to 14% of patients with resistant virus.[54–57] Second-line treatment with foscarnet is typically used if acyclovir resistance is detected.[58]

VZV

VZV, the α-herpes virus responsible for chickenpox and shingles, causes symptomatic infection through reactivation or primary infection in approximately 1% to 20% of solid-organ transplant recipients, with lung transplant recipients having the highest rates.[2,59–61] The rate of VZV disease approaches more than 40% in hematopoetic stem cell transplant recipients.[62–66] Reactivation of VZV is the most common route of VZV disease in adult transplant recipients, with more than 90% of adults in the United States estimated to have antibodies against VZV.[67] In previous series, the median time frame for reactivation ranged from 9 to 23 months following solid-organ transplant.[68–70] In hematopoietic cell transplant recipients most cases of VZV disease tends to occur within the first 12 months following transplantation, with up to 26% of transplant recipients developing disease following discontinuation of antiviral prophylaxis.[63] Suggested risk factors for VZV disease in solid-organ transplant include mycophenolate use, recent treatment of rejection, induction therapy, and age greater than 50 years.[69,71] All solid-organ transplant candidates should be tested before transplantation for VZV antibodies in an effort to determine the risk for primary infection. Solid-organ transplant candidates with VZV IgG negative status should undergo vaccination with the live attenuated Oka strain VZV vaccine before solid-organ transplant.[58] The vaccine should not be given after transplant because it is a live vaccine and there are currently insufficient data to determine its safety in immunosuppressed transplant recipients.[72–77] The rate of VZV disease (primary and reactivation) in allogeneic stem cell transplant recipients remains high regardless of VZV serostatus before transplant.[66] An investigational inactivated varicella vaccine was successfully used to prevent disease in autologous hematopoetic stem cell transplant recipients; however it is currently not available.[78]

As with HSV, the clinical manifestations of VZV disease are wide ranging, but can be severe and associated with increased mortality, especially in the early posttransplant period. Primary infection with VZV in the posttransplant setting can be severe, with disseminated infection presenting with skin, lung, and visceral organ involvement.[79–81] Donor-derived VZV infections are rare, but have been reported.[82] The most common presentation of VZV is cutaneous infection, typically with single dermatomal involvement. However, multiple dermatome involvement occurs in a sizable minority of cases. In cases of disseminated disease, typical vesicular skin lesions remain a common marker of disease. It is notable that the rash is not always vesicular in immunosuppressed hosts; consequently biopsy of the skin may be required for viral identification either by direct fluorescence or nucleic acid detection or culture. Patients may present with other symptoms of disseminated disease, including abdominal pain or hepatitis before the onset of rash.[83] CNS involvement with VZV can present with encephalitis, myelitis, or meningoencephalitis. Unlike disseminated cutaneous infections, CNS VZV often presents without skin or other organ involvement.[84] The diagnosis of VZV CNS infection is typically made by detection of VZV in the CSF using nucleic acid testing in conjunction with a compatible clinical presentation.[85,86] CSF typically shows a lymphocyte predominant pleocytosis, moderately increased protein level and normal to low-normal glucose level.[87] All cases of disseminated zoster should be placed in isolation once the diagnosis is suspected in an effort to prevent spread to other immunocompromised patients and susceptible health care workers.

Treatment of VZV disease is generally recommended for all transplant recipients.[58] High-dose acyclovir or its analogues has been successfully used for the treatment of localized and disseminated VZV infections. In cases of disseminated disease and CNS infection, intravenous acyclovir (30 mg/kg/d in 3 divided doses) is preferred as initial therapy. Ganciclovir has not been studied specifically in the treatment of VZV, however it has been used successfully for treatment in several reports.[88] Oral agents, such as valacyclovir (1 g every 8 hours), acyclovir (800 mg 5 times each day) and famciclovir (500 mg every 8 hours) are reasonable choices for localized infections.[58,89] In rare cases where acyclovir resistance occurs, foscarnet can be used.[58]

Several studies have shown acyclovir and ganciclovir to be effective as prophylaxis against VZV reactivation in the posttransplant period.[1,11,12,14,15,18,21,53] Other methods of preventing primary infection in VZV-negative transplant recipients (who were not vaccinated before transplant or failed to mount a detectable VZV antibody titer) include vaccinating household and close contacts at risk for primary infection, preferably before transplant. VZV seronegative patients exposed to persons with active VZV (either chicken pox or shingles) should ideally be given postexposure prophylaxis with intravenous varicella zoster immunoglobulin (VZIG) given within the first 96 hours of exposure.[58,90,91] Unfortunately, VZIG is no longer available in the United States.[92] An intramuscularly dosed formulation of concentrated VZV IgG (VariZIG, Cangene Corp, Winnepeg, Canada) is available through an investigational new drug expanded access protocol from the Food and Drug Administration (http://www.fda.gov/BiologicsBloodVaccines/SafetyAvailability/ucm176029.htm). There are currently insufficient data to support the use of antiviral agents after VZV exposure, and it is currently not recommended by the Centers of Disease Control's Advisory Committee on Immunization Practices.[91]

EBV

EBV is a gammaherpes virus responsible for several clinical entities. In the general population, EBV is the causative agent of infectious mononucleosis, Burkitt lymphoma, and nasopharyngeal carcinoma. The role of EBV as a cause of posttransplant lymphoproliferative disorder (PTLD) is now well established, accounting for 90% of cases of PTLD.[93–95] Other rare disorders attributed to EBV in the posttransplant period include smooth muscle tumors and the hemophagocytic syndrome.[96,97] EBV is ubiquitous, with up to 90% seropositivity observed in the general community.[98] Infection in early childhood is common and often without significant symptoms.[99] The clinical entity of mononucleosis, characterized by pharyngitis, lymphadenopathy, and fatigue, is typically seen with primary infection in young immunocompetent adults. Rarely, neurologic manifestations of EBV infection, including encephalitis and optic neuritis, occur.[100] Like other herpes viruses, EBV is a chronic infection, with latent virus infecting B cells in the blood and lymphoid tissues. The virus is typically transmitted to naive individuals through saliva and respiratory secretions. Transmissions to naive transplant recipients through blood transfusion and organ transplant are also described.[95,101,102]

The clinical entity known as PTLD comprises a spectrum of disease characterized by the abnormal proliferation of lymphocytic cells, often with an invasive component, in patients following transplantation. The clinical manifestations of PTLD vary considerably. In some instances patients are asymptomatic and disease is only suggested by incidental imaging findings. Other cases may present with a mononucleosis-like syndrome, organ dysfunction secondary to tissue infiltration or septic-appearing febrile illness. Tissue infiltration from PTLD may present as extranodal masses, which can involve various organs, including the lungs, liver, spleen, bowels, and CNS.[95,103,104] In some instances, allografts are the primary site of PTLD, with resulting organ dysfunction mimicking rejection.[105] PTLD may present as an infiltrative process rather than a focal mass, mimicking such entities as pneumonia, lymphocele, and colitis.[106–109]

Numerous risk factors for the development of PTLD are described. Host EBV seronegative status has been shown to increase the risk of developing PTLD up to 76-fold, making the issue particularly troublesome for pediatric patients.[110–113] These patients, at risk for primary EBV infection, are most likely to present with disease within only a few months of transplant. Other risk factors in solid-organ transplant recipients, reflect a state of actual or potentially augmented immune suppression and include CMV disease, CMV donor/recipient mismatch, and intensity of pharmacologically mediated immune suppression.[112–116] Risk factors for PTLD in hematopoetic stem cell recipients include unrelated donor HLA mismatch, use of antithymocyte globulin, T-cell depletion, and use of anti-CD3 monoclonal antibodies for graft-versus-host disease prophylaxis.[117]

The initial diagnosis of PTLD is best made with tissue, ideally from an excisional biopsy specimen.[118] High serum levels of EBV DNA may be seen in PTLD, especially in younger recipients, and may precede clinical disease.[119,120] Currently, the incongruity in EBV DNA testing methods between centers and the need for tissue for pathologic grading, argue against the use of EBV viral load testing as replacement for histologic diagnosis, although it is estimated that up to 90% of PTLD is EBV-associated.[93] The Society of Hematopathology classification schema for PTLD divides lesions into 3 general categories: lymphoid hyperplasia (early lesions), polymorphic PTLD, and lymphomatous (monomorphic) PTLD.[121,122] Lymphoid hyperplasia, sometimes referred to as early PTLD, is subcharacterized into posttransplant infectious mononucleosis and reactive plasmacytic hyperplasia. A notable characteristic in both of these groups is the presence of polyclonal cell populations.[94,121] Polymorphic PTLD is characterized by more aggressive lesions that escape the normal lymphatic system boundaries and infiltrate underlying tissue. Although these lesions behave similarly to malignant lymphoma, the cell population involved remains heterogeneous in appearance, although they are all typically monoclonal at the molecular level. The term monomorphic PTLD is used to describe lymphomas in the posttransplant setting. Many are associated with EBV, although some are not. These lesions are generally categorized according to the Revised European American Lymphoma system with the suffix PTLD to note the correlation with transplant status.[121]

Treatment varies considerably depending on which variation of PTLD is diagnosed. A cornerstone of therapy is decreasing the level of immunosuppression whenever possible.[93,123,124] In 1 series of solid-organ transplant recipients treated for PTLD, 63% of patients treated by reducing immunosuppression alone had complete disease remission.[124] Risk factors for failing treatment with reduction of immunosuppression included a high baseline lactate dehydrogenase level, multiorgan involvement, presence of B symptoms, and organ dysfunction from disease.[124] The data for antiviral medications in the treatment of PTLD through suppression of EBV are limited. Although early reports suggested acyclovir and ganciclovir, which have some in vitro activity against EBV, might have a potential role in PTLD treatment there is no compelling clinical data to support their use.[125–128] Treatment with immunomodulatory agents such as anti-CD-20 (rituximab), interleukin 6 (IL-6) and interferon-α is described.[95,127,129–132] Infusions of cytotoxic EBV-specific T cells have also been used as a therapeutic and prophylactic treatment in solid-organ and hematopoetic stem cell transplant recipients.[133–140] As a treatment, results have been mixed and no controlled trials have been published on the subject.[133,136–138,140] The use of cytotoxic EBV-specific T cells as a prophylactic measure in individuals with high levels of circulating EBV DNA were also reported to be beneficial, but data are limited to small uncontrolled series.[133,134,139] In some cases treatment with chemotherapeutic agents used in nontransplant-associated lymphomas are also used, often in conjunction with rituximab.[141–144] Other strategies include resection of localized tumors, radiotherapy, and treatment of other infections, such as CMV, that may act to suppress the immune system further.[127,145] In cases where reduction of immunosuppression has resulted in graft loss, retransplantation can be successful.[146]

The use of antivirals gained some support as a prophylactic measure against EBV based on the results of some uncontrolled studies.[147–149] A randomized controlled trial exploring the use of ganciclovir and acyclovir as a prophylactic strategy for EBV and CMV did not show any decrease in PTLD, however.[150] The use of quantitative EBV viral load monitoring has been advocated as another method to prevent the development of PTLD in high-risk individuals.[93] In this approach regular quantitative EBV viral loads are obtained and immunosuppression is decreased when viral loads reach a predetermined threshold.[119,151]

HHV-6 AND HHV-7

HHV-6, the causative agent of the common childhood disease roseola infantum (exanthem sabitum), has received attention in the past several years as an opportunistic infection in the posttransplant population. The virus, first described in 1986, is a member of the β-herpes virus family, and establishes latency in CD4+ T lymphocytes.[152] Genetic sequencing has demonstrated 2 variants, A and B. The B variant has been linked to most disease in children and in the transplant population.[153] It is estimated that greater than 90% of children are seropositive for

HHV-6 by 1 year of age.[154,155] Therefore, most cases of HHV-6 viremia are believed to be caused by viral reactivation, although primary infection following transplantation has been described.[156,157]

Reactivation of HHV-6 is common in the immediate period following hematopoetic stem cell transplant, when immunosuppression is highest. A prospective study by Zerr and colleagues[158] detected HHV-6 viremia in 52 of 110 (47%) patients evaluated during the first 100 days after transplant. Numerous indirect effects have been suggested related to HHV-6 viremia in the hematopoetic stem cell transplant population. These include delayed engraftment, higher rates of graft-versus-host disease, cytomegalovirus disease, and all-cause mortality.[158–162] Estimates of HHV-6 viremia following solid-organ transplant range from 24% to 66%, although this is likely reduced in patients receiving ganciclovir for CMV prophylaxis.[163–167] Reported indirect effects associated with HHV-6 viremia include higher frequencies of allograft rejection, severe CMV disease, and invasive fungal infections.[163,164,168–170] Despite these associations, no causal link has been definitively established between HHV-6 reactivation and indirect effects. A recent prospective cohort study that included 298 solid-organ transplant recipients found no connection between severity or duration of CMV disease and HHV-6 coinfection.[171]

Several case series and reports have linked HHV-6 with encephalitis in solid-organ and hematopoetic stem cell transplant recipients.[156,158,172–176] Most of the cases reported in the literature occurred 30 to 90 days after transplant. Manifestations of neurologic disease include generalized confusion, amnesia, insomnia, seizures (often subclinical), and coma.[172,176,177] Magnetic resonance imaging imaging of the brain often reveals involvement of the basal ganglia.[100,176,177] The detection of HHV-6 in CSF through PCR or culture, in conjunction with compatible neuroradiology and clinical manifestations, is highly suggestive of HHV-6 encephalitis.[178] Nonetheless, other causes of encephalitis should be ruled out as HHV-6 has been detected in the CSF of asymptomatic patients and the symptoms of HHV-6 encephalitis may be strikingly similar to those of immunosuppression leukoencephalopathy.[172,179,180] Other manifestations of HHV-6 disease reported in the literature include gastroenteritis, pneumonitis, hepatitis, and myelosuppression.[181–183]

No prospective clinical trials have evaluated the use of antiviral medications in the treatment of HHV-6 associated disease. In vitro data suggest that HHV-6 is inhibited by ganciclovir, foscarnet, and cidofovir.[184–186] Most clinical experience has been with the treatment of HHV-6 encephalitis. Most reported cases used ganciclovir, foscarnet, or a combination of both with varying success.[156,172–176] Despite their in vitro activity against HHV-6, neither intravenous ganciclovir nor valganciclovir affected HHV-6 viral loads in a multicenter prospective clinical trial of CMV disease treatment.[171]

The β-herpes virus, HHV-7, is closely related to HHV-6 but its role in clinically relevant disease remains unclear. In children, HHV-7 has been associated with rare cases of exanthem subitum, febrile seizures, and encephalitis.[187] A few cases of encephalitis and myelitis have been attributed to HHV-7 among hematopoetic stem cell transplant recipients.[188,189] In comparison with HHV-6, however, little data exist supporting organ-specific infections with HHV-7 in transplant recipients. Like HHV-6, HHV-7 has been proposed to act as an immunomodulatory virus, potentially lowering the barrier to other opportunistic infections, including CMV.[190–192] A recent prospective multicenter cohort examined the effect of HHV-7 viremia in patients with diagnosed CMV disease and found no correlation with duration of CMV disease or CMV disease outcomes.[171]

HHV-8

HHV-8 also known as Kaposi sarcoma–associated herpes virus, is responsible for the malignant entities of Kaposi sarcoma (KS) and primary effusion lymphoma (PEL), as well as some forms of multicentric Castleman disease (MCD).[193–195] HHV-8 belongs to the γ-herpes virus family along with EBV and infects CD-19 positive B cells in its latent form.[196] Unlike the other herpes viruses discussed earlier, the seroprevalence to HHV-8 is highly variable, depending on geography and behavioral risk factors.[197–200] Of 13,984 Americans sampled in the National Health and Nutrition Survey, 1.5% were found to be seropositive for HHV-8.[201] The highest rate of HHV-8 seropositivity in the United States was found in men who have sex with men, with a prevalence rate estimated to be 8.2%.[201] Worldwide prevalence varies dramatically, with some areas of sub-Saharan Africa estimated to have 30% to 50% seropositivity.[199,202]

Transmission of HHV-8 is believed to occur through sexual activity and possibly through saliva.[197,199,201] In endemic regions both means of transmission probably occur.[196,199] Elsewhere, such as in North America, sexual activity is believed to be the primary mode of transmission.[201] Transmission of HHV-8 has also been documented through solid-organ and hematopoetic stem cell transplantation.[203–205]

Manifestations of HHV-8 disease in transplant recipients are variable. In the Middle East, where seroprevalence for HHV-8 reaches 25%, KS is the most common malignancy following renal transplant.[198] The incidence is lower in North America. Prior series describing KS following solid-organ transplant reported onset of disease ranging from 2 to 23 months after transplant.[205–207] Lesions may present as focal nodules on the skin, within organs (including allografts), or as disseminated disease with lymph node, bone marrow, and splenic infiltration.[203,204,207,208] The diagnosis of KS is made by pathologic examination of affected tissues.

As with EBV-associated PTLD, reduction in immunosuppression is the first-line therapy for KS and is often curative.[202] Some investigators have suggested that using sirolimus instead of other calcineurin inhibitors may provide additional treatment effect by inhibition of vascular endothelial cell growth factor.[209,210] Chemotherapy and radiation may also be necessary in cases where reduction of immunosuppression is ineffective or not possible.[202,208] Antiviral medications have not been shown to be useful in the treatment of KS.[211,212]

Other rare manifestations of HHV-8 reported in transplant recipients include MCD and PEL.[213–217] MCD is an aggressive lymphoproliferative disorder characterized by fever, diffuse lymphadenopathy, wasting, and hepatosplenomegaly.[218] HHV-8 is not always found in MCD, but is common, with virus detected in 75% of MCD lesions in 1 series.[219] The diagnosis of MCD is made by tissue biopsy. Other causes of diffuse lymphadenopathy, such as disseminated mycobacterial and fungal infections, should be ruled out. The reported outcomes of MCD in transplant recipients are poor, with rapidly fatal disease or allograft failure in several reports.[214,215,220,221] Treatments with immunomodulatory agents, chemotherapy, and antivirals have all been used with variable results.[218,222]

PEL, also known as body cavity lymphoma, typically presents with a refractory exudative effusion in 1 of several potential spaces within the body. Lymphomatous cells fill the affected cavity, with tumor foci often studding the serous membranes.[223] The most frequent location is the pleural space, however pericardial, peritoneal, and intracranial cases are also reported.[223] Diagnosis is made by pathologic evaluation of effusion cells. HHV-8 PCR of the effusion may also be helpful in making a diagnosis. Other causes of exudative effusions should be ruled out, including infectious entities such as tuberculosis and empyema. Treatment experience of transplant-associated

PEL is limited. Reduction in immunosuppression may be useful, as with KS and MCD.[202] Antivirals have not been shown to offer much benefit and chemotherapy remains the treatment of choice in most cases.[222,223]

SUMMARY

The herpes viruses are responsible for a wide range of diseases in patients following transplant. The development of effective antiviral prophylaxis against HSV and VZV has substantially reduced the morbidity and mortality associated with these infections. Nonetheless, primary disease and reactivation of HSV and VZV can cause significant harm if not treated promptly. The role of EBV as a major cause of PTLD continues to pose a significant challenge. Current therapies focus on reduction of immunosuppression, chemotherapy, and rituximab therapy. There are few data to support antiviral therapy for EBV-associated PTLD, however ganciclovir may have a prophylactic effect, either by indirect or direct means. HHV-6 and -7 may have several indirect effects on transplant patients, including increased risk of infections and rejection episodes. These effects may be related to the viruses' effect on immune cell function. The evidence for HHV-6 as a cause of posttransplant encephalitis is growing. Treatment with ganciclovir and/or foscarnet may be beneficial. The role of HHV-8 in posttransplant KS is well established. Reduction in immune suppression is the mainstay of therapy; in some cases alteration of immunosuppression to include sirolimus may be effective. Other manifestations of HHV-8 infection, including PEL and MCD may require chemotherapy in conjunction with reduction in immunosuppression. Antivirals have not been shown to be beneficial in the treatment of KS or PEL.

REFERENCES

1. Balfour HH Jr, Chace BA, Stapleton JT, et al. A randomized, placebo-controlled trial of oral acyclovir for the prevention of cytomegalovirus disease in recipients of renal allografts. N Engl J Med 1989;320(21):1381–7.
2. Snydman DR. Epidemiology of infections after solid-organ transplantation. Clin Infect Dis 2001;33(Suppl 1):S5–8.
3. Montoya J, Giraldo L, Efron B, et al. Infectious complications among 620 consecutive heart transplant patients at Stanford University Medical Center. Clin Infect Dis 2001;33:629–40.
4. Singh N, Dummer JS, Kusne S, et al. Infections with cytomegalovirus and other herpesviruses in 121 liver transplant recipients: transmission by donated organ and the effect of OKT3 antibodies. J Infect Dis 1988;158(1):124–31.
5. Dummer JS, Armstrong J, Somers J, et al. Transmission of infection with herpes simplex virus by renal transplantation. J Infect Dis 1987;155(2):202–6.
6. Koneru B, Tzakis AG, DePuydt LE, et al. Transmission of fatal herpes simplex infection through renal transplantation. Transplantation 1988;45(3):653–6.
7. Malkin J. Epidemiology of genital herpes simplex virus infection in developed countries. Herpes 2004;11(Suppl 1):24.
8. Malkin J, Morand P, Malvy D. Seroprevalence of HSV-1 and HSV-2 in the general French population. Sex Transm Dis 2002;78:201–3.
9. Vyse A, Gay N, Slomka M. The burden of infection with HSV-1 and HSV-2 in England and Wales: implications for the changing epidemiology of genital herpes. Sex Transm Dis 2000;76:183–7.
10. Xu F, Sternberg MR, Kottiri BJ, et al. Trends in herpes simplex virus type 1 and type 2 seroprevalence in the United States. JAMA 2006;296(8):964–73.

11. Gane E, Saliba F, Valdecasas GJ, et al. Randomised trial of efficacy and safety of oral ganciclovir in the prevention of cytomegalovirus disease in liver-transplant recipients. The Oral Ganciclovir International Transplantation Study Group [corrected]. Lancet 1997;350(9093):1729–33.

12. Lowance D, Neumayer HH, Legendre CM, et al. Valacyclovir for the prevention of cytomegalovirus disease after renal transplantation. International Valacyclovir Cytomegalovirus Prophylaxis Transplantation Study Group. N Engl J Med 1999; 340(19):1462–70.

13. Meyers JD, Flournoy N, Thomas ED. Infection with herpes simplex virus and cell-mediated immunity after marrow transplant. J Infect Dis 1980;142(3): 338–46.

14. Meyers JD, Wade JC, Mitchell CD, et al. Multicenter collaborative trial of intravenous acyclovir for treatment of mucocutaneous herpes simplex virus infection in the immunocompromised host. Am J Med 1982;73(1A):229–35.

15. Saral R, Burns WH, Laskin OL, et al. Acyclovir prophylaxis of herpes-simplex-virus infections. N Engl J Med 1981;305(2):63–7.

16. Seale L, Jones CJ, Kathpalia S, et al. Prevention of herpesvirus infections in renal allograft recipients by low-dose oral acyclovir. JAMA 1985;254(24): 3435–8.

17. Kusne S, Schwartz M, Breinig MK, et al. Herpes simplex virus hepatitis after solid organ transplantation in adults. J Infect Dis 1991;163(5):1001–7.

18. Pettersson E, Hovi T, Ahonen J, et al. Prophylactic oral acyclovir after renal transplantation. Transplantation 1985;39(3):279–81.

19. Naraqi S, Jackson GG, Jonasson O, et al. Prospective study of prevalence, incidence, and source of herpesvirus infections in patients with renal allografts. J Infect Dis 1977;136(4):531–40.

20. Corey L. Herpes simplex virus. In: Mandell G, Bennett J, Dolin R, editors. 6th edition, Principles and practice of infectious diseases, vol. 2. Philadelphia (PA): Elsevier; 2005. p. 1762–80.

21. Hann IM, Prentice HG, Blacklock HA, et al. Acyclovir prophylaxis against herpes virus infections in severely immunocompromised patients: randomised double blind trial. Br Med J (Clin Res Ed) 1983;287(6389):384–8.

22. Buss DH, Scharyj M. Herpesvirus infection of the esophagus and other visceral organs in adults. Incidence and clinical significance. Am J Med 1979;66(3):457–62.

23. Cunha BA, Eisenstein LE, Dillard T, et al. Herpes simplex virus (HSV) pneumonia in a heart transplant: diagnosis and therapy. Heart Lung 2007;36(1):72–8.

24. Herout V, Vortel V, Vondrackova A. Herpes simplex involvement of the lower respiratory tract. Am J Clin Pathol 1966;46(4):411–9.

25. Morgan HR, Finland M. Isolation of herpes virus from a case of atypical pneumonia and erythema multiforme exudativum with studies of four additional cases. Am J Med Sci 1949;217(1):92–5.

26. Nash G. Necrotizing tracheobronchitis and bronchopneumonia consistent with herpetic infection. Hum Pathol 1972;3(2):283–91.

27. Nash G, Foley FD. Herpetic infection of the middle and lower respiratory tract. Am J Clin Pathol 1970;54(6):857–63.

28. Ramsey PG, Fife KH, Hackman RC, et al. Herpes simplex virus pneumonia: clinical, virologic, and pathologic features in 20 patients. Ann Intern Med 1982; 97(6):813–20.

29. Bruynseels P, Jorens PG, Demey HE, et al. Herpes simplex virus in the respiratory tract of critical care patients: a prospective study. Lancet 2003;362(9395): 1536–41.

30. Camps K, Jorens PG, Demey HE, et al. Clinical significance of herpes simplex virus in the lower respiratory tract of critically ill patients. Eur J Clin Microbiol Infect Dis 2002;21(10):758–9.
31. Klainer AS, Oud L, Randazzo J, et al. Herpes simplex virus involvement of the lower respiratory tract following surgery. Chest 1994;106(Suppl 1):8S–14S [discussion: 34S–5S].
32. Liebau P, Kuse E, Winkler M, et al. Management of herpes simplex virus type 1 pneumonia following liver transplantation. Infection 1996;24(2):130–5.
33. Tuxen DV, Wilson JW, Cade JF. Prevention of lower respiratory herpes simplex virus infection with acyclovir in patients with the adult respiratory distress syndrome. Am Rev Respir Dis 1987;136(2):402–5.
34. Schuller D, Spessert C, Fraser VJ, et al. Herpes simplex virus from respiratory tract secretions: epidemiology, clinical characteristics, and outcome in immunocompromised and nonimmunocompromised hosts. Am J Med 1993;94(1):29–33.
35. Campsen J, Hendrickson R, Bak T, et al. Herpes simplex in a liver transplant recipient. Liver Transpl 2006;12(7):1171–3.
36. Basse G, Mengelle C, Kamar N, et al. Disseminated herpes simplex type-2 (HSV-2) infection after solid-organ transplantation. Infection 2008;36(1):62–4.
37. Duckro AN, Sha BE, Jakate S, et al. Herpes simplex virus hepatitis: expanding the spectrum of disease. Transpl Infect Dis 2006;8(3):171–6.
38. Kaufman B, Gandhi SA, Louie E, et al. Herpes simplex virus hepatitis: case report and review. Clin Infect Dis 1997;24(3):334–8.
39. Taylor RJ, Saul SH, Dowling JN, et al. Primary disseminated herpes simplex infection with fulminant hepatitis following renal transplantation. Arch Intern Med 1981;141(11):1519–21.
40. Bissig KD, Zimmermann A, Bernasch D, et al. Herpes simplex virus hepatitis 4 years after liver transplantation. J Gastroenterol 2003;38(10):1005–8.
41. Adler M, Goldman M, Liesnard C, et al. Diffuse herpes simplex virus colitis in a kidney transplant recipient successfully treated with acyclovir. Transplantation 1987;43(6):919–21.
42. Delis S, Kato T, Ruiz P, et al. Herpes simplex colitis in a child with combined liver and small bowel transplant. Pediatr Transplant 2001;5(5):374–7.
43. el-Serag HB, Zwas FR, Cirillo NW, et al. Fulminant herpes colitis in a patient with Crohn's disease. J Clin Gastroenterol 1996;22(3):220–3.
44. Fishbein PG, Tuthill R, Kressel H, et al. Herpes simplex esophagitis: a cause of upper-gastrointestinal bleeding. Dig Dis Sci 1979;24(7):540–4.
45. Howiler W, Goldberg HI. Gastroesophageal involvement in herpes simplex. Gastroenterology 1976;70(5 Pt 1):775–8.
46. Mosimann F, Cuenoud PF, Steinhauslin F, et al. Herpes simplex esophagitis after renal transplantation. Transpl Int 1994;7(2):79–82.
47. Naik HR, Chandrasekar PH. Herpes simplex virus (HSV) colitis in a bone marrow transplant recipient. Bone Marrow Transplant 1996;17(2):285–6.
48. Watts SJ, Alexander LC, Fawcett K, et al. Herpes simplex esophagitis in a renal transplant patient treated with cyclosporine A: a case report. Am J Gastroenterol 1986;81(3):185–8.
49. Gomez E, Melon S, Aguado S, et al. Herpes simplex virus encephalitis in a renal transplant patient: diagnosis by polymerase chain reaction detection of HSV DNA. Am J Kidney Dis 1997;30(3):423–7.
50. Raschilas F, Wolff M, Delatour F, et al. Outcome of and prognostic factors for herpes simplex encephalitis in adult patients: results of a multicenter study. Clin Infect Dis 2002;35(3):254–60.

51. Lakeman FD, Whitley RJ. Diagnosis of herpes simplex encephalitis: application of polymerase chain reaction to cerebrospinal fluid from brain-biopsied patients and correlation with disease. National Institute of Allergy and Infectious Diseases Collaborative Antiviral Study Group. J Infect Dis 1995;171(4):857–63.

52. Whitley RJ, Alford CA, Hirsch MS, et al. Vidarabine versus acyclovir therapy in herpes simplex encephalitis. N Engl J Med 1986;314(3):144–9.

53. Shepp DH, Dandliker PS, Flournoy N, et al. Once-daily intravenous acyclovir for prophylaxis of herpes simplex virus reactivation after marrow transplantation. J Antimicrob Chemother 1985;16(3):389–95.

54. Chen Y, Scieux C, Garrait V, et al. Resistant herpes simplex virus type 1 infection: an emerging concern after allogeneic stem cell transplantation. Clin Infect Dis 2000;31(4):927–35.

55. Erard V, Wald A, Corey L, et al. Use of long-term suppressive acyclovir after hematopoietic stem-cell transplantation: impact on herpes simplex virus (HSV) disease and drug-resistant HSV disease. J Infect Dis 2007;196(2):266–70.

56. Morfin F, Thouvenot D. Herpes simplex virus resistance to antiviral drugs. J Clin Virol 2003;26(1):29–37.

57. Nugier F, Colin JN, Aymard M, et al. Occurrence and characterization of acyclovir-resistant herpes simplex virus isolates: report on a two-year sensitivity screening survey. J Med Virol 1992;36(1):1–12.

58. Herpes simplex virus (HSV)-1 and -2, and varicella zoster virus (VZV). Am J Transplant 2004;4(s10):69–71.

59. Alcaide ML, Abbo L, Pano JR, et al. Herpes zoster infection after liver transplantation in patients receiving induction therapy with alemtuzumab. Clin Transplant 2008;22(4):502–7.

60. Arness T, Pedersen R, Dierkhising R, et al. Varicella zoster virus-associated disease in adult kidney transplant recipients: incidence and risk-factor analysis. Transpl Infect Dis 2008;10(4):260–8.

61. Manuel O, Kumar D, Singer LG, et al. Incidence and clinical characteristics of herpes zoster after lung transplantation. J Heart Lung Transplant 2008;27(1): 11–6.

62. Locksley RM, Flournoy N, Sullivan KM, et al. Infection with varicella-zoster virus after marrow transplantation. J Infect Dis 1985;152(6):1172–81.

63. Boeckh M, Kim HW, Flowers ME, et al. Long-term acyclovir for prevention of varicella zoster virus disease after allogeneic hematopoietic cell transplantation– a randomized double-blind placebo-controlled study. Blood 2006;107(5): 1800–5.

64. Han CS, Miller W, Haake R, et al. Varicella zoster infection after bone marrow transplantation: incidence, risk factors and complications. Bone Marrow Transplant 1994;13(3):277–83.

65. Leung TF, Chik KW, Li CK, et al. Incidence, risk factors and outcome of varicella-zoster virus infection in children after haematopoietic stem cell transplantation. Bone Marrow Transplant 2000;25(2):167–72.

66. Koc Y, Miller KB, Schenkein DP, et al. Varicella zoster virus infections following allogeneic bone marrow transplantation: frequency, risk factors, and clinical outcome. Biol Blood Marrow Transplant 2000;6(1):44–9.

67. Gnann J. Herpes simplex and varicella zoster virus infection after hemopoietic stem cell or solid organ transplantation. Philadelphia: Lippincott, Williams and Wilkins; 2003.

68. Fuks L, Shitrit D, Fox BD, et al. Herpes zoster after lung transplantation: incidence, timing, and outcome. Ann Thorac Surg 2009;87(2):423–6.

69. Gourishankar S, McDermid JC, Jhangri GS, et al. Herpes zoster infection following solid organ transplantation: incidence, risk factors and outcomes in the current immunosuppressive era. Am J Transplant 2004;4(1):108–15.
70. Herrero JI, Quiroga J, Sangro B, et al. Herpes zoster after liver transplantation: incidence, risk factors, and complications. Liver Transpl 2004;10(9):1140–3.
71. Lauzurica R, Bayes B, Frias C, et al. Disseminated varicella infection in adult renal allograft recipients: role of mycophenolate mofetil. Transplant Proc 2003; 35(5):1758–9.
72. Weinberg A, Horslen SP, Kaufman SS, et al. Safety and immunogenicity of varicella-zoster virus vaccine in pediatric liver and intestine transplant recipients. Am J Transplant 2006;6(3):565–8.
73. Khan S, Erlichman J, Rand EB. Live virus immunization after orthotopic liver transplantation. Pediatr Transplant 2006;10(1):78–82.
74. Kraft JN, Shaw JC. Varicella infection caused by Oka strain vaccine in a heart transplant recipient. Arch Dermatol 2006;142(7):943–5.
75. Levitsky J, Te HS, Faust TW, et al. Varicella infection following varicella vaccination in a liver transplant recipient. Am J Transplant 2002;2(9):880–2.
76. Sauerbrei A, Prager J, Hengst U, et al. Varicella vaccination in children after bone marrow transplantation. Bone Marrow Transplant 1997;20(5):381–3.
77. Merck. Varivax varicella virus vaccine live. 2009 [PDF file]. Available at: http://www.merck.com/product/usa/pi_circulars/v/varivax/varivax_pi.pdf. Accessed August 8, 2009.
78. Hata A, Asanuma H, Rinki M, et al. Use of an inactivated varicella vaccine in recipients of hematopoietic-cell transplants. N Engl J Med 2002;347(1):26–34.
79. Feldhoff CM, Balfour HH Jr, Simmons RL, et al. Varicella in children with renal transplants. J Pediatr 1981;98(1):25–31.
80. McGregor RS, Zitelli BJ, Urbach AH, et al. Varicella in pediatric orthotopic liver transplant recipients. Pediatrics 1989;83(2):256–61.
81. Parnham AP, Flexman JP, Saker BM, et al. Primary varicella in adult renal transplant recipients: a report of three cases plus a review of the literature. Clin Transplant 1995;9(2):115–8.
82. Fall AJ, Aitchison JD, Krause A, et al. Donor organ transmission of varicella zoster due to cardiac transplantation. Transplantation 2000;70(1):211–3.
83. Hyland JM, Butterworth J. Severe acute visceral pain from varicella zoster virus. Anesth Analg 2003;97(4):1117–8.
84. Koskiniemi M, Piiparinen H, Rantalaiho T, et al. Acute central nervous system complications in varicella zoster virus infections. J Clin Virol 2002;25(3):293–301.
85. Aberle SW, Puchhammer-Stockl E. Diagnosis of herpesvirus infections of the central nervous system. J Clin Virol 2002;25(Suppl 1):S79–85.
86. Puchhammer-Stockl E, Popow-Kraupp T, Heinz FX, et al. Detection of varicella-zoster virus DNA by polymerase chain reaction in the cerebrospinal fluid of patients suffering from neurological complications associated with chicken pox or herpes zoster. J Clin Microbiol 1991;29(7):1513–6.
87. Glaser CA, Honarmand S, Anderson LJ, et al. Beyond viruses: clinical profiles and etiologies associated with encephalitis. Clin Infect Dis 2006;43(12):1565–77.
88. Gilden D. Varicella zoster virus and central nervous system syndromes. Herpes 2004;11(Suppl 2):89A–94A.
89. Tyring S, Belanger R, Bezwoda W, et al. A randomized, double-blind trial of famciclovir versus acyclovir for the treatment of localized dermatomal herpes zoster in immunocompromised patients. Cancer Invest 2001;19(1):13–22.

90. American Academy of Pediatrics. Varicella zoster virus. 25th edition. Elk Grove (IL): American Academy of Pediatrics; 2000.

91. Marin M, Guris D, Chaves SS, et al. Prevention of varicella: recommendations of the Advisory Committee on Immunization Practices (ACIP). MMWR Recomm Rep 2007;56(RR-4):1–40.

92. A new product (VariZIG™) for postexposure prophylaxis of varicella available under an investigational new drug application expanded access protocol. MMWR Morb Mortal Wkly Rep 2006;55(8):209–10.

93. Epstein-Barr virus and lymphoproliferative disorders after transplantation. Am J Transplant 2004;4(Suppl 10):59–65.

94. Nalesnik MA. The diverse pathology of post-transplant lymphoproliferative disorders: the importance of a standardized approach. Transpl Infect Dis 2001;3(2):88–96.

95. Preiksaitis JK. New developments in the diagnosis and management of post-transplantation lymphoproliferative disorders in solid organ transplant recipients. Clin Infect Dis 2004;39(7):1016–23.

96. Karras A, Thervet E, Legendre C. Hemophagocytic syndrome in renal transplant recipients: report of 17 cases and review of literature. Transplantation 2004; 77(2):238–43.

97. Lee ES, Locker J, Nalesnik M, et al. The association of Epstein-Barr virus with smooth-muscle tumors occurring after organ transplantation. N Engl J Med 1995;332(1):19–25.

98. Jenkins FJ, Rowe DT, Rinaldo CR Jr. Herpesvirus infections in organ transplant recipients. Clin Diagn Lab Immunol 2003;10(1):1–7.

99. Johannsen E, Schooley R, Kaye K. Epstein-Barr virus (infectious mononucleosis). In: Mandell G, Bennett J, Dolin R, editors, Principles and practice of infectious diseases, vol. 2. Philadelphia (PA): Elsevier; 2005. p. 1801–20.

100. Baskin HJ, Hedlund G. Neuroimaging of herpesvirus infections in children. Pediatr Radiol 2007;37(10):949–63.

101. Alfieri C, Tanner J, Carpentier L, et al. Epstein-Barr virus transmission from a blood donor to an organ transplant recipient with recovery of the same virus strain from the recipient's blood and oropharynx. Blood 1996;87(2): 812–7.

102. Haque T, Thomas JA, Falk KI, et al. Transmission of donor Epstein-Barr virus (EBV) in transplanted organs causes lymphoproliferative disease in EBV-seronegative recipients. J Gen Virol 1996;77(Pt 6):1169–72.

103. Frizzera G, Hanto DW, Gajl-Peczalska KJ, et al. Polymorphic diffuse B-cell hyperplasias and lymphomas in renal transplant recipients. Cancer Res 1981; 41(11 Pt 1):4262–79.

104. Hanto DW, Gajl-Peczalska KJ, Frizzera G, et al. Epstein-Barr virus (EBV) induced polyclonal and monoclonal B-cell lymphoproliferative diseases occurring after renal transplantation. Clinical, pathologic, and virologic findings and implications for therapy. Ann Surg 1983;198(3):356–69.

105. Yousem SA, Randhawa P, Locker J, et al. Posttransplant lymphoproliferative disorders in heart-lung transplant recipients: primary presentation in the allograft. Hum Pathol 1989;20(4):361–9.

106. Diaz-Guzman E, Farver C, Kanne JP, et al. A 65-year-old man with odynophagia and a lung mass. Chest 2009;135(3):876–9.

107. Khan MS, Ahmed S, Challacombe B, et al. Post-transplant lymphoproliferative disorder (PTLD) presenting as painful lymphocele 12 years after a cadaveric renal transplant. Int Urol Nephrol 2008;40(2):547–50.

108. Lee WK, Lau EW, Duddalwar VA, et al. Abdominal manifestations of extranodal lymphoma: spectrum of imaging findings. AJR Am J Roentgenol 2008;191(1): 198–206.

109. Kunitomi A, Arima N, Ishikawa T. Epstein-Barr virus-associated post-transplant lymphoproliferative disorders presented as interstitial pneumonia; successful recovery with rituximab. Haematologica 2007;92(4):e49–52.

110. Ellis D, Jaffe R, Green M, et al. Epstein-Barr virus-related disorders in children undergoing renal transplantation with tacrolimus-based immunosuppression. Transplantation 1999;68(7):997–1003.

111. Ho M, Miller G, Atchison RW, et al. Epstein-Barr virus infections and DNA hybridization studies in posttransplantation lymphoma and lymphoproliferative lesions: the role of primary infection. J Infect Dis 1985;152(5):876–86.

112. Swinnen LJ, Costanzo-Nordin MR, Fisher SG, et al. Increased incidence of lymphoproliferative disorder after immunosuppression with the monoclonal antibody OKT3 in cardiac-transplant recipients. N Engl J Med 1990;323(25):1723–8.

113. Walker RC, Marshall WF, Strickler JG, et al. Pretransplantation assessment of the risk of lymphoproliferative disorder. Clin Infect Dis 1995;20(5):1346–53.

114. Keay S, Oldach D, Wiland A, et al. Posttransplantation lymphoproliferative disorder associated with OKT3 and decreased antiviral prophylaxis in pancreas transplant recipients. Clin Infect Dis 1998;26(3):596–600.

115. Cox KL, Lawrence-Miyasaki LS, Garcia-Kennedy R, et al. An increased incidence of Epstein-Barr virus infection and lymphoproliferative disorder in young children on FK506 after liver transplantation. Transplantation 1995;59(4):524–9.

116. Manez R, Breinig MC, Linden P, et al. Posttransplant lymphoproliferative disease in primary Epstein-Barr virus infection after liver transplantation: the role of cytomegalovirus disease. J Infect Dis 1997;176(6):1462–7.

117. Weinstock DM, Ambrossi GG, Brennan C, et al. Preemptive diagnosis and treatment of Epstein-Barr virus-associated post transplant lymphoproliferative disorder after hematopoietic stem cell transplant: an approach in development. Bone Marrow Transplant 2006;37(6):539–46.

118. Preiksaitis JK, Keay S. Diagnosis and management of posttransplant lymphoproliferative disorder in solid-organ transplant recipients. Clin Infect Dis 2001; 33(Suppl 1):S38–46.

119. Tsai DE, Douglas L, Andreadis C, et al. EBV PCR in the diagnosis and monitoring of posttransplant lymphoproliferative disorder: results of a two-arm prospective trial. Am J Transplant 2008;8(5):1016–24.

120. Wheless SA, Gulley ML, Raab-Traub N, et al. Post-transplantation lymphoproliferative disease: Epstein-Barr virus DNA levels, HLA-A3, and survival. Am J Respir Crit Care Med 2008;178(10):1060–5.

121. Harris NL. Posttransplant lymphoproliferative disorders (PTLD). In: Jaffe E, Harris N, Stein H, et al, editors. Pathology and genetics: tumours of haematopoietic and lymphoid tissues. WHO classification of tumours. Lyon (France): IARC Press; 2001. p. 264–9.

122. Harris NL, Ferry JA, Swerdlow SH. Posttransplant lymphoproliferative disorders: summary of Society for Hematopathology Workshop. Semin Diagn Pathol 1997; 14(1):8–14.

123. Starzl TE, Nalesnik MA, Porter KA, et al. Reversibility of lymphomas and lymphoproliferative lesions developing under cyclosporin-steroid therapy. Lancet 1984; 1(8377):583–7.

124. Tsai DE, Hardy CL, Tomaszewski JE, et al. Reduction in immunosuppression as initial therapy for posttransplant lymphoproliferative disorder: analysis of

prognostic variables and long-term follow-up of 42 adult patients. Transplantation 2001;71(8):1076–88.

125. Hanto DW, Frizzera G, Gajl-Peczalska KJ, et al. Epstein-Barr virus-induced B-cell lymphoma after renal transplantation: acyclovir therapy and transition from polyclonal to monoclonal B-cell proliferation. N Engl J Med 1982;306(15):913–8.

126. Andersson J, Skoldenberg B, Ernberg I, et al. Acyclovir treatment in primary Epstein-Barr virus infection. A double-blind placebo-controlled study. Scand J Infect Dis Suppl 1985;47:107–15.

127. Paya CV, Fung JJ, Nalesnik MA, et al. Epstein-Barr virus-induced posttransplant lymphoproliferative disorders. ASTS/ASTP EBV-PTLD Task Force and The Mayo Clinic Organized International Consensus Development Meeting. Transplantation 1999;68(10):1517–25.

128. Yao QY, Ogan P, Rowe M, et al. Epstein-Barr virus-infected B cells persist in the circulation of acyclovir-treated virus carriers. Int J Cancer 1989;43(1):67–71.

129. Choquet S, Leblond V, Herbrecht R, et al. Efficacy and safety of rituximab in B-cell post-transplantation lymphoproliferative disorders: results of a prospective multicenter phase 2 study. Blood 2006;107(8):3053–7.

130. Norin S, Kimby E, Ericzon BG, et al. Posttransplant lymphoma–a single-center experience of 500 liver transplantations. Med Oncol 2004;21(3):273–84.

131. Trappe RU, Choquet S, Reinke P, et al. Salvage therapy for relapsed posttransplant lymphoproliferative disorders (PTLD) with a second progression of PTLD after upfront chemotherapy: the role of single-agent rituximab. Transplantation 2007;84(12):1708–12.

132. Oertel SH, Verschuuren E, Reinke P, et al. Effect of anti-CD 20 antibody rituximab in patients with post-transplant lymphoproliferative disorder (PTLD). Am J Transplant 2005;5(12):2901–6.

133. Rooney CM, Smith CA, Ng CYC, et al. Infusion of cytotoxic T cells for the prevention and treatment of Epstein-Barr virus-induced lymphoma in allogeneic transplant recipients. Blood 1998;92(5):1549–55.

134. Gustafsson A, Levitsky V, Zou J-Z, et al. Epstein-Barr virus (EBV) load in bone marrow transplant recipients at risk to develop posttransplant lymphoproliferative disease: prophylactic infusion of EBV-specific cytotoxic T cells. Blood 2000;95(3):807–14.

135. Savoldo B, Goss JA, Hammer MM, et al. Treatment of solid organ transplant recipients with autologous Epstein Barr virus-specific cytotoxic T lymphocytes (CTLs). Blood 2006;108(9):2942–9.

136. Haque T, Taylor C, Wilkie GM, et al. Complete regression of posttransplant lymphoproliferative disease using partially HLA-matched Epstein Barr virus-specific cytotoxic T cells. Transplantation 2001;72(8):1399–402.

137. Haque T, Wilkie GM, Jones MM, et al. Allogeneic cytotoxic T-cell therapy for EBV-positive posttransplantation lymphoproliferative disease: results of a phase 2 multicenter clinical trial. Blood 2007;110(4):1123–31.

138. Haque T, Wilkie GM, Taylor C, et al. Treatment of Epstein-Barr-virus-positive post-transplantation lymphoproliferative disease with partly HLA-matched allogeneic cytotoxic T cells. Lancet 2002;360(9331):436–42.

139. Comoli P, Labirio M, Basso S, et al. Infusion of autologous Epstein-Barr virus (EBV)-specific cytotoxic T cells for prevention of EBV-related lymphoproliferative disorder in solid organ transplant recipients with evidence of active virus replication. Blood 2002;99(7):2592–8.

140. Khanna R, Bell S, Sherritt M, et al. Activation and adoptive transfer of Epstein-Barr virus-specific cytotoxic T cells in solid organ transplant patients with

posttransplant lymphoproliferative disease. Proc Natl Acad Sci U S A 1999; 96(18):10391–6.

141. Choquet S, Trappe R, Leblond V, et al. CHOP-21 for the treatment of post-transplant lymphoproliferative disorders (PTLD) following solid organ transplantation. Haematologica 2007;92(2):273–4.

142. Elstrom RL, Andreadis C, Aqui NA, et al. Treatment of PTLD with rituximab or chemotherapy. Am J Transplant 2006;6(3):569–76.

143. Garrett TJ, Chadburn A, Barr ML, et al. Posttransplantation lymphoproliferative disorders treated with cyclophosphamide-doxorubicin-vincristine-prednisone chemotherapy. Cancer 1993;72(9):2782–5.

144. Mamzer-Bruneel MF, Lome C, Morelon E, et al. Durable remission after aggressive chemotherapy for very late post-kidney transplant lymphoproliferation: a report of 16 cases observed in a single center. J Clin Oncol 2000;18(21):3622–32.

145. Everly MJ, Bloom RD, Tsai DE, et al. Posttransplant lymphoproliferative disorder. Ann Pharmacother 2007;41(11):1850–8.

146. Karras A, Thervet E, Le Meur Y, et al. Successful renal retransplantation after post-transplant lymphoproliferative disease. Am J Transplant 2004;4(11): 1904–9.

147. Darenkov IA, Marcarelli MA, Basadonna GP, et al. Reduced incidence of Epstein-Barr virus-associated posttransplant lymphoproliferative disorder using preemptive antiviral therapy. Transplantation 1997;64(6):848–52.

148. Davis CL, Harrison KL, McVicar JP, et al. Antiviral prophylaxis and the Epstein Barr virus-related post-transplant lymphoproliferative disorder. Clin Transplant 1995;9(1):53–9.

149. Funch DP, Walker AM, Schneider G, et al. Ganciclovir and acyclovir reduce the risk of post-transplant lymphoproliferative disorder in renal transplant recipients. Am J Transplant 2005;5(12):2894–900.

150. Green M, Kaufmann M, Wilson J, et al. Comparison of intravenous ganciclovir followed by oral acyclovir with intravenous ganciclovir alone for prevention of cytomegalovirus and Epstein-Barr virus disease after liver transplantation in children. Clin Infect Dis 1997;25(6):1344–9.

151. Bakker NA, Verschuuren EA, Erasmus ME, et al. Epstein-Barr virus-DNA load monitoring late after lung transplantation: a surrogate marker of the degree of immunosuppression and a safe guide to reduce immunosuppression. Transplantation 2007;83(4):433–8.

152. Salahuddin SZ, Ablashi DV, Markham PD, et al. Isolation of a new virus, HBLV, in patients with lymphoproliferative disorders. Science 1986;234(4776):596–601.

153. Gentile G. Post-transplant HHV-6 diseases. Herpes 2000;7(1):24–7.

154. Leach CT, Sumaya CV, Brown NA. Human herpesvirus-6: clinical implications of a recently discovered, ubiquitous agent. J Pediatr 1992;121(2):173–81.

155. Brown NA, Sumaya CV, Liu CR, et al. Fall in human herpesvirus 6 seropositivity with age. Lancet 1988;2(8607):396.

156. Lau YL, Peiris M, Chan GC, et al. Primary human herpes virus 6 infection transmitted from donor to recipient through bone marrow infusion. Bone Marrow Transplant 1998;21(10):1063–6.

157. Cervera C, Marcos MA, Linares L, et al. A prospective survey of human herpesvirus-6 primary infection in solid organ transplant recipients. Transplantation 2006;82(7):979–82.

158. Zerr DM, Corey L, Kim HW, et al. Clinical outcomes of human herpesvirus 6 reactivation after hematopoietic stem cell transplantation. Clin Infect Dis 2005; 40(7):932–40.

159. de Pagter PJ, Schuurman R, Meijer E, et al. Human herpesvirus type 6 reactivation after haematopoietic stem cell transplantation. J Clin Virol 2008;43(4): 361–6.
160. de Pagter PJ, Schuurman R, Visscher H, et al. Human herpes virus 6 plasma DNA positivity after hematopoietic stem cell transplantation in children: an important risk factor for clinical outcome. Biol Blood Marrow Transplant 2008; 14(7):831–9.
161. Wang LR, Dong LJ, Zhang MJ, et al. The impact of human herpesvirus 6B reactivation on early complications following allogeneic hematopoietic stem cell transplantation. Biol Blood Marrow Transplant 2006;12(10):1031–7.
162. Yamane A, Mori T, Suzuki S, et al. Risk factors for developing human herpesvirus 6 (HHV-6) reactivation after allogeneic hematopoietic stem cell transplantation and its association with central nervous system disorders. Biol Blood Marrow Transplant 2007;13(1):100–6.
163. DesJardin JA, Gibbons L, Cho E, et al. Human herpesvirus 6 reactivation is associated with cytomegalovirus infection and syndromes in kidney transplant recipients at risk for primary cytomegalovirus infection. J Infect Dis 1998; 178(6):1783–6.
164. Dockrell DH, Prada J, Jones MF, et al. Seroconversion to human herpesvirus 6 following liver transplantation is a marker of cytomegalovirus disease. J Infect Dis 1997;176(5):1135–40.
165. Lehto JT, Halme M, Tukiainen P, et al. Human herpesvirus-6 and -7 after lung and heart-lung transplantation. J Heart Lung Transplant 2007;26(1):41–7.
166. Ratnamohan VM, Chapman J, Howse H, et al. Cytomegalovirus and human herpesvirus 6 both cause viral disease after renal transplantation. Transplantation 1998;66(7):877–82.
167. Yoshikawa T, Suga S, Asano Y, et al. A prospective study of human herpesvirus-6 infection in renal transplantation. Transplantation 1992;54(5):879–83.
168. Humar A, Malkan G, Moussa G, et al. Human herpesvirus-6 is associated with cytomegalovirus reactivation in liver transplant recipients. J Infect Dis 2000; 181(4):1450–3.
169. Herbein G, Strasswimmer J, Altieri M, et al. Longitudinal study of human herpesvirus 6 infection in organ transplant recipients. Clin Infect Dis 1996;22(1):171–3.
170. Razonable RR, Paya CV. The impact of human herpesvirus-6 and -7 infection on the outcome of liver transplantation. Liver Transpl 2002;8(8):651–8.
171. Humar A, Asberg A, Kumar D, et al. An assessment of herpesvirus co-infections in patients with CMV disease: correlation with clinical and virologic outcomes. Am J Transplant 2009;9(2):374–81.
172. Singh N, Paterson DL. Encephalitis caused by human herpesvirus-6 in transplant recipients: relevance of a novel neurotropic virus. Transplantation 2000; 69(12):2474–9.
173. Bollen AE, Wartan AN, Krikke AP, et al. Amnestic syndrome after lung transplantation by human herpes virus-6 encephalitis. J Neurol 2001;248(7):619–20.
174. Mookerjee BP, Vogelsang G. Human herpes virus-6 encephalitis after bone marrow transplantation: successful treatment with ganciclovir. Bone Marrow Transplant 1997;20(10):905–6.
175. Mori T, Mihara A, Yamazaki R, et al. Myelitis associated with human herpes virus 6 (HHV-6) after allogeneic cord blood transplantation. Scand J Infect Dis 2007; 39(3):276–8.
176. Seeley WW, Marty FM, Holmes TM, et al. Post-transplant acute limbic encephalitis: clinical features and relationship to HHV6. Neurology 2007;69(2):156–65.

177. Vu T, Carrum G, Hutton G, et al. Human herpesvirus-6 encephalitis following allogeneic hematopoietic stem cell transplantation. Bone Marrow Transplant 2007;39(11):705–9.

178. Fotheringham J, Akhyani N, Vortmeyer A, et al. Detection of active human herpesvirus-6 infection in the brain: correlation with polymerase chain reaction detection in cerebrospinal fluid. J Infect Dis 2007;195(3):450–4.

179. Luppi M, Barozzi P, Maiorana A, et al. Human herpesvirus 6 infection in normal human brain tissue. J Infect Dis 1994;169(4):943–4.

180. Caserta MT, McDermott M, Dewhurst S, et al. Human herpesvirus 6 (HHV6) DNA persistence and reactivation in healthy children. J Pediatr 2004; 145(4):478–84.

181. Singh N, Carrigan DR, Gayowski T, et al. Variant B human herpesvirus-6 associated febrile dermatosis with thrombocytopenia and encephalopathy in a liver transplant recipient. Transplantation 1995;60(11):1355–7.

182. Revest M, Camus C, D'Halluin PN, et al. Fatal human herpes virus 6 primary infection after liver transplantation. Transplantation 2007;83(10):1404–5.

183. Randhawa PS, Jenkins FJ, Nalesnik MA, et al. Herpesvirus 6 variant A infection after heart transplantation with giant cell transformation in bile ductular and gastroduodenal epithelium. Am J Surg Pathol 1997;21(7):847–53.

184. Burns WH, Sandford GR. Susceptibility of human herpesvirus 6 to antivirals in vitro. J Infect Dis 1990;162(3):634–7.

185. Agut H, Aubin JT, Huraux JM. Homogeneous susceptibility of distinct human herpesvirus 6 strains to antivirals in vitro. J Infect Dis 1991;163(6):1382–3.

186. Reymen D, Naesens L, Balzarini J, et al. Antiviral activity of selected acyclic nucleoside analogues against human herpesvirus 6. Antiviral Res 1995;28(4): 343–57.

187. Ward KN. Human herpesviruses-6 and -7 infections. Curr Opin Infect Dis 2005; 18(3):247–52.

188. Ward KN, White RP, Mackinnon S, et al. Human herpesvirus-7 infection of the CNS with acute myelitis in an adult bone marrow recipient. Bone Marrow Transplant 2002;30(12):983–5.

189. Yoshikawa T, Yoshida J, Hamaguchi M, et al. Human herpesvirus 7-associated meningitis and optic neuritis in a patient after allogeneic stem cell transplantation. J Med Virol 2003;70(3):440–3.

190. Kidd IM, Clark DA, Sabin CA, et al. Prospective study of human betaherpesviruses after renal transplantation: association of human herpesvirus 7 and cytomegalovirus co-infection with cytomegalovirus disease and increased rejection. Transplantation 2000;69(11):2400–4.

191. Osman HK, Peiris JS, Taylor CE, et al. "Cytomegalovirus disease" in renal allograft recipients: is human herpesvirus 7 a co-factor for disease progression? J Med Virol 1996;48(4):295–301.

192. Tong CY, Bakran A, Williams H, et al. Association of human herpesvirus 7 with cytomegalovirus disease in renal transplant recipients. Transplantation 2000; 70(1):213–6.

193. Moore PS, Chang Y. Detection of herpesvirus-like DNA sequences in Kaposi's sarcoma in patients with and without HIV infection. N Engl J Med 1995; 332(18):1181–5.

194. Cesarman E, Chang Y, Moore PS, et al. Kaposi's sarcoma-associated herpesvirus-like DNA sequences in AIDS-related body-cavity-based lymphomas. N Engl J Med 1995;332(18):1186–91.

195. Antman K, Chang Y. Kaposi's sarcoma. N Engl J Med 2000;342(14):1027–38.

196. Moore PS. The emergence of Kaposi's sarcoma-associated herpesvirus (human herpesvirus 8). N Engl J Med 2000;343(19):1411–3.

197. Melbye M, Cook PM, Hjalgrim H, et al. Risk factors for Kaposi's-sarcoma-associated herpesvirus (KSHV/HHV-8) seropositivity in a cohort of homosexual men, 1981–1996. Int J Cancer 1998;77(4):543–8.

198. Ahmadpoor P, Ilkhanizadeh B, Sharifzadeh P, et al. Seroprevalence of human herpes virus-8 in renal transplant recipients: a single center study from Iran. Transplant Proc 2007;39(4):1000–2.

199. Butler LM, Dorsey G, Hladik W, et al. Kaposi sarcoma-associated herpesvirus (KSHV) seroprevalence in population-based samples of African children: evidence for at least 2 patterns of KSHV transmission. J Infect Dis 2009; 200(3):430–8.

200. Fu B, Sun F, Li B, et al. Seroprevalence of Kaposi's sarcoma-associated herpesvirus and risk factors in Xinjiang, China. J Med Virol 2009;81(8):1422–31.

201. Engels EA, Atkinson JO, Graubard BI, et al. Risk factors for human herpesvirus 8 infection among adults in the United States and evidence for sexual transmission. J Infect Dis 2007;196(2):199–207.

202. Human herpesvirus-8 (HHV-8, KSHV). Am J Transplant 2004;4(s10):67–9.

203. Dudderidge TJ, Khalifa M, Jeffery R, et al. Donor-derived human herpes virus 8-related Kaposi's sarcoma in renal allograft ureter. Transpl Infect Dis 2008; 10(3):221–6.

204. Luppi M, Barozzi P, Schulz TF, et al. Bone marrow failure associated with human herpesvirus 8 infection after transplantation. N Engl J Med 2000;343(19): 1378–85.

205. Parravicini C, Olsen SJ, Capra M, et al. Risk of Kaposi's sarcoma-associated herpes virus transmission from donor allografts among Italian posttransplant Kaposi's sarcoma patients. Blood 1997;90(7):2826–9.

206. Bergallo M, Costa C, Margio S, et al. Human herpes virus 8 infection in kidney transplant patients from an area of northwestern Italy (Piemonte region). Nephrol Dial Transplant 2007;22(6):1757–61.

207. Boeckle E, Boesmueller C, Wiesmayr S, et al. Kaposi sarcoma in solid organ transplant recipients: a single center report. Transplant Proc 2005;37(4): 1905–9.

208. Verucchi G, Calza L, Trevisani F, et al. Human herpesvirus-8-related Kaposi's sarcoma after liver transplantation successfully treated with cidofovir and liposomal daunorubicin. Transpl Infect Dis 2005;7(1):34–7.

209. Stallone G, Schena A, Infante B, et al. Sirolimus for Kaposi's sarcoma in renal-transplant recipients. N Engl J Med 2005;352(13):1317–23.

210. Lebbe C, Euvrard S, Barrou B, et al. Sirolimus conversion for patients with post-transplant Kaposi's sarcoma. Am J Transplant 2006;6(9):2164–8.

211. Robles R, Lugo D, Gee L, et al. Effect of antiviral drugs used to treat cytomegalovirus end-organ disease on subsequent course of previously diagnosed Kaposi's sarcoma in patients with AIDS. J Acquir Immune Defic Syndr Hum Retrovirol 1999;20(1):34–8.

212. Little RF, Merced-Galindez F, Staskus K, et al. A pilot study of cidofovir in patients with Kaposi sarcoma. J Infect Dis 2003;187(1):149–53.

213. Jones D, Ballestas ME, Kaye KM, et al. Primary-effusion lymphoma and Kaposi's sarcoma in a cardiac-transplant recipient. N Engl J Med 1998;339(7):444–9.

214. Al Otaibi T, Al Sagheir A, Ludwin D, et al. Post renal transplant Castleman's disease resolved after graft nephrectomy: a case report. Transplant Proc 2007;39(4):1276–7.

215. Cagirgan S, Cirit M, Ok E, et al. Castleman's disease in a renal allograft recipient. Nephron 1997;76(3):352–3.
216. Dotti G, Fiocchi R, Motta T, et al. Primary effusion lymphoma after heart transplantation: a new entity associated with human herpesvirus-8. Leukemia 1999; 13(5):664–70.
217. Melo NC, Sales MM, Santana AN, et al. Pleural primary effusion lymphoma in a renal transplant recipient. Am J Transplant 2008;8(4):906–7.
218. Stebbing J, Pantanowitz L, Dayyani F, et al. HIV-associated multicentric Castleman's disease. Am J Hematol 2008;83(6):498–503.
219. Soulier J, Grollet L, Oksenhendler E, et al. Kaposi's sarcoma-associated herpesvirus-like DNA sequences in multicentric Castleman's disease. Blood 1995; 86(4):1276–80.
220. Mandel C, Silberstein M, Hennessy O. Case report: fatal pulmonary Kaposi's sarcoma and Castleman's disease in a renal transplant recipient. Br J Radiol 1993;66(783):264–5.
221. Theate I, Michaux L, Squifflet JP, et al. Human herpesvirus 8 and Epstein-Barr virus-related monotypic large B-cell lymphoproliferative disorder coexisting with mixed variant of Castleman's disease in a lymph node of a renal transplant recipient. Clin Transplant 2003;17(5):451–4.
222. Casper C. Defining a role for antiviral drugs in the treatment of persons with HHV-8 infection. Herpes 2006;13(2):42–7.
223. Gaidano G, Carbone A. Primary effusion lymphoma: a liquid phase lymphoma of fluid-filled body cavities. Adv Cancer Res 2001;80:115–46.

Fungal Infections in Transplant and Oncology Patients

Anna K. Person, MD[a],*, Dimitrios P. Kontoyiannis, MD, ScD[b],
Barbara D. Alexander, MD, MHS[c]

KEYWORDS

• Invasive fungal infection • Transplant • Solid-organ transplant
• Hematopoietic stem cell transplant • Oncology • Fungus

Invasive fungal infections (IFIs) in oncology and transplant populations have been associated with significant morbidity and mortality. Research in this area remains in flux; as epidemiologic patterns shift, more is being learned about optimal treatment and the unique risks that predispose these special populations to such potentially devastating infections. This article highlights recent advances and important factors to consider when treating transplant and oncology patients with IFIs.

EPIDEMIOLOGY OF IFIS

Despite high associated morbidity and mortality, the epidemiology of IFIs in high-risk populations has not previously been well defined. Incidence estimates have been primarily based on single-center, retrospective studies.[1–3] The Transplant Associated Infections Surveillance Program (TRANSNET), a network of 23 transplant centers in the United States, prospectively studied the epidemiology of IFIs among solid-organ and stem cell transplant populations over a 5-year period (March 2001 to March 2006) and provided the first true approximation of the burden of fungal disease among transplant populations in the United States. Based on TRANSNET data, the overall incidence of IFIs in the hematopoietic stem cell transplant (HSCT) population was

---

This work was supported by Grant No. NIAID K24 AI072522 (BD Alexander) from the National Institutes of Health.

A version of this article was previously published in the *Infectious Disease Clinics of North America*, 24:2.

[a] Division of Infectious Diseases, Department of Medicine, Duke University Health System, Duke University School of Medicine, Box 102359, Durham, NC 27710, USA

[b] Department of Infectious Diseases, Infection Control and Employee Health, The University of Texas MD Anderson Cancer Center, 1515 Holcombe Boulevard, Houston, TX 77030, USA

[c] Division of Infectious Diseases, Department of Medicine, Duke University School of Medicine, PO Box 3035, Durham, NC 27710, USA

* Corresponding author.

E-mail address: perso006@mc.duke.edu

3.4%, somewhat lower than previous estimates (DP Kontoyiannis, unpublished data, July 2009). In addition, invasive aspergillosis (IA) surpassed invasive candidiasis (IC) as the most common IFI encountered in the HSCT population: *Aspergillus* accounted for 43% of infections and *Candida* accounted for 28%, followed by other or unspecified molds including *Fusarium* and *Scedosporium* (16%), and zygomycetes (8%). Pneumocystosis, endemic fungal infections, and cryptococcosis were rarely encountered in the HSCT population. Consistent with previous reports,[4–7] mortality was high and 1-year survival was low for HSCT patients with IFI. Fusarium infections and IA were associated with the lowest 1-year survival (6% and 25%, respectively); however, survival among patients with zygomycosis (28%) and IC (34%) was not substantially better.

Among solid-organ transplant (SOT) recipients, *Candida* infections were significantly more common than *Aspergillus* infections. This distribution held true for all solid-organ groups except lung transplant recipients. In lung transplant recipients, *Aspergillus* was the most common fungal pathogen, and, when coupled with other molds, invasive mold infections were responsible for 70% of IFIs (PG Pappas, unpublished data, July 2009). This distribution has also been shown in other studies of SOT recipients.[8,9] Less common overall, but seen more frequently than in the HSCT population, were infections due to *Cryptococcus* and endemic fungi, causing 8% and 5% of IFIs, respectively. Zygomycetes were responsible for 2% of infections (PG Pappas, unpublished data, July 2009). The mortality associated with IFIs in the SOT population is high, but lower overall than in HSCT and oncology patients.

There are no recent, multicenter studies describing the incidence and clinical outcome of IFIs among the general oncology population, and it is difficult to obtain an accurate estimate of the frequency of fungal infections in this population from the published literature because most reports do not provide sufficient information regarding the patients' underlying disease. In general, compared with patients with solid tumors, patients with hematologic malignancies are at increased risk for fungal disease and response to IFI treatment is lower.[10] A 1992 international autopsy survey of patients with cancer identified fungal infections in 25% of patients with leukemia, 12% with lymphoma, and 5% with solid tumors. Overall, *Candida* was the most common fungal pathogen, responsible for 58% of fungal infections, whereas 30% of fungal infections were caused by *Aspergillus*.[11] A more recent single-center survey of autopsies performed on patients with hematologic malignancy confirmed the increased risk for IFI among patients with leukemia. Consistent with trends among transplant populations, the prevalence of IFI remained high and constant throughout the study period (1989–2003); although the rate of IC decreased, the prevalence of invasive mold infections increased.[12]

TYPES OF IFIS
Aspergillus

Aspergillus fumigatus is the most frequent species of *Aspergillus* causing clinical disease, perhaps due to specific virulence factors unique to the organism.[13] However, other species, most commonly *Aspergillus flavus*, *Aspergillus terreus*, and *Aspergillus niger*, are also implicated in invasive infections in humans. *A terreus* has been associated with amphotericin B resistance and a higher mortality[14] than other *Aspergillus* species, although the data to support this claim were primarily gleaned from patients treated with amphotericin B as initial therapy and before use of triazoles as first-line treatment of IA.[15]

In immunocompromised hosts, *Aspergillus* most commonly presents as invasive pulmonary aspergillosis, often with subsequent dissemination.[16–18] In lung transplant recipients, *Aspergillus* may also cause tracheobronchitis and bronchial anastomotic infection. However, pulmonary infections can present with fever, hemoptysis, cough, dyspnea, reduction in pulmonary function, pleuritic chest pain, respiratory failure, and altered mental status,[19] and the immunosuppressed patient may have few, or only subtle, clinical signs and symptoms present early in the course of infection. The distinction between colonization and infection with *Aspergillus* can be difficult. For example, *Aspergillus* can be recovered from the lower respiratory tract of many patients after lung transplant, but, based on a review of the literature, progression from colonization to infection in lung transplant recipients is rare.[20] In contrast, recovery of *Aspergillus* from lower respiratory tract specimens in patients with hematologic malignancy or undergoing HSCT has a high positive predictive value for invasive disease.[21]

Candida

The overall decrease in *Candida* infections and the shift from *Candida albicans* to non-*albicans* Candida as the most common infecting *Candida* species in the past 2 decades are notable. Data from Brazil collected between 1997 and 2003 document that 79% of episodes of candidemia in patients with hematological malignancies, and 52% in those with solid tumors, were caused by non-*albicans* Candida (P = .034).[22] Similarly, between 2001 and 2007 at MD Anderson Cancer Center, non-*albicans* Candida species were responsible for 75% of IC cases occurring in patients with hematologic malignancy or undergoing HSCT.[23] The routine use of azole prophylaxis in high-risk cancer populations has contributed to the decreased incidence of IC in these populations,[24,25] and likely accounts in part for the increasing frequency of infections caused by non-*albicans* Candida.[23,26,27] Although *C albicans* remains the most frequently isolated *Candida* species among SOT recipients, a shift toward more non-*albicans* Candida infections also seems to be occurring in this population.[28]

Infections due to *Candida* can manifest as candidemia, peritonitis, empyema, endopthalmitis, esophagitis, and urinary tract or anastomotic infections. In lung transplant recipients, *Candida* can also cause tracheobronchitis.[29] Presenting clinical signs may be fever, leukocytosis, and, less commonly, hypothermia.[30]

Hyaline Hyphomycetes

The other molds responsible for IFIs in immunosuppressed patients are a heterogeneous group of organisms. More than 30 non-*Aspergillus* hyalohyphomycetes have been implicated in human disease, including species of *Acremonium*, *Fusarium*, *Paecilomyces*, and *Scedosporium*.[31] These organisms are typically opportunistic, causing invasive disease following environmental exposures. Several of the non-*Aspergillus* hyalohyphomycetes are unique in their capability to sporulate in vivo, which permits recovery of the organisms from the bloodstream and dissemination to other organs, particularly skin.[32]

Recently, a shift toward more non-*Aspergillus* mold infections has been noticed in SOT recipients. In a prospective multicenter study, 53 invasive mold infections were reported from liver and heart transplant recipients. Pathogens included *Aspergillus* species in 70%, non-*Aspergillus* hyalohyphomycetes in 9%, phaeohyphomycetes in 9%, zygomycetes in 6%, and other or unidentified molds in 6% of patients. Dissemination was significantly more likely with infection due to a non-*Aspergillus* mold compared with *Aspergillus*.[17]

Zygomycetes

Zygomycetes cause devastating invasive disease in a variety of different hosts. In one review of 929 reported cases of zygomycosis, 36% were seen in patients with diabetes mellitus, 7% in SOT recipients, and 5% in bone marrow transplant recipients. Among the bone marrow transplant group, slightly more than half (52%) had pulmonary zygomycosis, with 16% having infection in the sinuses. Outcome from zygomycosis varied based on the underlying condition, site of infection, and use of antifungal therapy. For patients with underlying malignancy, overall mortality was 66%.[33] Other studies cite mortalities up to 80% among those with hematologic malignancies.[34] The incidence of zygomycosis seems to be increasing in oncology centers and in HSCT populations specifically, possibly related to the use of voriconazole prophylaxis.[35–39]

Pneumocystis jiroveci

The risk of *Pneumocystis jiroveci* infection (previously *Pneumocystis carinii*) in HSCT and SOT recipients can be as high as 5% to 15% without prophylaxis.[40,41] In the era of routine *P jiroveci* prophylaxis, transplant recipients who develop infection typically do so after stopping their prophylactic regimen.[42] Similarly, patients with cancer who develop *Pneumocystis* infection typically do so in the absence of prophylaxis.[43] *Pneumocystis* has a worldwide distribution and the organism that infects humans has been recognized as unique and distinct from that infecting animals[44]; humans seem to acquire *Pneumocystis* only from other humans, but active pneumonia does not seem to be required for transmission to occur. Serologic data indicate that most humans are infected with *Pneumocystis* within the first 2 to 4 years of life.[45] Immunocompromised patients develop disease as a consequence of reinfection with a new strain, or possibly from reactivation of latent infection. However, it is believed that most cases of *P jiroveci* pneumonia develop following acquisition of a new strain shortly before clinical symptoms manifest.[46]

Particular attention was given to *P jiroveci* infection in SOT recipients in the 1980s given to high rates of infection in heart-lung transplant recipients.[47,48] However, in the era of routine prophylaxis for at least 6 months following the transplant procedure in all solid-organ groups,[41] *Pneumocystis* infections in the SOT population are rare. In one retrospective review of 32,757 kidney recipients transplanted between 2000 and 2004, the cumulative incidence was 0.4%. Patients receiving sirolimus as part of their immunosuppressive regimen had an increased risk of developing *P jiroveci* pneumonia that was associated with increased risk of graft loss and death.[49] The underlying mechanism by which sirolimus predisposes to *P jiroveci* infection is as yet undefined; however, it may ultimately be linked with the ability of sirolimus to cause interstitial pneumonia, a known side effect of the drug.

Cryptococcus

Cryptococcus neoformans and *Cryptococcus gatti*[50] represent the main pathogenic species in the genus *Cryptococcus*.[51] Although cryptococcosis has been most commonly encountered in the HIV-infected population,[52] a multicenter study reporting 306 cases of cryptococcosis in patients who are not infected with HIV found 0.7% of total cases occurred in HSCT recipients, 18% in SOT recipients, 9% in patients with hematologic malignancies, and 9% in patients with other malignancies.[53] Other studies in the United States have found similarly low rates of cryptococcal infection in the HSCT population,[1,5,54] most likely because of the use of routine fluconazole prophylaxis following HSCT. The overall mortality for cryptococcosis in the non-HIV population was 30%, attributable mortality 12%, and hematologic malignancy as an underlying diagnosis was associated with decreased survival.[53]

Cryptococcus infection most commonly involves the lungs and central nervous system, but cutaneous infection and disseminated disease also occur. In one study, heart transplant patients were more likely than other solid-organ groups to develop cryptococcosis, but kidney transplant recipients were most likely to have disseminated disease. This study also showed that serum cryptococcal antigen was not always helpful in identifying isolated pulmonary *Cryptococcus* infection; 82% of patients with cryptococcal pneumonia had a negative serum cryptococcal antigen.[55]

Endemic Fungi

Endemic fungi, including *Histoplasma capsulatum*, *Blastomyces dermatitidis*, and *Coccidioides immitus*, are present in the soil in certain geographic regions, and inhalation of conidia leads to systemic infection.[56] Disease may manifest after primary exposure or through reactivation of a latent focus when there is a decrease in cell-mediated immunity. Pulmonary involvement is common but clinical symptoms are nonspecific and may be subacute in onset.

Although endemic mycoses are rarely encountered in cancer and transplant populations, immunosuppression (defined as hematologic malignancy or treatment with immunosuppressive medications) has been identified as a risk for developing histoplasmosis. Among immunosuppressed patients with histoplasmosis, 74% had fatal or disseminated infections, compared with 7% of patients who were not immunosuppressed.[57] Histoplasmosis is the most frequent endemic mycosis reported in the SOT population[58,59] and it has been transmitted to SOT recipients via the transplanted allograft.[60] Information regarding *B dermatitidis* in transplant populations remains limited to individual case reports and small case series.[61] The largest series included 11 cases in SOT recipients; infection occurred a median of 26 months after SOT and rejection did not precede any case.[62] *B dermatitidis* pneumonia was frequently complicated by acute respiratory distress syndrome and accordingly high mortality (67%).[63] Even in endemic regions, *C immitus* infection is rarely encountered in the HSCT population,[64] and most descriptions are in SOT recipients.[65] As with the other endemic mycoses in the immunosuppressed population, dissemination is common, mortality is high (up to 72%), and infection can be transmitted via donated organs.[66]

TIMING OF IFIS
IFI Timeline: HSCT

Time to development of IFI after transplantation varies according to type of fungal infection, type of transplant, and the use/duration of antifungal prophylaxis. As shown in **Fig. 1**, the timeline for IFIs following HSCT is typically broken into 3 periods, early onset ($\leq$40 days after HSCT), late onset (41–180 days after HSCT), and very late onset (>180 days after HSCT). In the TRANSNET cohort, 66% of *Candida* infections among autologous HSCT recipients occurred within the first 30 days (DP Kontoyiannis MD, unpublished data, July 2009). Similarly, in a single-center study of 655 allogeneic HSCT recipients transplanted between 1994 and 1997 and receiving routine fluconazole prophylaxis, the median time to development of candidemia was day 28 after transplant.[25] A recent multicenter report of IFIs occurring between 2004 and 2007 reported the median timing of IC after HSCT to be 77 days; IC tended to occur earlier after autologous HSCT (median 28 days) compared with allogeneic HSCT (median 108 days).[67] In general, early-onset IC following HSCT is influenced by the presence of neutropenia and mucosal injury (mucositis), whereas later onset is more often seen in allogeneic HSCT recipients owing to the development of graft-versus-host disease (GVHD) and the need for chronic central venous catheters.

Aspergillus and other mold infections tend to occur later after HSCT. In a single-center study of allogeneic HSCT recipients transplanted between 1993 and 1998, 30% of IA diagnoses (N = 187) were early, 53% late, and 17% very late onset following

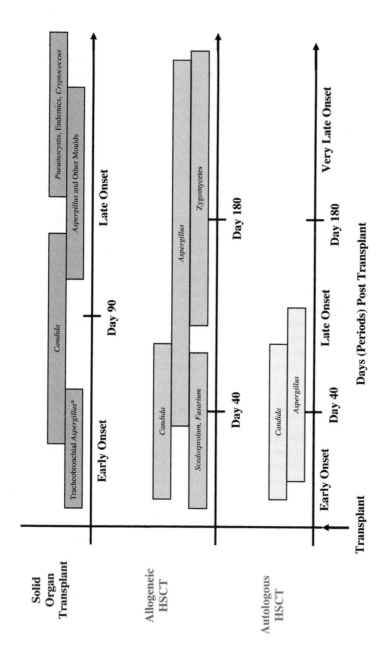

Fig. 1. Timing of IFIs based on transplant type.

*Unique to lung transplant

the procedure.[68] In the more recent TRANSNET cohort, 50% of IA cases among autologous HSCT recipients were early onset and 24% occurred more than 120 days after onset, whereas 22% of cases among allogeneic HSCT recipients were early onset and 47% occurred more than 120 days after transplant (DP Kontoyiannis, MD, unpublished data, July 2009). In general, IA occurs more frequently and is encountered later after allogeneic HSCT compared with autologous HSCT. Late IA has been associated with a higher mortality, possibly because of increased fungal burden accompanying a delay in diagnosis and the cumulative burden of immunosuppression in patients with chronic/refractory GVHD.[69]

The timing of non-*Aspergillus* mold infections such as zygomycetes, *Fusarium*, and *Scedosporium* seems to be organism specific. One large study of more than 5500 HSCT recipients showed that the majority (56%) of zygomycete infections occurred more than 90 days after transplant, and GVHD was associated with zygomycete infection. However, *Scedosporium* infections were more likely to occur within the first 30 days after transplant.[5] Similarly, nearly half (46%) of patients with fusariosis were neutropenic at the time of diagnosis, and the median time from transplant to diagnosis was 64 days.[6]

IFI Timeline: SOT

The timeline for infections following SOT has traditionally been divided into 3 phases: the first month, months 2 to 6, and more than 6 months after the transplant procedure.[70] Recent data regarding the epidemiology of IFIs following SOT suggest that the timing of fungal infections may no longer conform precisely with these risk windows.

Historically, infections due to *Candida* occurred early after SOT, typically during the transplant hospitalization.[9,71] However, TRANSNET data showed a somewhat later time to onset, with median time to diagnosis of IC of 103 days (PG Pappas MD, unpublished data, July 2009). In addition, a recent Australian study of candidemia in SOT recipients found that 54% of infections developed greater than 6 months after transplant, most of them in renal transplant recipients. Nearly all these patients were hospitalized at the time of diagnosis because of complications from various bacterial infections, and had been receiving broad-spectrum antibiotics.[72]

Most *Aspergillus* infections historically occurred within the first year following SOT.[20,73,74] Tracheobronchial or anastomotic *Aspergillus* infections typically occurred within the first 90 days after transplant, compared with invasive pulmonary aspergillosis that tended to occur later.[73,74] Most experts agree that the risk for IA is high enough immediately following lung transplant to warrant antifungal prophylaxis, and American Society of Transplantation guidelines recommend continuing prophylaxis following lung transplantation at least until bronchial anastomosis remodeling is complete.[75] A 2006 international survey of lung transplant centers revealed that 69% (30/43) used universal antifungal prophylaxis during the immediate posttransplant period as the anastomosis was healing, most commonly an aerosolized formulation of amphotericin B alone or in combination with itraconazole. The median durations of prophylaxis with aerosolized amphotericin B and itraconazole were 30 and 90 days, respectively.[76] In the current era of routine prophylaxis in high-risk organ transplant recipients, nearly one-half of *Aspergillus* infections in SOT recipients occur late (>90 days after SOT) and, as in the HSCT population, late-onset IA has been associated with a higher mortality compared with early-onset infection.[77]

Cryptococcus and the endemic mycoses tend to occur even later in the posttransplant period.[70] In one study of SOT recipients with cryptococcosis, the median time to diagnosis in lung, heart, and kidney transplant recipients was 210, 450, and 630 days, respectively.[55] In the TRANSNET cohort, median time to diagnosis of cryptococcosis was 575 days. Similarly, the median time to diagnosis of the endemic mycoses was 343 days (PG Pappas MD, unpublished data, July 2009), and *P jiroveci* infections are most often seen after routine prophylaxis is stopped, typically more than 180 days after transplant.[49,70,78]

RISK FACTORS DEVELOPING IFIS
Unique Risks for IFIs in HSCT Recipients

Many factors affect a patient's individual risk for fungal disease, including those associated with the host, the transplanted graft, and complications of the procedure. The influence of each factor fluctuates throughout the posttransplant course, creating a dynamic timeline. Host (eg, older age) and transplant variables (eg, human leukocyte antigen mismatch) tend to influence IFI risk early, whereas complications of the transplant procedure (eg, GVHD and cytomegalovirus [CMV] disease) tend to predominate later.[1,2,5,68] Certain biologic factors, such as malnutrition, iron overload, diabetes mellitus, and cytopenias, are influential throughout the posttransplant course.[79] Risk factors specific to early-onset IA have been identified as aplastic anemia, myelodysplastic syndrome, cord-blood transplantation, delayed neutrophil engraftment, and CMV disease. Risks for late-onset IA were multiple myeloma, neutropenia, GVHD, and CMV disease.[68] Iron overload has been shown to be a risk factor for severe bacterial infections in autologous HSCT recipients,[80] and also associated with IA and zygomycete infections.[81] Diabetes mellitus, voriconazole prophylaxis, and malnutrition have also been identified as risks for zygomycosis.[39]

Only a subset of patients who are at risk will actually develop IFI. This fact has led to a growing interest in host genetic differences that may contribute to the individual's risk of developing IFI. Recently, studies in HSCT populations have shown that polymorphisms in Toll-like receptor 4[82] and genetic variations within the plasminogen allele may influence susceptibility to IA after transplant.[83] More research is needed into host genetic influence on the risk of fungal disease following transplant.

Unique Risks for IFIs in Oncology Patients

In patients with acute leukemia, the risk for IC in published reports varies considerably. This is related to the status of leukemia (newly diagnosed, postremission, relapsed, or refractory to treatment), duration of neutropenia, and the types of antineoplastic agents used. Based on a study of patients from Brazil with cancer and with candidemia between 1997 and 2003, in comparison with patients with solid tumors, neutropenia and corticosteroid use were more frequent in the hematologic malignancy group. Only 22% of patients with solid tumors were neutropenic before candidemia. The presence of ileus and the use of anaerobicides were independent risk factors for candidemia in patients with solid cancers. Compared with candidemic patients without cancer, central venous catheters and gastrointestinal surgery were independently associated with candidemia in patients with solid tumor.[22]

Unique Risks for IFIs in SOT Recipients

Rejection and exogenous immunosuppressive agents, particularly high-dose steroids and antilymphocyte antibody treatment, lead to increased risk for IFIs in the SOT population.[84] However, within organ transplant groups, the risk for IFI is strongly influenced by medical and surgical factors including technical complexity. For example, prolonged operative time requiring multiple blood transfusions, reperfusion organ injury during transplantation, or multiple simultaneous organ transplants have all been associated with the development of fungal infections.[85] One study associated prolonged ischemia time with the development of IA in lung transplant recipients.[86] Liver transplant recipients have been shown to be at higher risk for IFIs if there is fulminant hepatic failure, a need to undergo retransplantation, or renal failure. Unique risks for renal transplant recipients include diabetes mellitus or need for prolonged hemodiaylsis before transplant.[87] Factors predisposing to IFI, primarily IC, in pancreas transplant recipients include older donor age, enteric (vs bladder) drainage, pancreas after kidney transplant (vs pancreas alone), the development of posttransplant pancreatitis, retransplantation, and preoperative peritoneal dialysis.[88]

Infection with certain viruses following SOT has also been associated with the development of IFIs. The most frequently implicated virus is CMV. In a prospective study of liver transplant recipients, 36% of patients with CMV disease developed IFIs within the first year after transplant, compared with 8% of those without CMV disease.[89] CMV prophylaxis seems to result in fewer IFIs, which further supports the association.

MANAGEMENT

Management of IFIs involves several components and is pathogen specific. Pharmacologic treatment requires consideration of first- and second-line therapies, potential drug interactions, and the value of combination therapies. The roles of immunomodulation, reversal of neutropenia, and surgery also need to be considered.

Aspergillus

Treatment of IA has evolved in the past decade, but few randomized controlled trials comparing various agents exist. The therapy of choice had historically been amphotericin B deoxycholate, its administration complicated by infusion reactions and renal dysfunction.[90] A randomized controlled trial documented superiority and decreased toxicity of voriconazole over amphotericin B deoxycholate. This landmark study also noted a 12-week survival advantage for patients treated with voriconazole.[91] As a result, voriconazole is now considered the drug of choice for IA.[92]

Complications of voriconazole therapy, as with other azoles, are mainly due to its drug interactions, which are particularly pertinent in transplant populations. Concomitant administration of cyclosporine, tacrolimus, or sirolimus with any azole requires preemptive dose adjustments of the immunosuppressants and subsequent close monitoring.[93] Voriconazole is metabolized through the cytochrome p450 system, and polymorphisms in the CYP2C19 gene can result in widely variable rates of drug metabolism.[94] In addition, response seems to be lower among patients with IA and low mean voriconazole plasma levels (<0.25 μg/mL). Because of these issues, voriconazole levels should be monitored during therapy.[95]

The appropriate choice for therapy in the setting of voriconazole intolerance or failure is a subject of debate. Current Infectious Diseases Society of America (IDSA) guidelines for treatment of IA include echinocandins (caspofungin and micafungin) as an option for salvage therapy, with lipid formulations of amphotericin B, itraconazole, and posaconazole.[92] Posaconazole, another triazole with activity against molds, is available in oral formulation only and shows moderate variability in absorption. In a salvage study for IA in patients previously treated with amphotericin products, favorable response was observed in 42%,[96] and among SOT recipients specifically, 58% had successful outcomes on treatment. As with voriconazole, drug interactions can frequently be seen with posaconazole, absorption is variable, and therapeutic drug level monitoring is encouraged. Treatment-related adverse events included nausea, vomiting, and increased liver function tests (the latter occurring in <3% of patients).[97] Visual disturbances and certain rashes experienced with voriconazole are not seen with posaconazole treatment. Thus, in some patients intolerant to voriconazole, posaconazole is an acceptable alternative. However, whether failure to respond to voriconazole should prompt the switch to a different antifungal class is a different issue. Research has shown that mutations in the Aspergillus cyp51A gene produces clinically significant resistance to the triazoles and different mutations confer unique patterns of azole activity.[98] For example, some mutations lead to high minimal inhibitory concentrations (MICs) for itraconazole and posaconazole, but not voriconazole and ravuconazole, whereas others result in high MICs for all 4 drugs.[99] Thus, in cases of voriconazole failure, susceptibility testing is recommended before switching to another triazole.

Echinocandins, which act by inhibiting the synthesis of β-D-glucan in the cell wall, are generally well tolerated and offer an appealing option for treatment if intolerance to, or failure of, voriconazole develops. Caspofungin was studied alone or in combination in 90 patients with IA refractory to, or intolerant of, other licensed therapy. Favorable response was achieved in 45% and only 2 patients discontinued the drug because of adverse events.[100] Micafungin, in contrast with caspofungin, does not have a formal indication as salvage treatment of IA, but it has been studied for this use. In an open-label, multicenter study of micafungin in the treatment of IA, an overall favorable response rate of 36% was reported.[101] The main drawback to echinocandin therapy is the narrow spectrum of activity and lack of an oral preparation.

There is a need for better outcomes in IA. Although it seems that combination antifungal therapy as primary therapy for IA may confer some benefit, this has not yet been rigorously tested in a controlled trial, and the decision regarding what combination to use is based primarily on in vitro data, retrospective cohort outcomes, and animal data.[102] Only 1, small, prospective randomized trial of combination anti-Aspergillus therapy has been published to date. This study included only 30 patients with hematologic malignancy and IA. Patients were randomized to caspofungin plus liposomal amphotericin B (3 mg/kg/d) versus monotherapy with high-dose liposomal amphotericin B (10 mg/kg/d). The combination therapy group had a 66% (10/15) favorable response, which was statistically superior to the 27% (4/15) clinical response in the monotherapy group. However, 12-week survival was not statistically different and there was significantly more nephrotoxicity in patients treated with the high-dose monotherapy. Thus, it is unclear whether the superiority of combination therapy was caused by the lower dose of liposomal amphotericin B or the addition of caspofungin.[103] Another study compared 40 SOT recipients with IA who received caspofungin plus voriconazole as primary therapy with a historical cohort of 47 SOTs treated with a lipid formulation of amphotericin B. Survival at 90 days, the primary end point, was not significantly different between the 2 groups.[104]

A phase III prospective, randomized, double-blind trial comparing voriconazole monotherapy with combination voriconazole plus anidulafungin as primary therapy for IA is currently enrolling and should help definitively establish the efficacy of azole-echinocandin combination therapy for this disease. Until such data are available, combination therapy should be reserved for patients in whom voriconazole monotherapy has failed or is contraindicated, and for patients who are high risk with unusual or resistant isolates.

Candida

Several randomized control trials comparing various antifungals have been performed and are summarized in **Table 1**. In 2009, the IDSA revised its guidelines on the treatment of Candida infections, reflecting new data on the use of echinocandins and the increasing prevalence of non-albicans Candida species. For non-neutropenic adults

Table 1
Major prospective randomized controlled trials of IC

Author, Year	Comparators	Number Enrolled[a]	Proportion Candidemic (%)	C albicans Infections (%)	End of Therapy Success (%)	Significance (P Value)	Comments
Rex 1994[122]	Fluconazole	113	100	70	72	0.17	Non-neutropenic population
	Amphotericin B	111	100	63	80		Less toxicity with fluconazole
Rex 2003[123]	Fluconazole plus placebo	107	100	68	56	0.043	Higher APACHE II scores in fluconazole arm
	Fluconazole plus amphotericin B	112	100	68	69		Mortality not improved with combination
							Higher nephrotoxicity with combination
Kullberg 2005[124]	Voriconazole	248	100	43	70	0.42	Nonblinded, non-neutropenic population
	Amphotericin B followed by fluconazole	122	100	51	74		More renal toxicity and SAEs with AmB
Mora-Duarte 2002[125]	Caspofungin	109	83	36	73	0.09	No difference in mortality
	Amphotericin B	115	79	54	62		More drug-related adverse events with AmB
Kuse 2007[126]	Micafungin	264	83	39	74	NS	12% of study population neutropenic
	LAMB	267	84	43	70		
Reboli 2007[127]	Anidulafungin	127	91	64	76	NS	3% of study population neutropenic
	Fluconazole	118	87	59	60		Microbiologic response higher with anidulafungin
Pappas 2007[128]	Caspofungin	188	86	44	72	NS	9% of study population neutropenic
	Micafungin 100 mg	191	85	48	76		
	Micafungin 150 mg	199	84	51	71		

Abbreviations: AmB, amphotericin B; LAMB, liposomal amphotericin B; NS, not significant; SAEs, serious adverse events.
[a] Modified intent to treat population.

with candidemia, fluconazole, or an echinocandin is recommended as initial therapy. For candidemia in neutropenic patients, initial therapy with a lipid formulation of amphotericin B or an echinocandin is recommended, unless the patient has had limited prior azole exposure, in which case initial therapy with fluconazole is appropriate. Once the infecting pathogen has been identified, treatment can be further tailored. For *Candida glabrata*, treatment with an echinocandin is recommended unless the isolate has been confirmed as susceptible to fluconazole or voriconazole, in which case transition to either drug is appropriate. For *Candida krusei*, which is intrinsically resistant to fluconazole, therapy with a lipid formulation of amphotericin B, voriconazole, or an echinocandin is recommended.[105]

Zygomycetes

Treatment of invasive zygomycosis has evolved to some extent; perhaps most importantly, lipid formulations of amphotericin B have replaced amphotericin B deoxycholate as the cornerstone of primary therapy.[106] Prompt initiation of amphotericin B–based therapy (ie, initiating treatment within 6 days of diagnosis) has been shown to significantly improve outcome.[107] Although it cannot be recommended as primary therapy for zygomycosis on the basis of available data, posaconazole has been increasingly studied as a therapeutic alternative. In one retrospective review of patients who had intolerance to, or progression of, infection on an amphotericin B–based regimen, 66% had a complete or partial response to posaconazole.[108] The zygomycetes include many pathogenic molds, and the MIC of posaconazole varies considerably between these organisms.[109]

Most recently, echinocandins have been shown in vitro to exhibit immunomodulatory activity and synergistic activity in combination with amphotericin B against the zygomycetes.[110,111] Clinical data supporting the addition of an echinocandin to an amphotericin B–based regimen are limited to a retrospective review of 34 diabetic patients with rhino-orbital-cerebral zygomycosis.[112] Treatment was successful for all evaluable patients (n = 6) who received amphotericin B–caspofungin combination therapy, compared with 41% (14/34) in patients treated with amphotericin B monotherapy ($P = .19$). Whether the addition of an echinocandin offers a significant advantage to the patient awaits further clinical study.

Other Molds

Although correlation between in vitro antifungal susceptibility testing of molds and clinical outcomes is limited, information regarding intrinsic patterns of resistance for the various non-*Asperigllus* hyalohyphomycetes has emerged.[31] Many of these molds are intrinsically resistant to available antifungal agents. Susceptibility to amphotericin B and triazoles is variable for *Fusarium*, and the echinocandins offer no activity against this pathogen. Currently, most experts consider voriconazole as first-line therapy for *Fusarium*.[93] Species of *Scedosporium* are considered intrinsically resistant to polyene antifungals and as with *Fusarium*, third generation triazoles are considered first-line therapy for *Scedosporium apiospermum*,[113] however, *Scedosporium prolificans* is intrinsically resistant to all antifungal agents. Data to support the use of combination antifungal therapy for the management of the hyalohyphomycoses are currently limited to those obtained in vitro and case reports.

P jiroveci

Trimethoprim-sulfamethoxazole (TMP/SMX) remains the treatment of choice for *P jiroveci* pneumonia. Oral administration is appropriate for those able to take medication by mouth, given good bioavailability of the TMP/SMX. One of the most problematic side effects of TMP/SMX in the transplant population is cytopenia; all cell lines can be affected and patients must be monitored for this side effect. Duration of therapy for *P jiroveci* pneumonia is generally accepted to be 14 to 21 days. Although data have shown that adding prednisone to the treatment regimen accelerates clinical improvement and improves survival in patients infected with HIV with moderate or severe *P jiroveci* infection, no randomized data are available in cancer or transplant patients to support this practice. However, assuming the patient was not already on corticosteroids at the time symptomatic infection developed, most clinicians presume efficacy based on data from the HIV literature and would consider adding corticosteroids in transplant and other patients who do not have HIV with severe disease. If allergic to, or intolerant of, TMP/SMX, atovaquone, dapsone, or pentamidine have been used as alternative agents.[114]

Cryptococcosis

Treatment recommendations for cryptococcal disease in the transplant population are based largely on data extrapolated from clinical trials in other hosts and expert opinion. Current IDSA guidelines recommend amphotericin B plus flucytosine for 2 weeks, followed by fluconazole orally at 400 to 800 mg for up to 10 weeks, followed by a decreased dose of fluconazole (200 mg) for 6 to 12 months[115] for central nervous system or other severe disease. There are some data to suggest that, in SOT recipients with isolated pulmonary cryptococcosis, prolonged treatment with oral fluconazole is sufficient and induction therapy with amphotericin B may not be necessary.[116]

Several management issues unique to the transplant population need to be considered. Owing to concomitant use of calcineurin inhibitors, lipid formulations of amphotericin B are preferred. In addition, flucytosine levels need to be monitored closely to avoid toxicity and side effects.[117] A gradual decrease in corticosteroids is another common management strategy; however, development of immune reconstitution syndrome (IRIS) in this setting has been seen and may be difficult to distinguish from manifestations of the cryptococcal infection itself.

Other Management Strategies

Reducing immunosuppression requires a delicate balance between improving outcome from infection and inducing rejection of the graft or an accelerated inflammatory reaction. As noted, rapid reduction of immunosuppressive therapy in conjunction with initiation of antifungal therapy in SOT recipients may lead to the development of IRIS, the clinical manifestations of which mimic worsening disease.[118] Reversal of neutropenia is another strategy that is often used in managing IFIs. The updated 2008 IDSA guidelines for treatment of IA include considering the use of a granulocyte-macrophage colony stimulating factor in those with prolonged neutropenia.[92] Granulocyte infusions may also be used as a bridge to recovery from neutropenia, but data to support this practice are scant. In one study of neutropenic patients with hematologic malignancies and IFI refractory to treatment with amphotericin B, 15 patients received granulocyte transfusions from related donors and 8 of the 15 had favorable outcomes.[119]

Surgery

The role of surgery in the treatment of IFIs can be paramount, but its usefulness depends on the type of IFI present. The IDSA recommends that surgery be considered in patients with IA who have a solitary lung lesion before chemotherapy or HSCT, those with hemoptysis from a lung lesion, disease that invades the chest wall, or situations in which the infection involves the pericardium or great vessels.[92] For zygomycosis in particular, treatment often requires surgical intervention in addition to pharmacologic therapy.[120] In one review of 86 cases of pulmonary zygomycosis reported in the literature, mortality was higher (55%) in those not receiving adjuvant surgery compared with those who did (27%).[121] For infections with highly resistant fungi, particularly for localized infection, surgical debridement and debulking should be considered.

SUMMARY

Recent shifts in the epidemiology of IFIs among transplant and oncology populations have led to new recommendations on treatment; however, they have also brought new controversies. New pharmacologic therapies are being studied, alone and in combination, and guidelines for management of several IFIs have been changed accordingly. More information is being discovered about unique genetic factors that put some transplant recipients at greater risk than others for fungal infection. The role of immunomodulation continues to be investigated; as always, the delicate balance of maintaining some immune integrity while assuring protection of the graft remains critical. Despite advances in the field, further studies are needed. For transplant and oncology patients, the diagnosis and management of IFIs remain challenging, and improving outcomes depends on continued progress in all of these arenas.

REFERENCES

1. Martino R, Subira M, Rovira M, et al. Invasive fungal infections after allogeneic peripheral blood stem cell transplantation: incidence and risk factors in 395 patients. Br J Haematol 2002;116(2):475–82.
2. Fukuda T, Boeckh M, Carter RA, et al. Risks and outcomes of invasive fungal infections in recipients of allogeneic hematopoietic stem cell transplants after nonmyeloablative conditioning. Blood 2003;102(3):827–33.
3. Singh N. Antifungal prophylaxis for solid organ transplant recipients: seeking clarity amidst controversy. Clin Infect Dis 2000;31(2):545–53.
4. Gudlaugsson O, Gillespie S, Lee K, et al. Attributable mortality of nosocomial candidemia, revisited. Clin Infect Dis 2003;37(9):1172–7.
5. Marr KA, Carter RA, Crippa F, et al. Epidemiology and outcome of mould infections in hematopoietic stem cell transplant recipients. Clin Infect Dis 2002;34(7): 909–17.
6. Nucci M, Marr KA, Queiroz-Telles F, et al. Fusarium infection in hematopoietic stem cell transplant recipients. Clin Infect Dis 2004;38(9):1237–42.
7. Husain S, Munoz P, Forrest G, et al. Infections due to *Scedosporium apiospermum* and *Scedosporium prolificans* in transplant recipients: clinical characteristics and impact of antifungal agent therapy on outcome. Clin Infect Dis 2005; 40(1):89–99.
8. Pugliese F, Ruberto F, Cappannoli A, et al. Incidence of fungal infections in a solid organ recipients dedicated intensive care unit. Transplant Proc 2007; 39(6):2005–7.
9. Grossi P, Farina C, Fiocchi R, et al. Prevalence and outcome of invasive fungal infections in 1,963 thoracic organ transplant recipients: a multicenter retrospective study. Italian Study Group of Fungal Infections in Thoracic Organ Transplant Recipients. Transplantation 2000;70(1):112–6.
10. DiNubile MJ, Hille D, Sable CA, et al. Invasive candidiasis in cancer patients: observations from a randomized clinical trial. J Infect 2005;50(5):443–9.

11. Bodey G, Bueltmann B, Duguid W, et al. Fungal infections in cancer patients: an international autopsy survey. Eur J Clin Microbiol Infect Dis 1992;11(2):99–109.

12. Chamilos G, Luna M, Lewis RE, et al. Invasive fungal infections in patients with hematologic malignancies in a tertiary care cancer center: an autopsy study over a 15-year period (1989–2003). Haematologica 2006;91(7):986–9.

13. Latge JP. *Aspergillus fumigatus* and aspergillosis. Clin Microbiol Rev 1999; 12(2):323–6.

14. Lass-Florl C, Kofler G, Kropshofer G, et al. In vitro testing of susceptibility to amphotericin B is a reliable predictor of clinical outcome in invasive aspergillosis. J Antimicrob Chemother 1998;42:497–502.

15. Steinbach WJ, Perfect JR, Schell WA, et al. In vitro analyses, animal models, and 60 clinical cases of invasive *Aspergillus terreus* infection. Antimicrobial Agents Chemother 2004;48(9):3217–25.

16. Munoz P, Rodriguez C, Bouza E, et al. Risk factors of invasive aspergillosis after heart transplantation: protective role of oral itraconazole prophylaxis. Am J Transplant 2004;4(4):636–43.

17. Husain S, Alexander BD, Munoz P, et al. Opportunistic mycelial fungal infections in organ transplant recipients: emerging importance of non-*Aspergillus* mycelial fungi. Clin Infect Dis 2003;37(2):221–9.

18. Minari A, Husni R, Avery RK, et al. The incidence of invasive aspergillosis among solid organ transplant recipients and implications for prophylaxis in lung transplants. Transpl Infect Dis 2002;4(4):195–200.

19. Marr KA, Patterson T, Denning D. Aspergillosis. Pathogenesis, clinical manifestations, and therapy. Infect Dis Clin North Am 2002;16(4):878–83.

20. Mehrad B, Paciocco G, Martinez FJ, et al. Spectrum of *Aspergillus* infection in lung transplant recipients: case series and review of the literature. Chest 2001;119(1):169–75.

21. Perfect JR, Cox GM, Lee JY, et al. The impact of culture isolation of *Aspergillus* species: a hospital-based survey of aspergillosis. Clin Infect Dis 2001;33(11): 1824–33.

22. Pasqualotto AC, Rosa DD, Medeiros LR, et al. Candidaemia and cancer: patients are not all the same. BMC Infect Dis 2006;6:50.

23. Sipsas NV, Lewis RE, Tarrand J, et al. Candidemia in patients with hematologic malignancies in the era of new antifungal agents (2001–2007): stable incidence but changing epidemiology of a still frequently lethal infection. Cancer 2009.

24. Goodman JL, Winston DJ, Greenfield RA, et al. A controlled trial of fluconazole to prevent fungal infections in patients undergoing bone marrow transplantation. N Engl J Med 1992;326(13):845–51.

25. Marr KA, Seidel K, White TC, et al. Candidemia in allogeneic blood and marrow transplant recipients: evolution of risk factors after the adoption of prophylactic fluconazole. J Infect Dis 2000;181(1):309–16.

26. Van Burik JH, Leisenring W, Myerson D, et al. The effect of prophylactic fluconazole on the clinical spectrum of fungal diseases in bone marrow transplant recipients with special attention to hepatic candidiasis. An autopsy study of 355 patients. Medicine 1998;77:246–54.

27. Wingard JR. Importance of *Candida* species other than *C. albicans* as pathogens in oncology patients. Clin Infect Dis 1995;20(1):115–25.

28. Horn DL, Neofytos D, Anaissie EJ, et al. Epidemiology and outcomes of candidemia in 2019 patients: data from the prospective antifungal therapy alliance registry. Clin Infect Dis 2009;48(12):1695–703.

29. Palmer SM, Perfect JR, Howell DN, et al. Candidal anastomotic infection in lung transplant recipients: successful treatment with a combination of systemic and inhaled antifungal agents. J Heart Lung Transplant 1998;17(10):1029–33.

30. Fraser VJ, Jones M, Dunkel J, et al. Candidemia in a tertiary care hospital: epidemiology, risk factors, and predictors of mortality. Clin Infect Dis 1992; 15(3):414–21.

31. Alexander BD, Schell WA. Hyalohyphomycosis. In: Kauffman CA, Mandell GL, editors. Atlas of fungal infections. 2nd edition. Philadelphia: Current Medicine Group, Inc; 2006. p. 253–66.

32. Schell WA. New aspects of emerging fungal pathogens. A multifaceted challenge. Clin Lab Med 1995;15(2):365–87.

33. Roden MM, Zaoutis TE, Buchanan WL, et al. Epidemiology and outcome of zygomycosis: a review of 929 reported cases. Clin Infect Dis 2005;41(5):634–53.

34. Kontoyiannis DP, Wessel VC, Bodey GP, et al. Zygomycosis in the 1990s in a tertiary-care cancer center. Clin Infect Dis 2000;30(6):851–6.

35. Trifilio SM, Bennett CL, Yarnold PR, et al. Breakthrough zygomycosis after voriconazole administration among patients with hematologic malignancies who receive hematopoietic stem-cell transplants or intensive chemotherapy. Bone Marrow Transplant 2007;39(7):425–9.

36. Marty FM, Cosimi LA, Baden LR. Breakthrough zygomycosis after voriconazole treatment in recipients of hematopoietic stem-cell transplants. N Engl J Med 2004;350(9):950–2.

37. Siwek GT, Dodgson KJ, de Magalhaes-Silverman M, et al. Invasive zygomycosis in hematopoietic stem cell transplant recipients receiving voriconazole prophylaxis. Clin Infect Dis 2004;39(4):584–7.

38. Imhof A, Balajee SA, Fredricks DN, et al. Breakthrough fungal infections in stem cell transplant recipients receiving voriconazole. Clin Infect Dis 2004;39(5): 743–6.

39. Kontoyiannis DP, Lionakis MS, Lewis RE, et al. Zygomycosis in a tertiary-care cancer center in the era of *Aspergillus*-active antifungal therapy: a case-control observational study of 27 recent cases. J Infect Dis 2005;191(8): 1350–60.

40. Sepkowitz KA. Opportunistic infections in patients with and patients without Acquired Immunodeficiency Syndrome. Clin Infect Dis 2002;34(8):1098–107.

41. *Pneumocystis jiroveci* (formerly *Pneumocystis carinii*). Am J Transplant 2004; 4(Suppl 10):135–41.

42. De Castro N, Neuville S, Sarfati C, et al. Occurrence of *Pneumocystis jiroveci* pneumonia after allogeneic stem cell transplantation: a 6-year retrospective study. Bone Marrow Transplant 2005;36(10):879–83.

43. Torres HA, Chemaly RF, Storey R, et al. Influence of type of cancer and hematopoietic stem cell transplantation on clinical presentation of *Pneumocystis jiroveci* pneumonia in cancer patients. Eur J Clin Microbiol Infect Dis 2006;25(6): 382–8.

44. Kovacs JA, Halpern JL, Swan JC, et al. Identification of antigens and antibodies specific for *Pneumocystis carinii*. J Immunol 1988;140(6):2023–31.

45. Meuwissen JH, Tauber I, Leeuwenberg AD, et al. Parasitologic and serologic observations of infection with *Pneumocystis* in humans. J Infect Dis 1977; 136(1):43–9.

46. Stringer JR. *Pneumocystis*. Int J Med Microbiol 2002;292(5–6):391–404.

47. Dummer JS, Montero CG, Griffith BP, et al. Infections in heart-lung transplant recipients. Transplantation 1986;41(6):725–9.

48. Gryzan S, Paradis IL, Zeevi A, et al. Unexpectedly high incidence of *Pneumocystis carinii* infection after lung-heart transplantation. Implications for lung defense and allograft survival. Am Rev Respir Dis 1988;137(6):1268–74.

49. Neff RT, Jindal RM, Yoo DY, et al. Analysis of USRDS: incidence and risk factors for *Pneumocystis jiroveci* pneumonia. Transplantation 2009;88(1):135–41.

50. MacDougall L, Kidd SE, Galanis E, et al. Spread of *Cryptococcus gattii* in British Columbia, Canada, and detection in the Pacific Northwest, USA. Emerg Infect Dis 2007;13(1):42–50.

51. Chayakulkeeree M, Perfect JR. Cryptococcosis. Infect Dis Clin North Am 2006; 20(3):507–44, v-vi.

52. Mirza SA, Phelan M, Rimland D, et al. The changing epidemiology of cryptococcosis: an update from population-based active surveillance in 2 large metropolitan areas, 1992–2000. Clin Infect Dis 2003;36(6):789–94.

53. Pappas PG, Perfect JR, Cloud GA, et al. Cryptococcosis in human immunodeficiency virus-negative patients in the era of effective azole therapy. Clin Infect Dis 2001;33(5):690–9.

54. Baddley JW, Stroud TP, Salzman D, et al. Invasive mold infections in allogeneic bone marrow transplant recipients. Clin Infect Dis 2001;32(9):1319–24.

55. Vilchez R, Shapiro R, McCurry K, et al. Longitudinal study of cryptococcosis in adult solid-organ transplant recipients. Transpl Int 2003;16(5):336–40.

56. Kauffman CA. Endemic mycoses: blastomycosis, histoplasmosis, and sporotrichosis. Infect Dis Clin North Am 2006;20(3):645–62, vii.

57. Wheat LJ, Slama TG, Norton JA, et al. Risk factors for disseminated or fatal histoplasmosis. Analysis of a large urban outbreak. Ann Intern Med 1982; 96(2):159–63.

58. Peddi VR, Hariharan S, First MR. Disseminated histoplasmosis in renal allograft recipients. Clin Transplant 1996;10(2):160–5.

59. Freifeld AG, Iwen PC, Lesiak BL, et al. Histoplasmosis in solid organ transplant recipients at a large Midwestern university transplant center. Transpl Infect Dis 2005;7(3-4):109–15.

60. Limaye AP, Connolly PA, Sagar M, et al. Transmission of *Histoplasma capsulatum* by organ transplantation. N Engl J Med 2000;343(16):1163–6.

61. Serody JS, Mill MR, Detterbeck FC, et al. Blastomycosis in transplant recipients: report of a case and review. Clin Infect Dis 1993;16(1):54–8.

62. Bradsher RW, Chapman SW, Pappas PG. Blastomycosis. Infect Dis Clin North Am 2003;17(1):21–40, vii.

63. Gauthier GM, Safdar N, Klein BS, et al. Blastomycosis in solid organ transplant recipients. Transpl Infect Dis 2007;9(4):310–7.

64. Glenn TJ, Blair JE, Adams RH. Coccidioidomycosis in hematopoietic stem cell transplant recipients. Med Mycol 2005;43(8):705–10.

65. Blair JE, Logan JL. Coccidioidomycosis in solid organ transplantation. Clin Infect Dis 2001;33(9):1536–44.

66. Wright PW, Pappagianis D, Wilson M, et al. Donor-related coccidioidomycosis in organ transplant recipients. Clin Infect Dis 2003;37(9):1265–9.

67. Neofytos D, Horn D, Anaissie E, et al. Epidemiology and outcome of invasive fungal infection in adult hematopoietic stem cell transplant recipients: analysis of Multicenter Prospective Antifungal Therapy (PATH) Alliance registry. Clin Infect Dis 2009;48(3):265–73.

68. Marr KA, Carter RA, Boeckh M, et al. Invasive aspergillosis in allogeneic stem cell transplant recipients: changes in epidemiology and risk factors. Blood 2002;100(13):4358–66.

69. Upton A, Kirby KA, Carpenter P, et al. Invasive aspergillosis following hemato-poietic cell transplantation: outcomes and prognostic factors associated with mortality. Clin Infect Dis 2007;44(4):531–40.

70. Fishman JA, Rubin RH. Infection in organ-transplant recipients. N Engl J Med 1998;338(24):1741–51.

71. Patel R. Infections in recipients of kidney transplants. Infect Dis Clin North Am 2001;15(3):901–52, xi.

72. van Hal SJ, Marriott DJ, Chen SC, et al. Candidemia following solid organ trans-plantation in the era of antifungal prophylaxis: the Australian experience. Transpl Infect Dis 2009;11(2):122–7.

73. Singh N, Husain S. *Aspergillus* infections after lung transplantation: clinical differences in type of transplant and implications for management. J Heart Lung Transplant 2003;22(3):258–66.

74. Sole A, Morant P, Salavert M, et al. *Aspergillus* infections in lung transplant recipients: risk factors and outcome. Clin Microbiol Infect 2005;11(5):359–65.

75. Fungal infections. Am J Transplant 2004;4(Suppl 10):110–34.

76. Husain S, Zaldonis D, Kusne S, et al. Variation in antifungal prophylaxis strate-gies in lung transplantation. Transpl Infect Dis 2006;8(4):213–8.

77. Singh N, Limaye AP, Forrest G, et al. Late-onset invasive aspergillosis in organ transplant recipients in the current era. Med Mycol 2006;44(5):445–9.

78. Zaas AK, Alexander BD. Prevention of fungal infections in lung transplant patients. Current Fungal Infection Reports 2008;2:103–11.

79. Garcia-Vidal C, Upton A, Kirby KA, et al. Epidemiology of invasive mold infec-tions in allogeneic stem cell transplant recipients: biological risk factors for infection according to time after transplantation. Clin Infect Dis 2008;47(8):1041–50.

80. Miceli MH, Dong L, Grazziutti ML, et al. Iron overload is a major risk factor for severe infection after autologous stem cell transplantation: a study of 367 myeloma patients. Bone Marrow Transplant 2006;37(9):857–64.

81. Maertens J, Demuynck H, Verbeken EK, et al. Mucormycosis in allogeneic bone marrow transplant recipients: report of five cases and review of the role of iron overload in the pathogenesis. Bone Marrow Transplant 1999;24(3):307–12.

82. Bochud PY, Chien JW, Marr KA, et al. Toll-like receptor 4 polymorphisms and aspergillosis in stem-cell transplantation. N Engl J Med 2008;359(17):1766–77.

83. Zaas AK. Plasminogen alleles influence susceptibility to invasive aspergillosis. PLoS Genet 2008;4(6):e1000101.

84. Issa NC, Fishman JA. Infectious complications of antilymphocyte therapies in solid organ transplantation. Clin Infect Dis 2009;48(6):772–86.

85. Gabardi S, Kubiak DW, Chandraker AK, et al. Invasive fungal infections and antifungal therapies in solid organ transplant recipients. Transpl Int 2007;20(12):993–1015.

86. Iversen M, Burton CM, Vand S, et al. *Aspergillus* infection in lung transplant patients: incidence and prognosis. Eur J Clin Microbiol Infect Dis 2007;26(12):879–86.

87. Singh N. Fungal infections in the recipients of solid organ transplantation. Infect Dis Clin North Am 2003;17(1):113–34, viii.

88. Benedetti E, Gruessner AC, Troppmann C, et al. Intra-abdominal fungal infec-tions after pancreatic transplantation: incidence, treatment, and outcome. J Am Coll Surg 1996;183(4):307–16.

89. George MJ, Snydman DR, Werner BG, et al. The independent role of cytomeg-alovirus as a risk factor for invasive fungal disease in orthotopic liver transplant

recipients. Boston Center for Liver Transplantation CMVIG-Study Group. Cyto-gam, MedImmune, Inc. Gaithersburg, Maryland. Am J Med 1997;103(2): 106–13.

90. Bowden R, Chandrasekar P, White MH, et al. A double-blind, randomized, controlled trial of amphotericin B colloidal dispersion versus amphotericin B for treatment of invasive aspergillosis in immunocompromised patients. Clin Infect Dis 2002;35(4):359–66.

91. Herbrecht R, Denning DW, Patterson TF, et al. Voriconazole versus amphotericin B for primary therapy of invasive aspergillosis. N Engl J Med 2002;347(6):408–15.

92. Walsh TJ, Anaissie EJ, Denning DW, et al. Treatment of aspergillosis: clinical practice guidelines of the Infectious Diseases Society of America. Clin Infect Dis 2008;46(3):327–60.

93. VFend. Package insert. New York: Pfizer Inc; 2008.

94. Weiss J, Ten Hoevel MM, Burhenne J, et al. CYP2C19 genotype is a major factor contributing to the highly variable pharmacokinetics of voriconazole. J Clin Pharmacol 2009;49(2):196–204.

95. Denning DW, Ribaud P, Milpied N, et al. Efficacy and safety of voriconazole in the treatment of acute invasive aspergillosis. Clin Infect Dis 2002;34(5):563–71.

96. Walsh TJ, Raad I, Patterson TF, et al. Treatment of invasive aspergillosis with posaconazole in patients who are refractory to or intolerant of conventional therapy: an externally controlled trial. Clin Infect Dis 2007;44(1):2–12.

97. Alexander BD, Perfect JR, Daly JS, et al. Posaconazole as salvage therapy in patients with invasive fungal infections after solid organ transplant. Transplantation 2008;86(6):791–6.

98. Pfaller MA, Messer SA, Boyken L, et al. In vitro survey of triazole cross-resistance among more than 700 clinical isolates of *Aspergillus* species. J Clin Microbiol 2008;46(8):2568–72.

99. Rodriguez-Tudela JL, Alcazar-Fuoli L, Mellado E, et al. Epidemiological cutoffs and cross-resistance to azole drugs in *Aspergillus fumigatus*. Antimicrobial Agents Chemother 2008;52(7):2468–72.

100. Maertens J, Glasmacher A, Herbrecht R, et al. Multicenter, noncomparative study of caspofungin in combination with other antifungals as salvage therapy in adults with invasive aspergillosis. Cancer 2006;107(12):2888–97.

101. Denning DW, Marr KA, Lau WM, et al. Micafungin (FK463), alone or in combination with other systemic antifungal agents, for the treatment of acute invasive aspergillosis. J Infect 2006;53(5):337–49.

102. Steinbach WJ, Stevens DA, Denning DW. Combination and sequential antifungal therapy for invasive aspergillosis: review of published in vitro and in vivo interactions and 6281 clinical cases from 1966 to 2001. Clin Infect Dis 2003;37(Suppl 3):S188–224.

103. Caillot D, Thiebaut A, Herbrecht R, et al. Liposomal amphotericin B in combination with caspofungin for invasive aspergillosis in patients with hematologic malignancies: a randomized pilot study (Combistrat trial). Cancer 2007; 110(12):2740–6.

104. Singh N, Limaye AP, Forrest G, et al. Combination of voriconazole and caspofungin as primary therapy for invasive aspergillosis in solid organ transplant recipients: a prospective, multicenter, observational study. Transplantation 2006;81(3):320–6.

105. Pappas PG, Kauffman CA, Andes D, et al. Clinical practice guidelines for the management of candidiasis: 2009 update by the Infectious Diseases Society of America. Clin Infect Dis 2009;48(5):503–35.

106. Spellberg B, Walsh TJ, Kontoyiannis DP, et al. Recent advances in the management of mucormycosis: from bench to bedside. Clin Infect Dis 2009;48(12): 1743–51.

107. Chamilos G, Lewis RE, Kontoyiannis DP. Delaying amphotericin B-based frontline therapy significantly increases mortality among patients with hematologic malignancy who have zygomycosis. Clin Infect Dis 2008;47(4):503–9.

108. van Burik JA, Hare RS, Solomon HF, et al. Posaconazole is effective as salvage therapy in zygomycosis: a retrospective summary of 91 cases. Clin Infect Dis 2006;42(7):e61–5.

109. Almyroudis NG, Sutton DA, Fothergill AW, et al. In vitro susceptibilities of 217 clinical isolates of zygomycetes to conventional and new antifungal agents. Antimicrobial Agents Chemother 2007;51(7):2587–90.

110. Lamaris GA, Lewis RE, Chamilos G, et al. Caspofungin-mediated beta-glucan unmasking and enhancement of human polymorphonuclear neutrophil activity against *Aspergillus* and non-*Aspergillus* hyphae. J Infect Dis 2008;198(2): 186–92.

111. Perkhofer S, Locher M, Cuenca-Estrella M, et al. Posaconazole enhances the activity of amphotericin B against hyphae of zygomycetes in vitro. Antimicrobial Agents Chemother 2008;52(7):2636–8.

112. Reed C, Bryant R, Ibrahim AS, et al. Combination polyene-caspofungin treatment of rhino-orbital-cerebral mucormycosis. Clin Infect Dis 2008;47(3):364–71.

113. Perfect JR, Marr KA, Walsh TJ, et al. Voriconazole treatment for less-common, emerging, or refractory fungal infections. Clin Infect Dis 2003;36(9):1122–31.

114. Kovacs JA, Masur H. Evolving health effects of Pneumocystis: one hundred years of progress in diagnosis and treatment. JAMA 2009;301(24):2578–85.

115. Saag MS, Graybill RJ, Larsen RA, et al. Practice guidelines for the management of cryptococcal disease. Infectious Diseases Society of America. Clin Infect Dis 2000;30(4):710–8.

116. Singh N, Alexander BD, Lortholary O, et al. *Cryptococcus neoformans* in organ transplant recipients: impact of calcineurin-inhibitor agents on mortality. J Infect Dis 2007;195(5):756–64.

117. Dromer F, Mathoulin-Pelissier S, Launay O, et al. Determinants of disease presentation and outcome during cryptococcosis: the CryptoA/D study. PLoS Med 2007;4(2):e21.

118. Singh N, Lortholary O, Alexander BD, et al. An immune reconstitution syndrome-like illness associated with *Cryptococcus neoformans* infection in organ transplant recipients. Clin Infect Dis 2005;40(12):1756–61.

119. Dignani MC, Anaissie EJ, Hester JP, et al. Treatment of neutropenia-related fungal infections with granulocyte colony-stimulating factor-elicited white blood cell transfusions: a pilot study. Leukemia 1997;11(10):1621–30.

120. Ribes JA, Vanover-Sams CL, Baker DJ. Zygomycetes in human disease. Clin Microbiol Rev 2000;13(2):236–301.

121. Lee FY, Mossad SB, Adal KA. Pulmonary mucormycosis: the last 30 years. Arch Intern Med 1999;159(12):1301–9.

122. Rex JH, Bennett JE, Sugar AM, et al. A randomized trial comparing fluconazole with amphotericin B for the treatment of candidemia in patients without neutropenia. Candidemia Study Group and the National Institute. N Engl J Med 1994; 331(20):1325–30.

123. Rex JH, Pappas PG, Karchmer AW, et al. A randomized and blinded multicenter trial of high-dose fluconazole plus placebo versus fluconazole plus

amphotericin B as therapy for candidemia and its consequences in nonneutropenic subjects. Clin Infect Dis 2003;36(10):1221–8.

124. Kullberg BJ, Sobel JD, Ruhnke M, et al. Voriconazole versus a regimen of amphotericin B followed by fluconazole for candidaemia in non-neutropenic patients: a randomised non-inferiority trial. Lancet 2005;366(9495):1435–42.

125. Mora-Duarte J, Betts R, Rotstein C, et al. Comparison of caspofungin and amphotericin B for invasive candidiasis. N Engl J Med 2002;347(25):2020–9.

126. Kuse ER, Chetchotisakd P, da Cunha CA, et al. Micafungin versus liposomal amphotericin B for candidaemia and invasive candidosis: a phase III randomised double-blind trial. Lancet 2007;369(9572):1519–27.

127. Reboli AC, Rotstein C, Pappas PG, et al. Anidulafungin versus fluconazole for invasive candidiasis. N Engl J Med 2007;356(24):2472–82.

128. Pappas PG, Rotstein CM, Betts RF, et al. Micafungin versus caspofungin for treatment of candidemia and other forms of invasive candidiasis. Clin Infect Dis 2007;45(7):883–93.

Immunotherapy and Vaccination After Transplant: The Present, the Future

Vincent C. Emery, PhD[a],*, Hermann Einsele, PhD[b],
Sowsan Atabani, PhD[a,c], Tanzina Haque, PhD[c]

KEYWORDS

- Cytomegalovirus • Papillomavirus • Epstein-Barr virus
- Varicella-zoster virus

Despite the progress in immunosuppressive drugs to manage and minimize organ rejection after transplantation, infectious complications remain a major cause of morbidity.[1] Infections such as herpes simplex virus 1 (HSV-1) and varicella-zoster virus (VZV) have been successfully controlled through the deployment of prophylactic acyclovir or its prodrug valaciclovir,[2,3] whereas prophylactic and preemptive therapy with valganciclovir has been instrumental in managing human cytomegalovirus (HCMV) infections.[4,5] However, the management of Epstein-Barr virus (EBV), human herpes virus-6 (HHV-6), adenovirus, hepatitis C virus (HCV), hepatitis B virus (HBV), papillomavirus, and BK virus infections remains challenging. In addition, the side effect profile of ganciclovir and the possibility that drug resistance may develop with long-term prophylactic use in high-risk patients, such as those needing lung transplants, have stimulated interest in other management strategies.[6] This article focuses on advances in the area of vaccinology for some of these infections and in the use of adoptive immunotherapy. At present, many of these approaches in transplant recipients have focused on infections such as HCMV, but the opportunity to using these examples as proof of concept for other infections is discussed.

A version of this article was previously published in the *Infectious Disease Clinics of North America*, 24:2.
[a] Department of Infection (Royal Free Campus), University College London, Rowland Hill Street, Hampstead, London, NW3 2QG, UK
[b] Department of Medicine, University of Wuerzburg, Klinikstrasse 6 97070, Wuerzburg, Germany
[c] Department of Virology, Royal Free Hampstead NHS Trust, London Street, Hampstead, London, NW3 2QG, UK
* Corresponding author.
E-mail address: v.emery@ucl.ac.uk

VACCINATION
HCMV Vaccines

The earliest vaccine deployed for HCMV infections was the low-passage, live, attenuated Towne strain of HCMV by Plotkin and colleagues.[7,8] The results of a trial in kidney transplant recipients showed that immunization was unable to prevent infection but was associated with a reduction in the severity of HCMV disease.[9] Despite these encouraging findings, progress on an HCMV vaccine has been slow in the intervening years, with several vaccine preparations being formulated but, until recently, few showing sufficient protection to warrant further study.[10–13] These vaccine preparations are summarized in **Table 1**. A fundamental question relating to the use of vaccination to control and potentially eradicate HCMV infection is the level of vaccine coverage required to induce herd immunity in the general population, and of the vaccine efficacy required to control replication and disease after transplantation. A key study by Griffiths and colleagues[14] showed that, in high resource countries such as the United Kingdom and United States where HCMV seroprevalence rates are approximately 60%, the basic reproductive number (Ro; the number of new infections arising from 1 infected individual) for HCMV in women of child-bearing age was approximately 2.4. Thus, a vaccine coverage of around 62% would be sufficient to lead to herd immunity and eradication of HCMV without a significant effect on the incidence of congenital HCMV infection/disease. In the transplant setting, vaccination could be deployed in high-risk patients who are seronegative or as a prophylactic vaccine in patients who are already seropositive for HCMV. One study provided an estimate of the basic reproductive number for HCMV in these 2 clinical settings for liver transplant recipients.[15] These data indicate that in the D+R− setting, the Ro for HCMV is approximately 15, meaning that a vaccine would need to have an efficacy against replication of approximately 93% if it was to fully control replication. In contrast, the Ro for HCMV in the D+R+ group was reduced to 2.4, indicating that an HCMV vaccine deployed as an immunotherapeutic in these patients would only need to achieve an efficacy of about 60% to successfully control HCMV replication. The ability to affect the probability of HCMV disease is intimately linked to the relationship between viral load and disease. In all cases to date, viral load and probability of HCMV disease follow a sigmoidal pattern whereby the risk of HCMV disease increases substantially at certain viral-load thresholds.[16] In the context of vaccination, a vaccine that did not eradicate infection/replication but which induced a sufficient level of immunity to partially control HCMV replication could still have a profound effect on

Table 1		
HCMV vaccines currently undergoing human trials		
Vaccine	**Description**	**Status**
Towne	Live attenuated	Being used in prime boost with DNA vaccines
gB	Recombinant, soluble	Phase II studies complete in healthy; undergoing phase I in solid-organ transplant recipients
Canarypox pp65	Live single-cycle expression	Phase I
pp65, gB	DNA plasmid	Phase I
AlphaVax	Alphavirus expressing gB and pp65-IE1 fusion protein Single-cycle expression	Phase I

the incidence and severity of HCMV disease. This concept is summarized in **Fig. 1** and is consistent with the findings of the Towne vaccine study described earlier.

At present, the most encouraging results for an HCMV vaccine have come from the recombinant glycoprotein B (gB) vaccine. gB is a major site for neutralizing antibodies and can adsorb up to 80% of the serum-neutralizing antibodies in healthy seropositive individuals.[17] In addition, purified and recombinant gB has been shown to elicit high-level humoral immunity in animal models and protect against fetal loss in a guinea pig model.[18,19] Recombinant gB consisting of the extracellular domain and the intracellular domain, but with a truncated transmembraneous domain, has been expressed in mammalian cell culture and subjected to phase I and II clinical trials.[20–22] The vaccine is highly immunogenic when administered with the adjuvant MF59 (3 doses at months 0, 1, and 6) yielding neutralizing titers in seronegative volunteers that were in excess of those found with natural immunity. In addition, the vaccine boosted neutralizing titers when given to seropositive individuals. The results of a randomized double-blind, placebo-controlled, phase II study in 464 seronegative women within 1 year of them giving birth have recently been reported.[23] The vaccine efficacy was 50%, reducing the number of seroconversions from 31 in the placebo group to 18 in the vaccine group. These results are encouraging and have rekindled interest in the HCMV vaccine area by small and large pharma.

Do these results have any effect on the vaccination of transplant patients against HCMV? One of the challenges in the transplant setting is the need for the gB vaccine to be given as 3 doses over a period of 6 months. Many patients proceed to transplant before the full course of vaccination can be given, and so the likelihood of protection may be reduced. Nevertheless, one study ongoing at the Royal Free Hospital, London, and coordinated by scientists at University College London, has recruited renal and liver transplant patients (seropositive and seronegative before transplant) into a placebo-controlled trial of the gB-MF59 vaccine with an end point of viral replication (incidence and kinetics) after transplantation. At the time of writing, this trial has not reported its results, but these should be available in 2010.

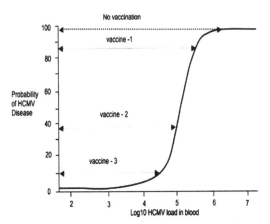

Fig. 1. The relationship between HCMV load and probability of disease and the potential effects of vaccination. In the scenario shown, in the absence of vaccination the patient would reach a viral load of $6\log_{10}$ genomes/mL of blood with an associated disease probability of 97%. The 3 vaccines 1, 2 and 3 have increasing efficacy by reducing viral load in blood by 0.5, 1.0, and $1.5\log_{10}$, which reduces disease probability to 86%, 37%, and 10% respectively. Comparable reductions can be modeled if the patient was destined to experience a maximum viral load of $5\log_{10}$ genomes/mL blood.

Human Papillomavirus Vaccines

Papillomavirus infections remain an important pathogen in immunocompromised men and women with HIV or in transplant recipients, for whom the risks for common warts and anogenital lesions attributable to human papillomavirus (HPV) are substantially increased compared with healthy individuals.[24] In particular, female renal transplant recipients have a substantially increased risk for HPV-associated anogenital cancers and cervical intraepithelial neoplasia. The development of HPV-related anal tumors has also been documented after liver transplantation in a retrospective analysis.[25] Anal HPV-DNA was detectable in 23% of men and women before the induction of immunosuppression for a liver or kidney transplant.[26] The recent licensing of recombinant HPV vaccines based on the L1 protein of HPV types 6, 11, 16, and 18 for the prevention of genital warts, cervical dysplasia, and cervical cancer[27,28] has now provided opportunities to deploy such vaccines in the transplant setting. Because these vaccines work best in individuals before HPV exposure, it is likely that the first deployment may occur in the pediatric transplant setting. In the setting of immunosuppression, the safety of HPV vaccines has yet to be determined. However, extrapolation from the use of other nonlive vaccines suggests that HPV vaccine would be safe and induce effective, if diminished, immune responses, with no associated graft rejection or other serious adverse effects. In addition, given the risks of anogenital lesions, the ability to boost preexisting immunity to reduce or prevent anogenital lesions is also likely to be an important consideration in adult populations, especially in women receiving renal transplants. However, it is interesting that a recent cost-effectiveness analysis suggests that a program of HPV vaccination before transplantation is unlikely to be cost-effective.[29] Nothwithstanding this, clinical trials of HPV vaccines are underway in centers in North America.[30]

VZV Vaccine

To date, a prophylactic vaccine against VZV is the only live, attenuated herpes virus vaccine to be licensed in any country. It was initially tested, and has been widely used for the past few decades, in Japan. The currently available vaccine consists of attenuated virus from the Oka strain of VZV and has been in use safely and successfully in healthy children and adults in many other parts of the world.[31]

Among immunocompromised patients, including transplant recipients, varicella infections may be severe and even fatal. The clinical presentation may be atypical in immunocompromised patients, in whom the rash may be nonvesicular or even absent. Immunocompromised children and adults may present with abdominal zoster, characterized by abdominal and back pain, which may precede or occur in the absence of skin lesions,[32,33] posing a diagnostic challenge. VZV-associated cerebral vasculitis has also been described in the setting of immunocompromised patients.[34] In addition, recovery from VZV infection may be slow, with individuals remaining infectious for up to several weeks following initial clinical presentation. It is therefore important to consider protection of these susceptible populations with the use of the VZV vaccine, 2 doses of which provide 75% protection against any disease and at least 95% protection against severe disease and its complications among immunocompetent adults.[35]

The use of the live, attenuated varicella vaccine has been most extensively studied in children with acute lymphoblastic leukemia (ALL), but studies involving other immunocompromised populations are limited.[36] In a multicenter trial, the vaccine was shown to be safe and immunogenic when administered to children with ALL who had suspended maintenance chemotherapy for at least 1 week before and 1 week after vaccination.[37] Seroconversion rates varied from 42% to 96% and were, on average, lower than in healthy children. Incidence of recurrent varicella (herpes zoster) was also found to be less in immunocompromised vaccine recipients compared with that observed following natural infection.[38] In children with asymptomatic or mild symptoms of HIV infection, the VZV vaccine was found to be safe but less immunogenic than in healthy children, with seroconversion rates of approximately 60%.[39] A recent phase II trial determined the VZV vaccine to be safe and immunogenic among HIV-infected children with a history of varicella,[40] and no child had developed herpes zoster 2 years later. Fewer vaccine efficacy studies have been performed among HIV-infected adults: a boost in VZV-specific immunoglobulin G (IgG) was observed in HIV-infected patients on stable antiretroviral therapy for at least 3 months, with a nadir CD4 count greater than 400 cells/mL.[41]

Among children who have received liver and intestine transplants and are on maximum dosages of 0.3 mg/kg prednisolone on alternate days and trough tacrolimus levels of less than 10 ng/mL for more than 1 month, the varicella vaccine was found to be safe, immunogenic, and protective.[42] In the latter study, 16 children who were VZV IgG seronegative and aged between 13 and 76 months were immunized, and 87% and 86% of children developed humoral and cellular immunity, respectively. Five of the children developed a mild pain and erythema at the site of the injection, and another 4 developed fever and disseminated rash. Among 11 children with follow-up of 6 months or more after vaccination, there were 5 subsequent reported exposures to chickenpox (1 child with 2 exposures), none of which resulted in chickenpox.

A severe but nonfatal vaccine-associated disease has been reported in some children with an undiagnosed immunodeficiency.[43] However, no fatalities have been observed in this group, in whom mortality associated with natural infection is known to occur. Hence, overall, it is believed that the potential benefits of vaccination against VZV in the immunocompromised host far outweigh the risks.

Other Viral Vaccines

Although HBV vaccination has been available for many years it has not been widely deployed in the setting of HBV infection in patients transplanted for chronic HBV. However, in the context of dialysis patients, HBV vaccination is recommended, although the immune response to vaccination can be suboptimal, especially if given intramuscularly.[44] Recently, the use of the adjuvant 3-O-desacyl-4'-monophosphoryl lipid A (AS04) in conjunction with standard hepatitis B recombinant vaccine has led to enhanced immunogenicity (earlier and higher antibody titers) in dialysis patients.[45]

At the time of writing, the prospects for viral vaccines against adenoviruses, BK virus, and HCV remain poor. It is therefore unlikely that prototype vaccines will be forthcoming for these infectious complications in transplant and oncology patients. Nevertheless, the experience and data generated from studies of HCMV and papillomavirus vaccines should provide important information concerning the likely immunogenicity of new vaccines in the context of dialysis and the immunocompromised state following transplantation.

ADOPTIVE IMMUNOTHERAPY
Cytomegalovirus Immunotherapy

Antigen-specific T cells are essential for control of cytomegalovirus infection,[46] and HCMV has evolved several mechanisms to overcome this component of the immune response.[47] Immunotherapy offers an attractive way to improve immune reconstitution in transplanted patients, leading to control of viral replication without major side effects. As a consequence, this approach may reduce the use of antiviral chemotherapy and hence the adverse effects such as myelo- or nephrotoxicity and, furthermore, the evolutionary pressure on HCMV to develop drug resistance.

Various strategies to generate HCMV-specific T lymphocytes have been developed (these are reviewed in Ref.[48]). One of the most effective approaches for the ex vivo induction of HCMV-specific T cells is using CMV-infected fibroblasts, but the potential biologic risk that results from the use of live virus particles does not permit the use of infected antigen-presenting cells (APCs) for T cell stimulation under current good management practice (GMP) standards. Other approaches used to generate HCMV-specific T cells include HCMV peptide-pulsed dendritic cells (DCs),[49] HCMV antigen–pulsed DCs,[50] or using genetically modified APCs.[51] All of these methods are effective in producing HCMV-specific T cells in high yield, but the process is expensive and time consuming to produce a product that can be deployed clinically.

Riddell and colleagues[52] and Walter and colleagues[53] were the first to show that adoptive immunotherapy for HCMV-specific CD8+ T cell clones into patients at risk of HCMV disease protected them from CMV-related complications. In these studies, 1×10^9 to 2×10^9 CMV-specific CD8+ T cells were administered and these cells persisted in patients' blood for at least 8 weeks. HCMV prophylaxis was effective despite the progressive decline of these HCMV CD8 T cells in patients who did not develop a concomitant HCMV-specific CD4+ T_{Helper} response. Although these results were groundbreaking, they suffered from the use of historical controls.

In an alternative study, patients lacking HCMV immunity were reconstituted by the adoptive transfer of HCMV-specific T cell lines which were generated by 4 repetitive weekly stimulations with HCMV lysate in vitro.[54] These cells could be infused without any side effects, even in patients receiving their graft from a donor mismatched in 1 to 3 HLA antigens, implicating a potential use of this strategy even after haploidentical transplantation. This approach has advantages in the context of time compared with the generation of the CD8+ CMV–specific clones described earlier, and provides a more flexible application of the technique in patients with HCMV DNAemia at high risk for HCMV disease, without a loss of specificity and safety. These findings show that HCMV-specific adoptive immune transfer is a therapeutic option in patients who are DNAemic after stem cell transplantation and can be achieved by infusion of low numbers of CD4+ HCMV–specific T cell lines.

To facilitate the enrichment of virus-specific T cells, novel selection using the IFN-γ secretion assay conforming to current GMP regulations can be deployed.[55] HCMV-Ag can also be used to elicit a combined HCMV-specific CD4+ and CD8+ T cell response. Stimulation of HCMV-specific CD4+ and CD8+ T cells was similarly effective when using HCMV antigen compared with the costimulation with HCMV antigen and HCMV peptides.[56] As a result, an average of 1.3×10^8 CMV-specific stimulated, selected, and expanded T cells from 8/8 randomly selected HCMV-seropositive donors were generated in 10 days from a single 500-mL blood donation using only autologous cellular and humoral components compatible with current GMP regulations. The adoptively transferred T cells may then undergo further expansion in vivo if they are stimulated by HCMV-Ag–presenting cells providing an in vivo amplification step rather than relying on in vitro expansion.

Important questions remain with respect to the number of HCMV-specific T cells required for an effective adoptive transfer and their composition in respect to CD4+/CD8+ ratio and antigen specificity required for prevention or treatment of HCMV DNAemia after allogeneic stem cell transplantation. Further work is needed to define these parameters. However, improvements in immunologic assays have enabled direct quantification of HCMV-specific T cells. Analysis of phenotype and activity of antigen-specific T cells have contributed to a substantial improvement in understanding of the role and function of immune responses in vivo.[57–59] Thus, phenotypic analysis with HLA-peptide multimers and functional assays can now be used in the setting of adoptive T cell therapy. Peptide-HLA multimers allow an easy visualization and isolation of antigen-specific cytotoxic T lymphocytes (CTLs). T cells that bind multimeric HLA complexes can be isolated to high purity using magnetic beads or fluorescent antibody cell separation (FACS) sorting.[60] There are several reasons why the adoptive transfer of HCMV-specific CTLs freshly isolated from peripheral blood might be more efficient than the infusion of in vitro expanded and manipulated T cells. The process of in vitro expansion may increase the expression of the proapoptotic FAS molecule (CD95) and reduce telomere length of specific T cells, leading to a shorter survival of the adoptive transferred T cells[61] similar to that observed in aging human populations.[62] Various methods of cell generation result in different stages of T cell senescence. Freshly isolated and specifically selected T cells have greater expansion potential in vivo compared with repetitive in vitro stimulated T cells. However, specific stimulation ex vivo might reduce the risk for alloreactivity. In addition, the in vitro cell culture process increases not only the risk for contamination of the CTL preparation but also the costs for adoptive immunotherapy.

Although the availability of clinical-grade reagents for the selection of antigen-specific T cells has improved greatly in the last few years, not enough is known about the ideal composition of a cellular product that will be highly effective in use for adoptive transfer. The optimal targets for HCMV-specific T cell control have not been defined precisely despite evidence suggesting that the host makes a broad CD4 and CD8 response to most proteins in the HCMV proteome.[63] However, there is still controversy about the benefit of transferring different T cell subsets for adoptive immunotherapy: namely, should only CD4+ T cells or CD8+ T cells be transferred, or a combination of both?

In view of the many different methods of generating T cells, future studies must address the following questions, preferably in placebo-controlled studies: (1) which are the best T cell subpopulations to be used for antiviral T cell therapy; (2) what differentiation/activation stage or stages are associated with efficient expansion and antiviral control; (3) what is the ideal range of antigen specificities of the T cells; and (4) what is the optimal cell dose required to control replication, and does it depend on the viral load and net state of immunosuppression of the patient?

EBV Immunotherapy

EBV is associated with posttransplant lymphoproliferative disease (PTLD), a common complication after hematopoietic stem cell and solid-organ transplantations.[64] PTLD occurs in up to 15% of patients depending on the transplant type, age of the recipient, and the intensity of immunosuppression. With conventional treatments (reduction of immunosuppression, rituximab, radiotherapy, chemotherapy, surgery),[65–67] relapses are common and the overall mortality remains high (around 50%).[68]

The search for an optimum treatment has led to recent trials of adoptive transfer of T cell immunity directed against EBV. These studies should be compared with those on HCMV discussed in the previous section. More than 90% of PTLD are EBV positive and most tumor cells express full latent cycle proteins (EB nuclear antigens [EBNAs] 1, 2, 3a, 3b, 3c, and leader protein [LP]; latent membrane proteins [LMPs] 1, 2), with a few cells expressing lytic cycle proteins.[69] Some of these proteins, particularly the EBNA 3 family, are immunodominant targets for virus-specific CTL, thus making PTLD an ideal candidate for adoptive immunotherapy.[70] EBV readily infects and transforms B lymphocytes in vitro giving rise to a continually growing lymphoblastoid cell line (LCL) in which each cell expresses all EBV latent antigens. Irradiated LCL cells can then be used as

APCs to stimulate and expand autologous peripheral blood mononuclear cells (PBMCs) into an EBV-specific CTL line.[71] Using this method, CTLs were grown ex vivo from HLA-matched hematopoietic stem cell donors and were used successfully to prevent and treat PTLD in respective stem cell recipients.[71,72] However, this approach is not feasible in solid-organ transplantation because the organ donor is not generally available to provide blood, and the donor and the recipients are not closely HLA matched. Attempts have been made to generate autologous CTL from patients before transplantation and from patients with PTLD.[73–75] However, the approach of generating autologous CTL from each transplant patient is prohibitively labor intensive and expensive for wide-scale use, and often there is not sufficient time to generate CTLs once PTLD has been diagnosed. An alternative strategy is to establish a bank of well-characterized EBV-specific CTL grown from EBV-seropositive healthy blood donors and provide these off-the-shelf CTLs to PTLD patients on a best HLA match basis (**Fig. 2**).[76] This third-party CTL strategy has several advantages: fully characterized CTLs are available for immediate use; 1 CTL line can be used for more than 1 PTLD patient, making it cost-effective; and these cells can be used to treat EBV-driven lymphomas in nontransplant immunosuppressed patients. A research team in Edinburgh University, Scotland, established a frozen bank of 100 EBV-specific CTL lines generated from Scottish blood donors selected to cover more than 99% of the HLA types of the UK population.[77] In a pilot study, the first of its kind in the United Kingdom, 8 patients with progressive PTLD were infused with these allogeneic CTLs, selected on the basis of best HLA matches between the CTL donor and PTLD patient, with 3 patients achieving a complete remission.[78] This CTL bank was then used in a multicenter phase II clinical trial to treat 33 PTLD patients (31 solid-organ and 2 stem cell transplant recipients in the

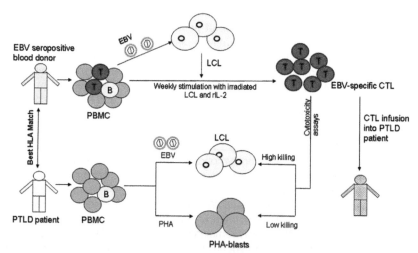

Fig. 2. Study design for the selection of partially HLA-matched third-party CTL for the treatment of PTLD. EBV-seropositive healthy blood donors were selected to cover most HLA types in the United Kingdom. PBMCs from blood donors were infected with EBV to obtain a LCL and irradiated LCL were used as APCs to stimulate and expand EBV-specific CTL from autologous PBMC in the presence of recombinant interleukin 2 (rIL2). PBMC from PTLD patients were collected to generate LCL and phytohemagglutinin blasts. Available CTL lines with the best HLA matches between the CTL donor and the PTLD patient were tested with in vitro cytotoxicity assays, and the CTL line showing the highest lysis of patient's LCL (EBV targets) and the lowest lysis of patient's PHA-blasts (non-EBV targets) was selected for infusion into the patient.

United Kingdom, Sweden, France, and Australia) who had failed to respond to conventional treatments.[79] At 6 months after treatment, 52% of patients had responded to the CTL infusions, with 14 achieving complete remission. A significantly better response was noted in patients receiving CTL with higher HLA matching ($P = .001$) and with higher numbers of CD4+ T cells ($P = .001$). No infusion-related toxicity or features of CTL-versus-host disease occurred in any of the infused patients and the third-party allogeneic CTL was considered a safe and effective form of treatment of PTLD.

A wide range of protocols have been used to generate CTL with specificities against individual EBV antigens (eg, LMP-1, LMP-2) by using APCs loaded with EBV peptides, or transfected with vaccinia or adenoviral vectors expressing selected EBV proteins.[80–82] An alternate approach is to redirect T cells to antigens on tumor cells using the recently developed chimeric T cell receptor (TCR) technology.[83] T cells expressing chimeric receptors with the antigen-binding domains of monoclonal antibodies fused to the downstream signal transducing elements of TCR can effectively target any tumor expressing that particular antigen without the need of major histocompatibility complex restriction.[84] Research is ongoing to generate T cells expressing the chimeric TCR containing the single variable chains of monoclonal antibodies against EBV latent membrane antigen, LMP-1 and LMP-2, fused to the CD3ζ chain, and to explore the possibility of their future use in clinical trials of targeting LMP-1 and LMP-2 expressing EBV-driven malignancies without the requirement of HLA restriction.

Adenovirus Immunotherapy

Although adoptive immunotherapy has been predominantly directed against HCMV and EBV infection, the lack of effective antiviral chemotherapy against adenovirus and the high morbidity and mortality associated with disseminated infection have resulted in interest in using T cells to control infection. Effective T cell function seems to be crucial in the control of adenovirus replication and reduction of immunosuppression and donor lymphocyte infusions have been shown to lead to a reduction in viral replication.[85,86] At present, one trial in pediatric stem cell transplant recipients has been reported using ex vivo isolated IFN-γ–producing T cells.[87] Infusions of between 1.2×10^3 and 50×10^3 T cells/kg were well tolerated in most patients, and in 5/6 patients, adenovirus loads decreased and replication resolved. Further controlled trials will be needed to judge the effectiveness of adoptive transfer of T cells against adenovirus and to optimize the initiation of therapy. The identification of several other potential T cell targets within the adenovirus proteome will also allow more complex T cell specificities to be generated, which should also allow more effective control of replication.[88] The ongoing experience with HCMV and EBV immunotherapy will be invaluable in the context of adoptive immunotherapy for adenovirus.

Researchers have also generated a multivirus-specific CTL line containing a mixture of cells that are capable of killing HCMV, adenovirus, and EBV target cells in in vitro cytotoxicity assays.[89,90] DCs and LCL, transduced with a clinical-grade recombinant adenovirus type 5 vector pseudotyped with an adenovirus type 35 fiber encoding CMVpp65 (Ad5f35CMVpp65), were used as APCs. These multivirus-specific CTL lines may be beneficial in treating transplant patients with combined HCMV, EBV, and adenoviral diseases.

SUMMARY

Vaccination and adoptive immunotherapy for herpes virus infections has become an attractive option for the control of a virus family that negatively affects transplantation. In the future, enhanced ability to select antigen-specific T cells without significant in vitro manipulation should provide new opportunities for refining and enhancing adoptive immunotherapeutic approaches. In addition, the trials of HCMV vaccine that are currently underway provide significant hope that these and other viral vaccines will soon be deployed in the transplant population.

REFERENCES

1. Fischer SA. Emerging viruses in transplantation: there is more to infection after transplant than CMV and EBV. Transplantation 2008;86(10):1327–39.
2. Saral R, Burns WH, Laskin OL, et al. Acyclovir prophylaxis of herpes-simplex-virus infections. N Engl J Med 1981;305(2):63–7.
3. Sempere A, Sanz GF, Senent L, et al. Long-term acyclovir prophylaxis for prevention of varicella zoster virus infection after autologous blood stem cell transplantation in patients with acute leukemia. Bone Marrow Transplant 1992;10(6):495–8.
4. Khoury JA, Storch GA, Bohl DL, et al. Prophylactic versus preemptive oral valganciclovir for the management of cytomegalovirus infection in adult renal transplant recipients. Am J Transplant 2006;6(9):2134–43.
5. Paya C, Humar A, Dominguez E, et al. Efficacy and safety of valganciclovir vs. oral ganciclovir for prevention of cytomegalovirus disease in solid organ transplant recipients. Am J Transplant 2004;4(4):611–20.
6. Boivin G, Goyette N, Rollag H, et al. Cytomegalovirus resistance in solid organ transplant recipients treated with intravenous ganciclovir or oral valganciclovir. Antivir Ther 2009;14(5):697–704.
7. Plotkin SA, Huygelen C. Cytomegalovirus vaccine prepared in WI-38. Dev Biol Stand 1976;37:301–5.
8. Glazer JP, Friedman HM, Grossman RA, et al. Live cytomegalovirus vaccination of renal transplant candidates. A preliminary trial. Ann Intern Med 1979;91(5):676–83.
9. Plotkin SA, Smiley ML, Friedman HM, et al. Towne-vaccine-induced prevention of cytomegalovirus disease after renal transplants. Lancet 1984;1(8376):528–30.
10. Pass RF, Duliege AM, Boppana S, et al. A subunit cytomegalovirus vaccine based on recombinant envelope glycoprotein B and a new adjuvant. J Infect Dis 1999;180(4):970–5.
11. Adler SP, Plotkin SA, Gonczol E, et al. A canarypox vector expressing cytomegalovirus (CMV) glycoprotein B primes for antibody responses to a live attenuated CMV vaccine (Towne). J Infect Dis 1999;180(3):843–6.
12. Reap EA, Dryga SA, Morris J, et al. Cellular and humoral immune responses to alphavirus replicon vaccines expressing cytomegalovirus pp65, IE1, and gB proteins. Clin Vaccine Immunol 2007;14(6):748–55.
13. Temperton NJ. DNA vaccines against cytomegalovirus: current progress. Int J Antimicrob Agents 2002;19(3):169–72.
14. Griffiths PD, McLean A, Emery VC. Encouraging prospects for immunisation against primary cytomegalovirus infection. Vaccine 2001;19(11–12):1356–62.
15. Emery VC, Hassan-Walker AF, Burroughs AK, et al. Human cytomegalovirus (HCMV) replication dynamics in HCMV-naive and -experienced immunocompromised hosts. J Infect Dis 2002;185(12):1723–8.
16. Emery VC. Viral dynamics during active cytomegalovirus infection and pathology. Intervirology 1999;42(5–6):405–11.
17. Wagner B, Kropff B, Kalbacher H, et al. A continuous sequence of more than 70 amino acids is essential for antibody binding to the dominant antigenic site of glycoprotein gp58 of human cytomegalovirus. J Virol 1992;66(9):5290–7.

18. Marshall GS, Li M, Stout GG, et al. Antibodies to the major linear neutralizing domains of cytomegalovirus glycoprotein B among natural seropositives and CMV subunit vaccine recipients. Viral Immunol 2000;13(3):329–41.
19. Schleiss MR, Bourne N, Stroup G, et al. Protection against congenital cytomeg-alovirus infection and disease in guinea pigs, conferred by a purified recombi-nant glycoprotein B vaccine. J Infect Dis 2004;189(8):1374–81.
20. Pass RF, Burke RL. Development of cytomegalovirus vaccines: prospects for preven-tion of congenital CMV infection. Semin Pediatr Infect Dis 2002;13(3):196–204.
21. Mitchell DK, Holmes SJ, Burke RL, et al. Immunogenicity of a recombinant human cytomegalovirus gB vaccine in seronegative toddlers. Pediatr Infect Dis J 2002; 21(2):133–8.
22. Pass RF. Development and evidence for efficacy of CMV glycoprotein B vaccine with MF59 adjuvant. J Clin Virol 2009;46:S73–6.
23. Pass RF, Zhang C, Evans A, et al. Vaccine prevention of maternal cytomegalo-virus infection. N Engl J Med 2009;360(12):1191–9.
24. Tan HH, Goh CL. Viral infections affecting the skin in organ transplant recipients: epidemiology and current management strategies. Am J Clin Dermatol 2006;7(1): 13–29.
25. Albright JB, Bonatti H, Stauffer J, et al. Colorectal and anal neoplasms following liver transplantation. Colorectal Dis 2009. [Epub ahead of print].
26. Roka S, Rasoul-Rockenschaub S, Roka J, et al. Prevalence of anal HPV infection in solid-organ transplant patients prior to immunosuppression. Transpl Int 2004; 17:366–9.
27. Harper DM, Franco EL, Wheeler CM, et al. Sustained efficacy up to 4.5 years of a bivalent L1 virus-like particle vaccine against human papillomavirus types 16 and 18: follow-up from a randomised control trial. Lancet 2006;367(9518):1247–55.
28. FUTURE II Study Group. Quadrivalent vaccine against human papillomavirus to prevent high-grade cervical lesions. N Engl J Med 2007;356(19):1915–27.
29. Wong G, Howard K, Webster A, et al. The health and economic impact of cervical cancer screening and human papillomavirus vaccination in kidney transplant recipients. Transplantation 2009;87(7):1078–91.
30. Safety and immunogenicity of human papillomavirus (HPV) vaccine in solid organ transplant recipients; 2009. Available at: www.clinicaltrials.gov/ct2/show/ NCT00677677. Accessed January 26, 2010.
31. Gershon AA, Katz SL. Perspective on live varicella vaccine. J Infect Dis 2008; 197(Suppl 2):242–5.
32. Milone G, Di Raimondo F, Russo M, et al. Unusual onset of severe varicella in adult immunocompromised patients. Ann Hematol 1992;64:155–6.
33. Yagi T, Karasumo T, Hasegawa T, et al. Acute abdomen without cutaneous signs of varicella zoster virus infection as a late complication of allogeneic bone marrow transplantation: importance of empiric therapy with aciclovir. Bone Marrow Trans-plant 2000;25:1003–5.
34. Hovens MMC, Vaessen N, Sijpkens YWJ, et al. Unusual presentation of central nervous system manifestations of varicella zoster virus vasculopathy in renal transplant recipients. Transpl Infect Dis 2007;9:237–40.
35. Varicella. In: The green book: immunization against infectious disease. London (UK): Department of Health 2006, chapter 34.
36. Sartori AMC. A review of the varicella vaccine in immunocompromised individ-uals. Int J Infect Dis 2004;8:259–70.
37. Gershon AA, Steinbert SP, Gelb L, et al. Live attenuated varicella vaccine, effi-cacy for children with leukemia in remission. The national institute of allergy

and infectious diseases varicella vaccine collaborative study group. JAMA 1984; 252:355–62.

38. Hardy IB, Gershon A, Steinberg S, et al. The incidence of zoster after immunization with live attenuated varicella vaccine: a study in children with leukemia. N Engl J Med 1991;325:1545–50.

39. Levin MJ, Gershon AA, Weingberg A, et al. Immunization of HIV-infected children with varicella vaccine. J Pediatr 2001;139:305–10.

40. Gershon AA, Levin MJ, Weinberg A, et al. A phase II study of live attenuated varicella-zoster virus vaccine to boost immunity in human immunodeficiency virus infected children with previous varicella. Pediatr Infect Dis J 2009;28:653–5.

41. Geretti AM, BHIVA Immunization Writing Committee. British HIV Association guidelines for immunization of HIV-infected adults in 2008. HIV Med 2008;9: 795–848.

42. Weinberg A, Horslen SP, Kaufmann SS, et al. Safety and immunogenicity of varicella-zoster virus vaccine in pediatric liver and intestine transplant recipients. Am J Transplant 2006;6:565–8.

43. Gershon AA. Varicella vaccine: rare serious problems: but the benefits still outweigh the risks. J Infect Dis 2003;188:945–7.

44. Barraclough KA, Wiggins KJ, Hawley CM, et al. Intradermal versus intramuscular hepatitis B vaccination in hemodialysis patients: a prospective open-label randomized controlled trial in nonresponders to primary vaccination. Am J Kidney Dis 2009;54(1):95–103.

45. Beran J. Safety and immunogenicity of a new hepatitis B vaccine for the protection of patients with renal insufficiency including pre-haemodialysis and haemodialysis patients. Expert Opin Biol Ther 2008;8(2):235–47.

46. Gandhi MK, Khanna R. Human cytomegalovirus: clinical aspects, immune regulation, and emerging treatments. Lancet Infect Dis 2004;4(12):725–38.

47. Lilley BN, Ploegh HL. Viral modulation of antigen presentation: manipulation of cellular targets in the ER and beyond. Immunol Rev 2005;207:126–44.

48. Peggs KS. Adoptive T cell immunotherapy for cytomegalovirus. Expert Opin Biol Ther 2009;9(6):725–36.

49. Einsele H, Rauser G, Grigoleit U, et al. Induction of CMV-specific T-cell lines using Ag-presenting cells pulsed with CMV protein or peptide. Cytotherapy 2002;4(1): 49–54.

50. Peggs K, Verfuerth S, Mackinnon S. Induction of cytomegalovirus (CMV)-specific T-cell responses using dendritic cells pulsed with CMV antigen: a novel culture system free of live CMV virions. Blood 2001;97(4):994–1000.

51. Koehne G, Gallardo HF, Sadelain M, et al. Rapid selection of antigen-specific T lymphocytes by retroviral transduction. Blood 2000;96(1):109–17.

52. Riddell SR, Watanabe KS, Goodrich JM, et al. Restoration of viral immunity in immunodeficient humans by the adoptive transfer of T cell clones. Science 1992;257(5067):238–41.

53. Walter EA, Greenberg PD, Gilbert MJ, et al. Reconstitution of cellular immunity against cytomegalovirus in recipients of allogeneic bone marrow by transfer of T-cell clones from the donor. N Engl J Med 1995;333(16):1038–44.

54. Einsele H, Roosnek E, Rufer N, et al. Infusion of cytomegalovirus (CMV)-specific T cells for the treatment of CMV infection not responding to antiviral chemotherapy. Blood 2002;99(11):3916–22.

55. Cobbold M, Khan N, Pourgheysari B, et al. Adoptive transfer of cytomegalovirus-specific CTL to stem cell transplant patients after selection by HLA-peptide tetramers. J Exp Med 2005;202(3):379–86.

56. Fujita Y, Leen AM, Sun J, et al. Exploiting cytokine secretion to rapidly produce multivirus-specific T cells for adoptive immunotherapy. J Immunother 2008; 31(7):665–74.

57. Nebbia G, Mattes FM, Smith C, et al. Polyfunctional cytomegalovirus-specific CD4+ and pp65 CD8+ T cells protect against high-level replication after liver transplantation. Am J Transplant 2008;8:2590–9.

58. La RC, Krishnan A, Longmate J, et al. Programmed death-1 expression in liver transplant recipients as a prognostic indicator of cytomegalovirus disease. J Infect Dis 2008;197(1):25–33.

59. Egli A, Binet I, Binggeli S, et al. Cytomegalovirus-specific T-cell responses and viral replication in kidney transplant recipients. J Transl Med 2008;6:29.

60. Szmania S, Galloway A, Bruorton M, et al. Isolation and expansion of cytomegalovirus-specific cytotoxic T lymphocytes to clinical scale from a single blood draw using dendritic cells and HLA-tetramers. Blood 2001;98(3): 505–12.

61. Tan R, Xu X, Ogg GS, et al. Rapid death of adoptively transferred T cells in acquired immunodeficiency syndrome. Blood 1999;93(5):1506–10.

62. Fletcher JM, Vukmanovic-Stejic M, Dunne PJ, et al. Cytomegalovirus-specific CD4+ T cells in healthy carriers are continuously driven to replicative exhaustion. J Immunol 2005;175(12):8218–25.

63. Sylwester AW, Mitchell BL, Edgar JB, et al. Broadly targeted human cytomegalovirus-specific CD4+ and CD8+ T cells dominate the memory compartments of exposed subjects. J Exp Med 2005;202(5):673–85.

64. Burns DM, Crawford DH. Epstein-Barr virus-specific cytotoxic T-lymphocytes for adoptive immunotherapy of post-transplant lymphoproliferative disease. Blood Rev 2004;18(3):193–209.

65. Starzl TE, Nalesnik MA, Porter KA, et al. Reversibility of lymphomas and lymphoproliferative lesions developing under cyclosporin-steroid therapy. Lancet 1984; 1(8377):583–7.

66. Swinnen LJ, Mullen GM, Carr TJ, et al. Aggressive treatment for postcardiac transplant lymphoproliferation. Blood 1995;86(9):3333–40.

67. Choquet S, Leblond V, Herbrecht R, et al. Efficacy and safety of rituximab in B-cell post-transplantation lymphoproliferative disorders: results of a prospective multicenter phase 2 study. Blood 2006;107(8):3053–7.

68. Opelz G, Dohler B. Lymphomas after solid organ transplantation: a collaborative transplant study report. Am J Transplant 2004;4(2):222–30.

69. Timms JM, Bell A, Flavell JR, et al. Target cells of Epstein-Barr-virus (EBV)-positive post-transplant lymphoproliferative disease: similarities to EBV-positive Hodgkin's lymphoma. Lancet 2003;361(9353):217–23.

70. Khanna R, Burrows SR. Role of cytotoxic T lymphocytes in Epstein-Barr virus-associated diseases. Annu Rev Microbiol 2000;54:19–48.

71. Rooney CM, Smith CA, Ng CY, et al. Use of gene-modified virus-specific T lymphocytes to control Epstein-Barr-virus-related lymphoproliferation. Lancet 1995;345(8941):9–13.

72. Rooney CM, Smith CA, Ng CY, et al. Infusion of cytotoxic T cells for the prevention and treatment of Epstein-Barr virus-induced lymphoma in allogeneic transplant recipients. Blood 1998;92(5):1549–55.

73. Haque T, Amlot PL, Helling N, et al. Reconstitution of EBV-specific T cell immunity in solid organ transplant recipients. J Immunol 1998;160(12):6204–9.

74. Khanna R, Bell S, Sherritt M, et al. Activation and adoptive transfer of Epstein-Barr virus-specific cytotoxic T cells in solid organ transplant patients with

posttransplant lymphoproliferative disease. Proc Natl Acad Sci U S A 1999; 96(18):10391–6.

75. Savoldo B, Huls MH, Liu Z, et al. Autologous Epstein-Barr virus (EBV)-specific cytotoxic T cells for the treatment of persistent active EBV infection. Blood 2002;100(12):4059–66.

76. Haque T, Taylor C, Wilkie GM, et al. Complete regression of posttransplant lymphoproliferative disease using partially HLA-matched Epstein Barr virus-specific cytotoxic T cells. Transplantation 2001;72(8):1399–402.

77. Wilkie GM, Taylor C, Jones MM, et al. Establishment and characterization of a bank of cytotoxic T lymphocytes for immunotherapy of Epstein-Barr virus-associated diseases. J Immunother 1997;27(4):309–16.

78. Haque T, Wilkie GM, Taylor C, et al. Treatment of Epstein-Barr-virus-positive posttransplantation lymphoproliferative disease with partly HLA-matched allogeneic cytotoxic T cells. Lancet 2002;360(9331):436–42.

79. Haque T, Wilkie GM, Jones MM, et al. Allogeneic cytotoxic T-cell therapy for EBV-positive posttransplantation lymphoproliferative disease: results of a phase 2 multicenter clinical trial. Blood 2007;110(4):1123–31.

80. Khanna R, Burrows SR, Nicholls J, et al. Identification of cytotoxic T cell epitopes within Epstein-Barr virus (EBV) oncogene latent membrane protein 1 (LMP1): evidence for HLA A2 supertype-restricted immune recognition of EBV-infected cells by LMP1-specific cytotoxic T lymphocytes. Eur J Immunol 1998;28(2): 451–8.

81. Gottschalk S, Edwards OL, Sili U, et al. Generating CTLs against the subdominant Epstein-Barr virus LMP1 antigen for the adoptive immunotherapy of EBV-associated malignancies. Blood 2003;101(5):1905–12.

82. Sing AP, Ambinder RF, Hong DJ, et al. Isolation of Epstein-Barr virus (EBV)-specific cytotoxic T lymphocytes that lyse Reed-Sternberg cells: implications for immune-mediated therapy of EBV+ Hodgkin's disease. Blood 1997;89(6): 1978–86.

83. Eshhar Z, Waks T, Gross G, et al. Specific activation and targeting of cytotoxic lymphocytes through chimeric single chains consisting of antibody-binding domains and the gamma or zeta subunits of the immunoglobulin and T-cell receptors. Proc Natl Acad Sci U S A 1993;90(2):720–4.

84. Sadelain M, Brentjens R, Riviere I. The promise and potential pitfalls of chimeric antigen receptors. Curr Opin Immunol 2009;21(2):215–23.

85. Chakrabarti S, Mautner V, Osman H, et al. Adenovirus infections following allogeneic stem cell transplantation: incidence and outcome in relation to graft manipulation, immunosuppression, and immune recovery. Blood 2002;100(5): 1619–27.

86. Bordigoni P, Carret AS, Venard V, et al. Treatment of adenovirus infections in patients undergoing allogeneic hematopoietic stem cell transplantation. Clin Infect Dis 2001;32(9):1290–7.

87. Feuchtinger T, Matthes-Martin S, Richard C, et al. Safe adoptive transfer of virus-specific T-cell immunity for the treatment of systemic adenovirus infection after allogeneic stem cell transplantation. Br J Haematol 2006;134(1):64–76.

88. Feuchtinger T, Richard C, Joachim S, et al. Clinical grade generation of hexon-specific T cells for adoptive T-cell transfer as a treatment of adenovirus infection after allogeneic stem cell transplantation. J Immunother 2008;31(2): 199–206.

89. Karlsson H, Brewin J, Kinnon C, et al. Generation of trispecific cytotoxic T cells recognizing cytomegalovirus, adenovirus, and Epstein-Barr virus: an approach

for adoptive immunotherapy of multiple pathogens. J Immunother 2007;30(5): 544–56.

90. Hanley PJ, Cruz CR, Savoldo B, et al. Functionally active virus-specific T cells that target CMV, adenovirus, and EBV can be expanded from naive T-cell populations in cord blood and will target a range of viral epitopes. Blood 2009;114(9): 1958–67.

Index

Note: Page numbers of article titles are in **boldface** type.

A

Abatacept, infectious complications of therapy with, 126–127
Acyclovir, prophylaxis in children undergoing HSCT, 145
    prophylaxis in children undergoing solid organ transplantation, 143
Adalimumab, infectious complications of therapy with, 120–123
Adaptive immune system, gene therapy for other primary immunodeficiencies of, 94–95
Adenosine deaminase deficiency, gene therapy for, 92–93
Adenovrius immunotherapy, after transplant, 223
Adoptive immunotherapy, after transplant, **215–229**
        adenovirus, 223
        cytomegalovirus, 219–221
        Epstein-Barr virus, 221–223
    for cytomegalovirus in HSCT recipients, 159
Alefacept, infectious complications of therapy with, 128
Alemtuzumab, infectious complications of therapy with, 124–125
Allogeneic hematopoietic stem cell transplantation, cytomegalovirus in recipients,
    153–154
        late infection, 154
    for severe combined immunodeficiency disease, 18–21
        related donors, 18–20
        related non-sibling donors, 20
        unrelated donors, 20–21
Anakinra, infectious complications of therapy with, 123–124
Anti-TNF-α therapies, infectious complications of therapy with, 120–123
Antiviral agents, prevention of cytomegalovirus in HSCT recipients, 155–157
    resistance to, 158
Antiviral prophylaxis, against cytomegalovirus in HSCT recipients, 155
Aspergillus infection, invasive, in transplant and oncology patients, 194–195
        management of, 201–202
Autoimmune diseases, purified HSCT for, 78–79
Autologous hematopoietic stem cell transplantation, cytomegalovirus in recipients,
    154–155

B

B-cell recovery, after T-cell depletion HSCT for primary immunodeficiency diseases, 55
B-lymphocyte depletion, infectious complications of, 118–120
Basliximab, infectious complications of therapy with, 126
Belatacept, infectious complications of therapy with, 126–127
Biologic therapies, immunomodulating, infectious complications of, **117–138**
        alefacept, 128
        alemtuzumab, 124–125

Hematol Oncol Clin N Am 25 (2011) 231–240
doi:10.1016/S0889-8588(10)00178-4
0889-8588/11/$ – see front matter © 2011 Elsevier Inc. All rights reserved.

hemonc.theclinics.com

Moving?

Make sure your subscription moves with you!

To notify us of your new address, find your **Clinics Account Number** (located on your mailing label above your name), and contact customer service at:

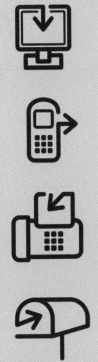

Email: journalscustomerservice-usa@elsevier.com

800-654-2452 (subscribers in the U.S. & Canada)
314-447-8871 (subscribers outside of the U.S. & Canada)

Fax number: 314-447-8029

Elsevier Health Sciences Division
Subscription Customer Service
3251 Riverport Lane
Maryland Heights, MO 63043

*To ensure uninterrupted delivery of your subscription, please notify us at least 4 weeks in advance of move.

Printed and bound by CPI Group (UK) Ltd, Croydon, CR0 4YY

03/10/2024

01040458-0006